MISSING THE MARK?

Women and the Millennium Development Goals in Africa and Oceania

EDITED BY
Naomi M. McPherson

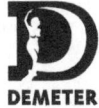

DEMETER PRESS, BRADFORD, ONTARIO

Copyright © 2016 Demeter Press

Individual copyright to their work is retained by the authors. All rights reserved. No part of this book may be reproduced or transmitted in any form by any means without permission in writing from the publisher.

Funded by the Government of Canada
Financé par la gouvernement du Canada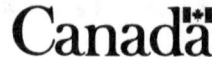

Demeter Press
140 Holland Street West
P. O. Box 13022
Bradford, ON L3Z 2Y5
Tel: (905) 775-9089
Email: info@demeterpress.org
Website: www.demeterpress.org

Demeter Press logo based on the sculpture "Demeter" by Maria-Luise Bodirsky <www.keramik-atelier.bodirsky.de>

Front cover photograph: "Young mother and newborn, Papua New Guinea." Photo©Naomi M. McPherson, 2009.

Printed and Bound in Canada

Library and Archives Canada Cataloguing in Publication

    Missing the mark? : women and the millennium development goals in Africa and Oceania / Naomi McPherson, editor.

Includes bibliographical references.
ISBN 978-1-77258-004-4 (paperback)

    1. Women — Africa — Social conditions — Case studies. 2. Women — Oceania — Social conditions — Case studies. 3. Women — Health and hygiene — Africa — Case studies. 4. Women — Health and hygiene — Oceania — Case studies. I. McPherson, Naomi, 1945–, editor

HQ1787 M58 2016   305.42096   C2016-900871-1

To all the women among whom the contributors to this volume have lived and have learned from, especially those women who shared their maternal experiences with us.

Table of Contents

Acknowledgements
xi

Introduction:
Cosmopolitan Obstetrics and Women's Lived Realities
Naomi M. McPherson
1

1.
Integrating Western Medicine and Local Practice:
Contributions of a Mission-Based Maternity Clinic to
Maternal and Child Health in the Lower Sepik
Region of Papua New Guinea
Kathleen Barlow
41

2.
Second Chance:
Caring for Infected Mothers and Their Children in
Mendi, Papua New Guinea
Philip Gibbs and Winnie William
74

3.
Faith, Hope, and Charity:
Barriers to Condom Use among Women in Southern Malawi
Nicole C. Hayes
96

4.
Shortages, Priorities, and Maternal Health:
Muddled *Kastom* and the Changing Status of Women in Malaita, Solomon Islands
Stephanie Hobbis
126

5.
Maternal Health (In)Equity in Mursi (Mun), Southern Ethiopia:
Behind the Hype of "Harmful Cultural Practices"
Shauna LaTosky
153

6.
Maternal Health Services Miss the Mark:
An Ethnographic Case Study in Rural Ghana
Vida Nygare Yakong and Naomi M. McPherson
176

7.
Giving Birth in Douala, Cameroon:
A Real Challenge
Jeannette Wogaing
212

8.
Throwing the Mother Out with the Bathwater:
Vanuatu's Breastfeeding Initiative in Theory and Practice
Chelsea Wentworth
234

9.
Reproductive Anomalies in the Marshall Islands
Nancy J. Pollock
264

10.
Examining the Intersections of Gender and
Reproduction in Chuuk:
Reflections on the Relevance and Utility of MDG Goals
in a Small Island(s) Community
Sarah A. Smith
286

Contributor Notes
315

Acknowledgements

On behalf of all the anthropologists whose ethnographic work is represented here in their respective chapters, I would like to acknowledge the women with whom we live and work in our various field site settings in Africa and Oceania. These women took us into their lives and into their confidence to share with us their thoughts, feelings, and reproductive experiences.

Introduction

Cosmpolitan Obstetrics and Women's Lived Realities

NAOMI M. MCPHERSON

MY INTENT IN THIS INTRODUCTORY OVERVIEW is to briefly present the "birth" of the 2000-2015 Millennium Development Goals (MDGs) to provide a framework for understanding how these goals and targets evolved. Briefly put, the Millennium Development Goals 2000–2015 constituted a global plan focused on improving the living conditions of the world's poorest peoples. The eight MDGs are the following:

Eradicate extreme poverty and hunger
Achieve universal primary education
Promote gender equality and empower women
Reduce child mortality
Improve maternal health
Combat HIV/AIDS, malaria, and other diseases
Ensure environmental sustainability
Develop global partnerships for development.

The MDGs were a universal response to local social, cultural, and economic issues to be applied in all developing countries, and as "the majority of the MDGs refer to improvements in the well-being of individuals, they are thus final goals of human development (education, health, access to water) to be measured at the micro-level" (Loewe 1). Our analytic lenses are trained squarely on the micro-level of women's lived experiences to grasp how gender equality and women's empowerment (or lack thereof) and women's maternal and reproductive health intersect. Gender equality, women's empowerment, women's well-being as mothers, and their sexual and reproductive health are culturally complex phenomena. We suggest that the achievement of MDG 3 and MDG 5 is less dependent upon women's access and uptake of biomedical services than upon the history, politics, and culture of the particular societies in which the women live.

The studies in this volume are grounded in specific cultural contexts in which the authors have conducted ethnographic research to understand women's lived realities and their maternal and reproductive health. In particular, the authors scrutinize the impact of a biomedical approach to illness and disease that has become a universal model, a one-size-fits-all approach to human health. Here, I replace the descriptor "biomedical" with the term "cosmopolitan medicine," a concept originated by Frederick L. Dunn in 1976. Dunn saw Euro-Western biomedicine becoming a global system of medicine and worried that this medical philosophy, with its urban based, technologically dependent practices, would eclipse other systems of medical philosophy and practice. Cosmopolitan medicine was a term later taken up by Brigitte Jordan in her original analysis of "Birth in Four Cultures" (10 n5), which she later expanded to include a concept of "cosmopolitan obstetrics" as the "official health care system" (214) for women's maternal and reproductive health care.

People all around the globe are subjected to a universal model of biomedicalization and women, in particular, to cosmopolitan obstetrics (Rapp; Ginsberg and Rapp). MDG 5 is aimed at improving maternal and reproductive health globally, especially in so-called developing countries. The women in Africa and Oceania, whose experiences this volume shares, fall under the UN mandate expressed in the MDG preferred medical model of cosmopolitan obstetrics and thus the women share similar experiences of reproductive health care delivery. The women do not, however, come to this cosmopolitan model of obstetrics from a shared cultural framework of understanding and experiencing reproduction. The studies in this volume situate the women's experiences of cosmopolitan obstetrics within their specific cultural contexts.

Throughout this introduction, I refer to the ethnographic case studies presented here as illustrative of the issues pertaining to that global system expressed in local contexts. These studies are drawn from African and Oceanic contexts, but they are not meant to be regional exemplars. Rather, they aim to show that the issues brought forward are not specific to any African or Oceanic society or culture but cut across all these societies and their cultures, including our own.

In June 2013, the United Nations published its Millennium Development Goals (MDGs) Report. With only one thousand days left before the September 2015 MDG deadline, UN Secretary-General Ban Ki-Moon noted in his foreword to this report that only *some* targets of the eight MDGs had been or were close to being achieved (*The Millennium Development Report* 3). According to Wu Hongbo, other goals, in particular those goals aimed at and designed for women, required either "accelerated" or "bolder action" merely to improve maternal and reproductive health care, never mind to actually meet their objectives by the intended deadline (4). The Millennium Development Goals have now expired, and the UN issued its 2015 *Millennium Development Goals Report* that reviewed the status of the goals and their stated objectives. Clearly, for some MDGs, positive changes have been made; other MDGs have not been so successful or only moderately so. The papers in this collection focus primarily on MDG 3, which is aimed at the promotion of gender equality and the empowerment of women, and on MDG 5, which is aimed at improving maternal health. In doing so, we consider in the ethnographic studies presented here whether MDG 3 and MDG 5 "made" or "missed" the mark. But first, how did we get here from there?

CONSIDERING WOMEN AND THE G-77

The inclusion of issues in the Millennium Development Goals specific to women's human right to equality, to sexual and reproductive health, and to make decisions about their bodies and their sexual and reproductive health has a lengthy and controversial history. As Crossette points out that in "the 1979 convention on the *Elimination of All forms of Discrimination Against Women*, there is no direct mention in the Secretary General's report of a woman's rights over her own reproductive life and why these rights matter in the battle against poverty" (73). It appears that women's reproductive rights, which must be considered human rights, were forced out of the final 1979 document due to opposition from members of the G-77, which was "a loosely organized association of developing nations." Under pressure from conservative anti-choice lobbyists in the U.S., these members refused to engage with reproductive rights because, they argued, reproductive rights and reproductive health were shorthand for a "feminist agenda" that "included the right to abortion" (73).[1]

Crossette quotes from her 2004 interview with Jacqueline Sharpe, then president of the Family Planning Association of Trinidad and Tobago, who pointed out that the G-77, which by 2004 numbered in excess of 130 members, was "deeply divided on issues involving women's health and reproductive rights ... [and] in most of these meetings involving women's health and reproductive rights ... there were only diplomats or government officials with no expertise in the issues being discussed" (75). Sharpe pointed out that the 1979 precursor to the MDGs was "shorn of reproductive rights" because women's rights were not high among governmental priorities in the G-77 and women's bodies "get to be the pawns in the [political] chess game.... They get traded away" (qtd. in Crossette, 74). Brolan and Hill point out that the "drafters of the MDGs were a select cluster of technocrats from the UN and other multilateral agencies, mainly the International Monetary Fund, World Bank and the Organisation for Economic Cooperation and Development's Development Assistance Committee (OECD-DAC)" (66). Influence also came from the Holy See (Coates et al.).

I posit that these technocrats, like the G-77 members before them, were predominantly male and assumed patriarchal privilege to usurp women's rights to determine their sexual and reproductive health and well-being. Even in the 2000–2015 redraft of the MDGs, an "explicit commitment to the reproductive rights of women was [still] nowhere to be found" (Brolan and Hill 71) and "the formal addition of a reproductive health target in 2007... depended on a huge advocacy effort" (66). Women's sexual and reproductive health were seen to be a necessary condition for eradicating extreme poverty and hunger (MDG 1), yet the realization of MDG 5 and MDG 1 was impossible without at the same time realizing

MDG 3, gender equity and the empowerment of women. It must always be kept in mind that universal access to health care means health care according to universal model of medicalization that has a long history of pathologizing women's bodies and childbearing (Arnup et al.).

Finally, in 2007, half way to the end date set to achieve the MDGs, women were included. However, enhancing women's equality and empowerment, and improving women's sexual and reproductive health has not been very successful. The studies here help to suggest some reasons why this is the case.

MDG 3 GOALS AND INDICATORS

Addressing the United Nations for International Women's Day 2014, Hillary Clinton stated that

> there is one lesson from the past, in particular, that we cannot afford to ignore: You cannot make progress on gender equality [MDG 3] or broader human development [MDG 1 to eradicate poverty], without safeguarding women's reproductive health and rights [MDG 5]. That is a bedrock truth. (qtd. in Merica)

Clinton's observation might seem self-evident; however, it assumes a domino effect such that eradication of poverty will assure gender equality that will, in turn, assure women's sexual and reproductive health rights. In other words, there is a false assumption here that inequitable gender relations and women's lack of empowerment are structured by poverty per se. This assumption is reflected in the indicators for successful achievement of MDG 3 that include ensuring girls (like boys) have access to all levels of education; that education will enable women's access to a share of wage earning employment outside agriculture and women will enter the labour market, earn cash, and purchase food rather than produce food. Education and engagement in the market will ensure an equitable number of seats among women and men so that women are better represented in national parliaments, where state decisions affecting women's lives are made. I explore each of these below.

Education

The way to achieve educational goals would thus appear to be ensuring that as many girls as boys have access to education, which would pave the way for women to access cash employment and to have a degree of economic independence and political power as representatives of their constituents in various governmental institutions of their countries. This is a very ethnocentric and neo-colonial approach to gender concepts and gender roles beyond the boundaries of cosmopolitan countries whose (mostly male) representatives designed the MDGs. It is necessary to at least recognize the fact that educational opportunities for *both* boys *and* girls are affected by many things, not least of all by gender inequities and women's lack of empowerment. Indeed, as Smith points out in chapter ten in this volume, in the Federated States of Micronesia the issue is not simply getting more girls in schools: "the issue in Chuuk is that the whole school system is deteriorating, so it is more an issue of the elite getting educated (in private schools) versus the rest, not girls versus boys."

This lack of material and human resources, as well as the inability to pay school fees and other requirements, does affect girls more severely than boys. Parents with little access to a cash income make decisions about who among their children gets to go to school when money for school fees, uniforms, and books is hard to come by. Usually these decisions favour boy children over girl children because educated girls are less valued than girls who become producers and reproducers. Not only must ideas and beliefs that inform gendered inequities be overcome so that families will consider sending their girls to school, but families also need financial resources to be able to support their sons *and* their daughters in their educational pursuits.

For example, the Bariai, with whom I live and work during research in Papua New Guinea (PNG), are subsistence horticulturalists who, among other things, grow taro, yams, and sweet potatoes. They engage in pig husbandry and augment their diet with seafood, tree fruits and nuts. As of this writing, there still is no cash economy in the area, despite demand for money to pay taxes, medical fees, to purchase various items of modern necessity (e.g., soap, clothes, metal pots), luxury items, such as radios and, recently, cell phones. Money is made on a contingency basis as needed. For example, women (and sometimes men) gather, dry, and sell sea cucumber [*bêche de mer*] to local representatives of exporters who resell them to traders for the international Asian specialty food market. To earn cash for school fees, women—whose garden labours feed their families—also grow extra garden produce or cut and carry firewood for smoking fish caught by their husbands to sell to teachers and workers in the nearest settlement 50 km away. Village parents reported to me that, in 2009, annual school fees were PGK 70 per child in grades one to four, PGK 100 for grade five and PGK 150 for grades six to eight. High school fees are higher yet at PGK 600.[2] Plus, all families pay a health fee of PGK 10 per family. Women who give birth in their village or along the foot path on their way to the health centre and later take their infants for a check-up at the clinic, are penalized with a further fine of PGK 5 for not coming to the health centre to birth their babies. These are considerable expenses for people who have no ready access to a cash income.[3]

In 2009, during a village meeting at which I was present, a teacher reprimanded parents for not maintaining the building and grounds of the local community school; this was not, she argued, something that the school children should have to do. She pointed out that children were coming to school with their homework assignments not done and without lunch food and, consequently, couldn't concentrate. She went on to chastise parents for treating their children as "parental slaves," by sending children off to do "chores" after school rather than ensuring their homework was completed. Finally, she reproached mothers who worked in the gardens all day for keeping their girl children home from school so that the girls could help work in the gardens, mind their younger siblings, and prepare the family's evening meal. Her speech was eloquent and heartfelt as she reminded parents they were "throwing away" their schools and "the future of their children" with this behaviour.[4]

Bariai women's lives are extremely overburdened, and they do need their daughters' assistance with gardening labour, carrying water and firewood, and child minding; they cannot do it all themselves, which is an issue rarely discussed. When I brought up women's labour burdens to the men, who, in fact, do a great deal of child minding, they pointed to their traditional gendered division of labour. Although they agreed that women had plenty to do and worked long, arduous hours, they argued that girls are brought up to be able to do this work; they are "trained" to endure hard work. In contrast, boys and men were not trained for gardening labour, carrying water, cutting and carrying firewood, and daily domestic chores of housecleaning, laundry, and care of children and pigs. Women who faltered in their roles and their work could be beaten with impunity (McPherson, "Black and Blue"). Education for Bariai children, especially for girls, is a complex undertaking entangled in a cashless economy, gender roles, gendered concepts of value, masculine privilege, and a gendered division of labour, among other considerations.

My particular Bariai example is not unique. Sub-Saharan Africa is "home to more than half the world's out-of-school children" (UN *MDG Report* 15). Even when some girls do go to school, the biggest educational gender disparity in both Africa and Oceania appears at the secondary level when most girls fall behind boys, which leads to a larger gender disparity at the secondary and tertiary level of education. Girls reaching secondary school are most likely to fall behind boys because these girls are more often than not removed from school by their parents, who see no point to investing scarce school fees in daughters who will just get married and her husband's family would reap any benefits from her education. Parental investment in raising and educating their daughter plus the loss of a daughter's labour would not be reciprocated as social security in their old age. Girls in both Africa and Oceania fall behind boys because mothers require their daughters' labour for subsistence work and child minding, or parents seek to marry off their daughters in order to realize her bridewealth (Yakong; Yakong and McPherson, this volume).

Employment and Governance

Without education, girls clearly have less access to training for cash employment and less of a chance to afford the lifestyle that a cash economy seems to promise. Without education, women are unable to take on the responsibilities of or to be involved in government—whether at the local, state, or federal levels—assuming, of course, their culturally relevant concepts of gender should imagine the possibility of such a role for a woman. Recent statistics on women's global representation in politics, compiled by the Inter-Parliamentary Union (IPU) and UN Women, clearly show the "sluggish progress" in gender equality and women's empowerment (IPU, Women in Politics Map). In Table 1 below, I list statistics specifically pertaining to the countries represented in the chapters herein. I also include examples from cosmopolitan countries of Canada, the UK and Australia for comparison.

Table 1: Based on Data from *Women in Politics Map 2014*.

Country	% Women in Parliament	Number of Seats	Global Rank Out of 145
Cameroon	31.1	56/180	33
Ethiopia	27.8	152/547	40
Ghana	10.9	30/275	113
Malawi	22.3	43/193	66
Marshall Islands	3.0	1/33	140
Micronesia	0.0	0/14	145
Papua New Guinea	2.7	3/111	141
Solomon Islands	2.0	1/50	142
Vanuatu	0.0	0/52	145
Australia	26.0	39/150	48
Canada	25.1	77/147	54
United Kingdom	22.6	147/650	64

The indicator of success for MDG 3 seems framed in a loose concept of female empowerment as a function of education and literacy. Although education is a necessary component of women's empowerment, it is not always a sufficient component. Crossette points out that "even educated, politically active women can have very low personal status and virtually no rights in making reproductive decisions.... They also face widespread violence, much of it linked to personal relationships" (75). Women's lack of empowerment is also evident in women's decision-making processes. In the studies of rural areas of Africa and Oceania presented in this collection, women have little or no say in money-related decisions, in inheritance and property rights matters and, most critically, in terms of their own health, especially when it comes to control over their reproductive choices. In the World Bank 2011 report *Reproductive Health at a Glance: Papua New Guinea* "gender equality and women's empowerment" are *finally* recognized as "important for improving reproductive health" (1). But it must be stated, this same empowerment can be hazardous to women's health "when men realise the implications for their authority" (Mcintyre 246). In PNG, masculine authority is a deeply entrenched sense of male entitlement and masculine privilege, and men resort to violence against women as a means of reclaiming their authority and control over women. As Mcintyre argues for PNG in particular, strategies thought to enable female empowerment and gender equality fail "because they do not confront the structural inequalities between men and women" (238; McPherson "Black and Blue").

MDG 5 TARGET AND INDICATORS

Generally, MDG 5 is focused on "improving maternal health," and the multiple indicators of success in improving maternal health globally are listed (UN MDG Indicators) as the following:

5.1 Reduce the rates of maternal mortality
5.2 Increase the presence of skilled birth attendants at a birth
5.3 Increase the contraception prevalence rate
5.4 Reduce the adolescent birth rate
5.5 Provide antenatal care coverage by at least one to four visits per pregnancy
5.6 Improve unmet need for family planning.

What do these points mean exactly? These targets or subcategories of MDG 5 suggest six interventions that are supposed to improve maternal health and, by extension, lower maternal and infant mortality. The targets in MDG 5 presume that MDG 3 has been accomplished and that women have power and control over their bodies and their reproductive decision making. The targets also assume that cosmopolitan obstetrics and the "authoritative knowledge" (Jordan 154) of health care delivery personnel trained in that knowledge and technology will prevent maternal deaths. Indeed, with trained personnel and appropriate equipment and medicines, some maternal deaths are prevented; however, not much attention is paid to the contributing factors in maternal deaths in the first place. Issues affecting women's maternal health include, among many others, poverty, overwork, anaemia due to endemic malaria (which is rife in many countries in Africa and Oceania), communicable diseases, poor nutrition, violence (e.g., spousal and familial abuse, beatings, and structural violence), too many pregnancies too close together, and sexually transmitted infections (STI). Although MDG indicators fit within a model of cosmopolitan obstetrics, at least two issues emerge from the studies presented in the following chapters. First, not all of these targets are in play at the same time or at all; and second, there is no indication of a relationship or correlation among these six "targets" that can be pointed to as causal for improved maternal health or reduced maternal mortality. If any one factor or a combination of these factors affecting women's daily lives can be identified as causal in a pregnant woman's death in childbirth, then antenatal care is not going to reduce maternal mortality rates; rather, changing those precipitating factors would be useful. This is a perspective found in the Papua New Guinea Report of 2009, which points out that "twenty percent of maternal deaths are due to an underlying disease that is aggravated by pregnancy—such as malaria, iron deficiency anaemia, hepatitis, tuberculosis or heart disease ... therefore a strong primary health care and prevention program is a necessary foundation for maternal health" (26-27).

In 2000, Luck reviewed thirty-four studies conducted in Africa under the Safe Motherhood Initiative and concluded that "there exists little evidence regarding which interventions will reduce maternal mortality levels in African settings" (599). Contra the high technology associated with cosmopolitan medicine, Luck further found that "several low-tech improvements in emergency obstetric services" were clearly identified as improving "maternal outcomes and deserve replication and testing" (599). Extrapolating from Luck's results, I find it interesting that there are no critical analyses of the MDGs drawing correlations between lower maternal mortality ratios and the presence of antenatal care, skilled birth attendants, contraceptive use, or a decline in adolescent pregnancies. In other words, there is no way of knowing what did or did not work to improve maternal mortality ratios or women's maternal and reproductive health according to the model of cosmopolitan obstetrics. As Smith rightly points out (this volume), the MDGs and their lists of targets exist in silos having no relationship with the other MDGs or even among the targets for individual MDGs, as I now briefly consider in relation to MDG 5.

5.1 Reduce the Rates of Maternal Mortality

Drawing on McCarthy and Maine, Luck outlines three steps to maternal death: first, there is a pregnancy, which is directly or indirectly related to the death; second, complications arise with that pregnancy due to "a pre-existing condition aggravated by pregnancy, from the pregnancy itself or from management of the pregnancy (including its termination)"; and third, "there must be no effective treatment of the complications, due to the absence of medical intervention or to inappropriate or insufficient intervention" (600). Thus, in order to prevent maternal mortality, intervention includes preventing the pregnancy in the first place, or preventing complications in a pregnancy, or preventing "complications from resulting in maternal death" (600).

Reduction of the number of maternal deaths is a quantifiable result, thus easily applied to measure progress or its lack. The maternal mortality ratio is the number of women who die during pregnancy, during birthing and up to forty-two days postpartum per 100,000 live births. A decrease in the number of maternal deaths previously recorded over a period of time is considered indicative of improvement in maternal health generally. Such statistics are notoriously incomplete. In many "challenging contexts countries" (Crichton and Onguko), maternal (and infant) deaths are not always reported or recorded, especially in rural areas where people do not keep written records and they have difficulty accessing local aid posts, district health centres, or regional hospital care where such records might be kept. It remains to be seen how accurately peri-urban and rural health care workers maintain their records and whether these statistical renderings take into account the women and neonates who die in rural villages. Indeed, with the pressure on rural health care workers to "produce" positive results, one wonders if some maternal and infant deaths are simply *not* recorded in order to provide a record of positive results for the clinic. The percentages of the maternal mortality rate (MMR) likely underrepresent the degree to which change has (or has not) occurred.

From 1994 to 2006, the maternal mortality rate in Papua New Guinea was 733/100,000 live births, the highest in the world (Papua New Guinea, *Ministerial Taskforce*, 1; World Bank, *Reproductive Health at a Glance: Papua New Guinea*). This number represents the "doubling of PNG's MMR as measured by the Demographic Health Surveys (DHS) ... a clear indication of the failure of access to and the delivery of quality health services over the last 10-15 years" (Papua New Guinea, *Ministerial Taskforce* v). The 2008 maternal mortality rate in PNG was given as 250/100,000 (a huge drop that is not explained) and, for Oceania generally, the MMR was about 200/100,000 live births (*Ministerial Taskforce* v). Another survey cited the MMR in Papua New Guinea as 312/100,000 (Dawson et al.). The MDG 5 target for PNG by 2015 was a rate of 85/100,000. MMRs in Sub-Saharan Africa reached 500/100,000 in 2010, and the MDG goal of approximately half that number was not achieved in 2015. Sub-Saharan Africa is a huge demographic and geographic area; nonetheless, the MMR for that demographic region was at 990/100,000 in 1990, dropped to 510 in 2013, but missed the 2015 target of 250/100,000 (UN Overview 29). Compare these rates to MMRs in Northern Africa at 78, Canada at 5, and the USA at 12 per 100,000, respectively.[5] In Oceania, a huge area of dispersed island states with relatively small populations and varying levels of health care provision and facilities, the MMR was 390/100,000 in 1990 and 190/100,000 in 2013, but missed the 2015 target aimed at less than 100/100,000. It is not made clear, if these statistics are accepted, how this drop in MMRs was actually accomplished.

A survey of seventeen Asian and four Pacific countries concludes that a Papua New Guinea woman has a 1/110 chance of dying in childbirth, only slightly better off than a woman in Laos at 1/74 and a woman in Afghanistan at 1/32 (Thanenthiran et al. 65). According to the UNDP report for Papua New Guinea, "the challenges of distance, isolation, lack of transport and an extreme shortage of skilled birth attendants, highlight the hazards of childbirth in PNG" ("About Papua New Guinea"). Even one maternal death is too many, but this last statement implies that women living in rurally isolated circumstances without transportation are somehow unable to birth without skilled personnel (i.e., technologically trained, cosmopolitan obstetrical practitioner) and thus have a high likelihood of dying. This is borne out by the next comment that there are "five women dying *every day* while giving birth [emphasis added]" and "currently a woman in rural PNG has a one in 25 chance of dying in her lifetime as a result of childbirth" ("About Papua New Guinea"). Clearly, any other conditions under which these women might live—known as the social determinants of health—are not deemed to contribute to maternal ill health or ability to birth successfully; circumstances of distance, lack of transport and inability to access skilled birth attendants are enough to seal the fate of the birthing woman.

Women do not die *because* of isolation or distance to urban areas. Their well-being and maternal health are jeopardized because of the conditions of their lived realities, such as I itemized above—malaria, poor nutrition, overwork, STIs, physical abuse, too many and too frequent pregnancies. These are the kinds of conditions that put women in mortal danger during pregnancy and birthing, not the mere biology of reproduction or distance and isolation. Although cosmopolitan obstetrics may well save them from death, cosmopolitan medicine does not prevent women from becoming seriously ill in the first place. This message comes across very clearly in the papers in this collection where, in some respects, cosmopolitan obstetrics creates more problems in women's lives than it alleviates (Hobbis; Smith; Wogaing, this volume).

5.2 Increase the Presence of Skilled Birth Attendants at a Birth

According to the World Health Organization, a skilled birth attendant is a midwife or doctor or nurse with technical training in midwifery, a category that excludes "traditional birth attendants and community health workers" (Kvernflaten 33) who have not been trained in cosmopolitan obstetrics. Furthermore, the World Health Organization (WHO) notes that, whether or not traditional birth attendants (TBAs) are trained, they are still "excluded from the category of skilled health workers" (Thanenthiran 68) by definition of their status as "traditional;" that is, they have not been educated in cosmopolitan obstetrics. Skilled birth attendants so defined represent a huge investment in education in order to train health care workers in biomedical technology and supply the expensive technology itself (Jordan 214). As Jordan points out, most developing countries have inadequate technology and technicians, such that

> the practice of scientific medicine suffers from chronically short health care resources, such as lack of adequately trained physicians and health care personnel, insufficient supplies of drugs, inadequate hospital facilities ... developing countries inherit not only the problems inherent in medicalized birth but also the problems inherent in doing obstetrics badly, that is, without the technological ... support [human, medicinal, facilities] for adequate functioning. (130-131)

Intervention suggests that a trained nurse or midwife not only is capable of dealing with obstetrical emergencies but also has the technological equipment to prevent a mother's death due to complications—obstructed birth, haemorrhage, transverse lie, sepsis and puerperal fever, and so forth. Some of the authors in this collection show that "skilled" personnel, who are or should be capable of dealing with obstetric emergencies, are not always available at rural health centres or clinics, and if they are, they often lack the tools—equipment, medicines, blood bank, and incubators—for obstetrical emergencies. These types of obstetrical emergencies are best treated at hospitals, where such facilities, supplies, and trained personnel are more likely (but still, not always) available; such facilities are certainly not readily available in rural areas, as the work presented in the following chapters illustrates.

5.3 Increase the Contraception Prevalence Rate

This target actually speaks to the notion that for a maternal death to occur there needs first of all to be a pregnancy. Access to and use of contraceptives, such as condoms, IUDs or injections could reduce the number of pregnancies a woman experiences in her reproductive lifetime. Interestingly, contraception as a form of birth spacing has only become "necessary" with the advent of colonial governance, global development, and cosmopolitan fears in the Global North of overpopulation. Women in Africa and Oceania have for ages traditionally spaced their pregnancies according to customary postpartum taboos. In my research sites in West New Britain, PNG, the postpartum taboo prohibits lactating women from engaging in sexual intercourse for as long as they breastfeed, which could be as long as two to four years. The taboo is based on a culturally defined female body that connects womb and breast; thus, if a lactating woman engages in sexual intercourse, sperm can travel from her uterus to her breasts causing her infant to experience respiratory problems as a consequence of ingesting sperm-contaminated milk. Husbands are under no such obligation to remain celibate, but they do (usually) refrain from sex with their wife, so as to protect their infants from respiratory disease and potential death. Such abstinence does not prevent husbands from having sex with other women. Bariai women reported to me that this strains their marriage, as they worry about their husbands going off with other women. Currently, this postpartum taboo is no longer observed in West New Britain because of the availability of antibiotics (primarily penicillin) administered for respiratory illnesses. Interestingly, however, the demise of this taboo has had an adverse effect on birth spacing for Bariai women. Thanks to antibiotics, the nursing infant's health is no longer considered to be at risk from its mother's sexual activities and as a result, husbands are demanding sex more often from their wives, with the effect that women are now having too many pregnancies too closely spaced (McPherson, "Black and Blue").

Besides providing contraception, using condoms can protect women from sexually transmitted infections linked to difficulties with conception, gestation to term, and a safe birthing process.

Condoms protect women from contracting infections from their sexual partner(s), including a woman's husband. Indeed, as Smith points out in this volume, male promiscuity is the leading source of married women contracting HIV (McPherson "*SikAids*;" Wardlow). But condom use is a fraught concept. As Pollock discusses in her chapter in this collection, Marshallese women have little interest in using condoms for contraception because they continue to experience interrupted pregnancies and stillbirths as a consequence of radiation contamination associated with U.S. nuclear testing in the Pacific. Marshallese women traditionally space their pregnancies two years apart with an expectation that they will give birth at least once every two years. For a Marshallese woman, bearing a child every two years is her contribution to her family and to the larger society. To not bear a child every two years is considered her personal failure. Contraceptive use is viewed negatively in many societies around the world due to a culture of pronatalism or to various religious tenets, such as the stance taken by the Catholic Church that the use of contraception (and abortion) is an immoral act. As the case studies in this volume suggest, women do not have decision-making control when it comes to contraceptives and birth spacing. Indeed, as Hayes points out in her chapter here, condom use in Malawi is associated with women who are sex workers, with foreign (that is, imported) sexual practices, and with infidelity.

In many societies, womanhood and social adulthood are conditional on a woman's ability to bear children. Bariai women who do not become pregnant after marriage are likely to beaten by their husbands who suspect them of using contraceptives or of infidelity, or both (McPherson, "Women, Childbirth and Change"). If women want to control the number of their pregnancies, they could, theoretically, seek contraceptive information and products at their local health centres and clinics. In West New Britain, a woman seeking contraception at a clinic must be accompanied by her husband who has to approve her request, a condition for access that usually blocks the process. Men generally do not approve of birth control in any form, as they assume a wife will be promiscuous without the consequence of pregnancy. Moreover, cultural concepts of masculinity include fathering of many children. Female and male health care workers might also hold beliefs about condom use as immoral and will act as gatekeepers or moral arbiters and refuse to dispense condoms. One health care worker in West New Britain who obtained a supply of condoms to give out to anyone who asked told me that in his experience, health workers will claim not to have condoms in order to avoid dispensing them. As a result, the condoms in stock rotted in the tropical heat and humidity. As shown in the studies in this collection (e.g., Hayes; Hobbis; Smith), it is very common for married women to be reluctant to seek contraceptives at clinics, as they rarely accommodate people's privacy concerns. Thus, women and adolescents do not access services or enter clinics as a strategy to avoid being gossiped about or shamed.

In sum, the MDG target to increase the prevalence rate of contraception does not consider women's lived realities. The MDG incorrectly assumes that female empowerment has been accomplished and that women have control over their reproductive decisions making. It also assumes that women's cultural belief systems permit them to use contraception, ignoring the fact that having children is closely tied to notions of womanhood and manhood. It also assumes that health clinics are culturally safe places and that health care workers do not act as gate keepers or monitors of the morality of others.

Access to family planning and birth control thus remains difficult if not impossible for most women who might seek it out. Luck points out that "conspicuously absent" in the Safe Motherhood Initiative is an "intervention to prevent unsafe abortions" (605). None of the thirty-four studies Luck reviewed "explicitly sought to prevent maternal morbidity and mortality caused by unsafe abortion, despite the growing evidence that unsafe abortion is responsible for a large proportion of maternal deaths in Africa" (605). Drawing on Benson et al (1996), Luck shows that "the contribution of unsafe abortion to maternal mortality [is] as high as 54 percent" (605). Luck also cites Likwa's 1993 study in Lesotho, Malawi, Uganda and Zambia where "30 percent of maternal deaths were a consequence of unsafe abortion" (605). Safe abortion is a conspicuously absent preventative of maternal morbidity and mortality in the MDGs, which do not acknowledge that abortion even occurs, or suggest interventions for obstetrical services and facilities for safe abortion for the prevention of maternal mortalities due to unsafe and clandestine abortions.

5.4 Reduce the Adolescent Birth Rate

The World Health Organization defines adolescents as the 10-19 age group, and in general terms, this period is considered a time of transition from childhood to adulthood, during which young people experience changes following puberty, but do not immediately assume the roles, privileges and responsibilities of adulthood (Thanenthiran et al. 107).

Calls to reduce adolescent birth rates do not address the reasons why there is an adolescent birth rate that needs to be curtailed. Adolescent sexual activity has been a reality forever and having babies at too young an age—before a woman is physically mature enough to carry to term and birth without complications and before she is socially mature enough to raise a child—is not something to be encouraged. However, why are adolescent girls getting pregnant? Among the several villages where I research in West New Britain, two adolescent girls I knew (fifteen years and sixteen years of age) had been repeatedly raped and were impregnated by a family member (an "uncle") in whose homes the girls boarded to attend high school. The potential for this kind of abuse is another reason parents are reluctant to send their daughters to attend distant high schools. Adolescent girls become pregnant because they are interested in or pressured into sex at an early age, because they are raped, and because they are married off much too young (see Yakong 2013 for a Ghanaian example of child marriage). In some Pacific countries, girls are by customary law permitted to marry as young as twelve or thirteen, and "young girls sold into marriage are often forced into domestic servitude for the husband's extended family" (Thanenthiran et al. 123).

If it is difficult for married women to access contraceptives, it is next to impossible for adolescent females to obtain them, since adolescent girls are expected not to engage in premarital sex. On the other hand, in many cultures there is a masculine prerogative when it comes to sexuality. The conundrum—the double standard—is that premarital sex is usually expected of adolescent males, but adolescent females are expected to remain chaste until marriage.

Smith's chapter in this collection discusses the gender-unequal standards in Chuuk. She finds that for girls, sexual activity is "not an accepted part of adolescence ... yet, sexual 'freedom' is an accepted part of boys' lives." Also in this collection, Hayes discusses how Malawian women must subordinate their desires to those of men and are unable to negotiate their sexual encounters or to request condoms. Hayes also notes that "Malawians are deeply suspicious of condoms because their dissemination is sponsored by the government and funded by the international donor community; the two groups most often blamed by locals for the introduction and spread of HIV." Hayes here provides another example of how women lack empowerment to make and carry through on decisions pertaining to their own sexuality and reproductive life.

5.5 Provide Antenatal Care Coverage by at Least One to Four Visits Per Pregnancy

Antenatal care can be beneficial in identifying and monitoring problems (e.g., gestational diabetes, heart conditions, high blood pressure, and STIs) that pregnancy is likely to aggravate. The studies presented in this volume show women's access to antenatal care is minimal at best and usually consists of measuring fundal height, fetal heartbeat, mother's weight, and dispensing of iron and calcium tablets. Because clinics are often far from where women live and women attend infrequently, if at all, clinic personnel—midwives, nurses, and orderlies—rarely have knowledge of their women clients, the circumstances of their lives, or even their languages and cultures. Ironically, in Luck's review of thirty-four studies, *not one study* "sought to assess the impact of antenatal care on maternal mortality. This may be due to the difficulties of establishing, even in industrialized societies, that standard antenatal practises improve maternal health [emphasis added]" (601). Even in cosmopolitan societies, it is not established that antenatal care improves maternal health outcomes. What does seem to be the case is that antenatal programs indoctrinate women into the beliefs, values and practices of cosmopolitan obstetrics.

In many societies, such as those presented in this volume, pregnancy is not something that women draw attention to or discuss. For example, where I study in West New Britain, people become aware of a woman's pregnancy by observing specific signs of bodily changes and, of course, when her pregnancy is advanced and, thus, physically unmistakable (McPherson, "Modern Obstetrics," "Women, Childbirth and Change"; Scaletta). To draw attention to her pregnancy (which also draws attention to her sexuality) could put mother and fetus at risk of jealous attack from sorcerers or spirit forces. Furthermore, pregnancy is not culturally defined as a pathological condition; thus, women are expected to be healthy and well during their pregnancies. In previously colonized societies, women have been taught about pregnancy as pathology during antenatal care provided by various missionaries, who, for the most part, disapproved of the existing indigenous system of reproductive care. Mission sites were far from most rural villages, as in West New Britain, and intrepid nursing sisters travelled to remote villages on foot or by outrigger canoe with or without small outboard motors (Barlow, this volume) on a monthly basis to weigh, measure, and immunize infants zero to five years of age. They also provided antenatal care to pregnant women who came forth (and not all presented at these clinics) to receive iron pills (to build "strong" blood), antimalarial tablets (not sufficient to be either prophylactic or curative doses in my field experience), and calcium tablets.

Since the construction in 1982 of a *haus karim* or "birthing house" in northwest coastal New Britain, women have been expected to attend the local health centre for antenatal care and birthing; however, few coastal women attend because it is too far to walk (McPherson "Modern Obstetrics;" "Women, Childbirth and Change"). Expectant mothers are enjoined to arrive at the health centre at least one month prior to the birthing due date to have the clinic nurse, "a skilled birth attendant," present at the birth (Scaletta). What the authors in this volume collectively show is that time, distance, and the availability and cost of transportation are usually prohibitive of a pregnant woman living in a rural area being able to attend at any kind of health care clinic. But as I pointed out above, distance and lack of transportation are not causes of a difficult birthing; what women do experience is much upheaval and distress trying to comply with the directive to attend a clinic with a trained birth attendant. Indeed, as

Pollock notes in her chapter, a Marshallese woman who wishes to birth at the hospital must plan on being away from her home village and family for up to six months because of the distance between islands and the unreliability of ships schedules that may or may not call at various ports. Ethnographers in this collection describe how women often travel to a rural health clinic only to find those facilities are closed or under-resourced by few, usually overworked, personnel who have little in the way of medicine or equipment to deal with complications that women face (Yakong and McPherson; Wogaing, this volume).

Few women in the studies included here have access to emergency obstetrical care at a hospital or even access to well-stocked and staffed rural clinics. Hospitals—rather than aid posts, local health centres, or clinics—are where one would hope to find trained personnel able to perform Caesarean sections and administer blood transfusions and other medications to deal with haemorrhage. Too often, clinics have no medication, their equipment is rudimentary, and emergency obstetrical care is non-existent or inefficient (see Wogaing, this volume; Yakong). Women's experience of the clinic is often not very welcoming or pleasant. In many instances, clinic nurses shout at women, are impatient with them, strike them, or treat rural women with disrespect (McPherson "Modern Obstetrics;" "Women, Childbirth and Change"; Scaletta). A pronounced lack of trust between pregnant women and health care workers is evident in all the studies in this volume.

Providing access to antenatal care and having a skilled attendant present at the birth are particularly problematic in rural areas of the world. In the African and insular Pacific nations discussed in this volume, the number of women whose birthing was assisted by a skilled attendant has increased. But the statistical uptick is primarily due to increased access to birth attendants in urban areas, where it is easier to practise cosmopolitan obstetrics. Generally, in Oceania, 31 percent fewer women in rural areas have skilled attendants at their births than do urban women; similarly, in Sub-Saharan Africa, rural women were attended for only 40 percent of births, which is a 36 percent gap compared to urban women, who were attended for 76 percent of births. Unless disaggregated for differences such as urban and rural, such statistics are overgeneralizations that misinform more than inform. These kinds of differences in services for women in rural areas and for women in urban areas are a function of the centralization of health care services in urban areas, where cosmopolitan obstetrics is more easily practised. It is, thus, not surprising that the 2009 Papua New Guinea Report notes that, "rural health has improved very little *in the last 30 years* [emphasis added]" (vii).

5.6 Improve Unmet Need for Family Planning

The site listing official MDG indicators defines "unmet need for family planning" as follows:

> Women with unmet need for family planning for limiting births are those who are fecund and sexually active but are not using any method of contraception, and report not wanting any more children. This is a subcategory of total unmet need for family planning, which also includes unmet need for spacing births. The concept of unmet need points to the gap between women's reproductive intentions and their contraceptive behaviour. For MDG monitoring, unmet need is expressed as a percentage based on women who are married or in a consensual union. ("Unmet Family Planning Needs")

What leaps out in the calculations to determine unmet family planning needs is that women have opinions about spacing their pregnancies, about having fewer pregnancies, and about preventing pregnancy altogether if they have enough children or simply do not want any more children. Key phrases in the above definition—"fecund and sexually active," "report not wanting any more children," and "the gap between women's reproductive intentions and their contraceptive behaviour"—suggest that women are being somewhat fickle or non-compliant here. In other words, women reportedly want to space or curtail their pregnancies but do not follow through on these "intentions" with an appropriate "contraceptive behaviour." The assumption again is that women freely make reproductive choices, and they can freely obtain contraceptives and control those choices with impunity. My discussion above regarding access to and use of condoms showed that married, fecund, and sexually active women (and adolescents) have few choices about "family planning." Surveys in the 2009 PNG *Ministerial Taskforce* note that more than half of women who already have two children do not wish to have more children; yet "despite this desire to have smaller families, fewer than 35.7 percent of women of reproductive age are using modern methods of family planning" (vii). The survey only selected married women and women in a consensual relationship. Rather naively, I think, the MDG target 5.6 assumes that by identifying women with unmet family planning needs, it is simply a matter of getting them to access and use an appropriate method of birth control. There is a general disregard for women's lack of empowerment not only in their personal lives but also in social, economic and political domains. The lack of empowerment is especially evident in women's desire to control their reproductive lives but their inability to do so.

Women in PNG are having more children than they wish to have (McPherson, "Black and Blue") but are constrained from using birth control by their customary and contemporary belief systems, their spouses, even their husband's kin—who culturally have a stake in the woman's fecundity, as she reproduces members of their kin group (Pollock, this volume; Yakong). In Sub-Saharan Africa, approximately 28 percent of women are unable to access family planning and may well be forbidden to do so by their husbands. The pronatalism in many patriarchal societies can have a hugely detrimental impact on women's physical and mental health (Yakong).

I have touched on some of the difficulties women (married, single, and adolescent) encounter when trying to obtain contraceptive information and products. Those difficulties include clinic gatekeepers, religious tenets that prohibit birth control, and the cultural negativity assigned to contraceptives and labelling women who use them as immoral, sinful, promiscuous or prostitutes. Infertility, pregnancy, and obstetric complications are also linked to sexually transmitted infections, but women are made continually vulnerable to contracting STIs, as they are unable to access condoms or, if they can access them, are unable to insist that a male sexual partner use them.

INTRODUCTION

A major barrier to improving maternal health is women's lack of empowerment due to cultural beliefs that inform gender asymmetry and assign masculine control over women's lives, including women's bodies and women's reproductive decision making. Customary gender hierarchy, reinforced by contemporary patriarchal institutions such as Christian churches and male-headed government at all levels, assigns masculine authority and control over women's bodies (McPherson, "Black and Blue"). This gendered power imbalance operates in the context of a nearly universal sexual double standard that gives men more sexual freedom and rights of sexual self-determination than women (Blanc 190; Mcintyre). Gender-based power inequities in sexual relationships highlight the question of "whose fertility preferences—the male partner's or the female partner's—carries more weight in the decision to practice contraception and ... in the decision regarding the number and timing of births" (Blanc 193). The chapters in this volume make the case that without gender equality and empowerment, women are unable to make and carry out decisions pertaining to their own (and their children's) health and well-being (Yakong). Clearly, women's human right to determine their sexual and reproductive health is disempowered by men, particularly husbands, who play a major role in a woman's decision-making processes. Brewis points out that "how men's and women's differing perspectives specifically operate in regard to each other in the process of reproductive decision-making has not been addressed" (391). For example, the role of men in promoting and empowering women's reproductive decision making is not part of the MDG indicators or interventions at all. Brewis records that "applied family planning research in the Pacific has very often ignored the potentially central role of men (usually husbands) to family planning dynamics and programmatic success" (397).

Interestingly, the "unmet family planning needs" in MDG 5.6 in no way suggest that there is any unmet need regarding women's *in*fertility needs. A 2003 WHO study determined that "more than 30 percent of women aged 25-49 suffer from secondary infertility," which means that a woman has had one successful birth but has been unable to become pregnant or to successfully carry to term another pregnancy ("Mother or Nothing: The Agony of Infertility").

But even more interesting is the statement that "although male infertility has been found to be the cause of a couple's failure to conceive in about 50 percent of cases, the social burden [of infertility] falls disproportionately on women" (Pollock, this volume; Van Balen and Inhorn, 19; Yakong). Typically, in cultures that mandate motherhood, women who are unable to conceive—for any number of reasons—can be divorced or put aside and made to endure a polygamous relationship in which their husband marries a second wife (Leonard). In a patrilineal society, an infertile, childless woman might never be considered a fully social adult and, therefore, has few or none of the privileges of adulthood. And because she has no rights to any resources in her husband's patrimony, her childlessness means that she will never have sons to assure her old age. Assisted reproductive technologies are available in Africa for treatment of infertility and

> the management of infertility is an important issue that demands the appropriate and judicious allocation of resources in Africa. However, we believe that from the public health perspective, African countries should invest in the prevention and conventional treatment of infertility, rather than on high-cost ART [assisted reproductive therapy]. The emphasis should be on prevention, since such programs will benefit other sexual and reproductive health problems and also free resources to address the mounting rate of ill-health from other diseases in Africa. The development of high-tech treatment of infertility in the public sector should be a long-term venture, when basic health and social issues have been adequately addressed. (Okonofua and Obi 11)

This statement suggests that until poverty, gender equality, excellent maternal and reproductive health facilities and outcomes, plus the treatment of the causes of infertility, are achieved (some of which fertility researchers argue are inexplicable), resources should not be invested in infertility treatments.

Thus, MDG 3 and MDG 5, despite being considered separate "goals," have foundational and intersecting social, cultural, and economic issues that affect all aspects of women's lives, especially their sexual, reproductive, and maternal health. The eight MDGs cannot be seem as standing alone but must be seen as a complex set of intersecting issues. It is the complexity that informs women's lived realities that is at heart of the articles in this volume.

ETHNOGRAPHIC STUDIES

Each of the studies presented here begins from a perspective of cultural complexity, an entanglement of beliefs, values, and behaviours. In this way, the authors acknowledge and explore the specific worldviews that inform cultural concepts of gender and gender relations, the culturally appropriate roles for women and men, the value of reproduction for women and men, and attitudes to health care, pregnancy, birthing, and contraception. Contributors ground their discussion in specific ethnographic examples in specific cultural worlds that the implementation of a universal health policy—a one MDG size fits all—will surely have to accommodate for any success in future. Cultures do not change overnight or even over decades; rather, cultural change is often resisted as people refuse to relinquish what they consider to be the "right way" or the "human way" to live their lives. Of particular importance to women's general health and their maternal and reproductive health is to address the "structural inequalities between men and women" (Mcintyre 239; McPherson, "Black and Blue").

Adopting cosmopolitan obstetrics assumes that any and all health care facilities are properly resourced with trained personnel, up-to-date technology, sufficient medical supplies, and drugs, and are easily accessible to all who need or want their services. In the chapters in this volume, it is clear that this is simply not something that governments, missionaries, or aid societies have been able to ensure.

Efforts are being made. However, as Wentworth shows, an overzealous breastfeeding campaign in Vanuatu often ends up "throwing the baby out with the bathwater." As a response to child malnutrition and poverty in Vanuatu, breastfeeding is promoted as a means to good growth and to prevent stunting and other outcomes of poor infant nutrition. In Vanuatu, as in all the societies presented here, breastfeeding is the norm; however, in the

Mother–Baby Friendly Hospital Initiative in Port Vila, mothers who have difficulty breastfeeding are stigmatized and portrayed as "inadequate mothers." The manner in which health care workers implement and carry out a breastfeeding only program that forbids bottle feeding and wet nursing regardless of circumstance, Wentworth (this volume) argues, "ultimately ends with alienating the mothers it is attempting to serve." Lack of trust is an all-too-frequent theme in the studies here. Wentworth concludes that "planting the seeds of distrust can lead to negative health outcomes for other MDGs as mothers exit the health care system with feelings of distrust and inadequacy and report not feeling confident that health care practitioners are really able to adequately serve them and their families in times of need."

Too often, women are enjoined to reject aspects of their cultural system, such as Mursi women's lip plates, because others perceive them to be "harmful cultural practices." As LaTosky points out, pregnant Mursi women are unable to access the small amount of money available to them to help pay for transportation to a health centre, unless they agree to have their lips surgically stitched. Mursi women's lip disks have nothing to do with reproductive health and in no way affect a woman's pregnancy or her ability to birth a baby. Pressure to change is a function of offended sensibilities of outsiders who disapprove of such body beautification practices. This theme of resistance to the invasive culture of cosmopolitan obstetrics, global capitalism, and neocolonialism sometimes whispers but more often shouts in the chapters here.

All the countries presented here have a history of colonialism, the aftermath of which continues to be prominent in their lives. Indeed, the Marshall Islands (Pollock) and the Federated States of Micronesian (FSM) (Smith) to this day remain tethered to the United States by a Compact of Free Association. Under this agreement, among other things, the U.S. is responsible for funding education and health care. This is especially poignant in Rongelap in the Marshall Islands, where people continue to suffer from exposure to radioactive fallout from U.S. atmospheric testing and the 1954 explosion of the nuclear bomb, *Bravo*. Pollock relates that Rongelap women still miscarry or birth horribly malformed fetuses, which they call "jelly babies." These "reproductive failures" affect women's lives as child-bearers for their kin groups but also underscores why Rongelap women view "family planning" and contraceptive use to be working against them rather than for them and their reproductive choices.

Health care is abysmal in the Marshalls and the FSM. Historically, Rongelap women's reproductive concerns were covered up by U.S. medical teams. In Chuuk, hospitals are dilapidated and women do not want to attend for birthing due to lack of supplies, lack of cleanliness, and poor quality of care. Nor do women, men, or young people attend hospital or health centres for tests for STIs or contraceptives because of the public nature of those places and the embarrassment or shame accrued simply by being seen to enter them (Smith this volume). The lack of privacy at clinics and health care facilities prevents people from accessing care or health information, which cripples people's decision-making processes about whether or not to access contraceptive methods or information and protection to avoid STIs that do affect women's reproductive health. As birth control devices, condoms have a mixed reputation, decried (by church and state) for promoting promiscuity and infidelity (Hayes this volume). As protection from disease, however, many women do not obtain condoms because they have no power to insist their partners use them, and they fear partner violence against them for being untrustworthy, too "worldly," sexually promiscuous, or immoral.

Another important aspect of maternal and reproductive care evident in these papers is the distance from where women live to the nearest health care facility and the costs in time and money, not only to get to a health centre but also to cover the financial and social expense incurred while at a health centre for treatments (Hobbis; Yakong and McPherson; Wentworth). Rural women are often hours if not days of travel away from a health care facility offering antenatal care and "skilled birth attendants." Transportation vehicles—cars, ambulances, and boats—are often mechanically broken, fuel or muscle power is often unavailable, and promised transportation may simply never materialize (Hobbis, LaTosky this volume). Rarely, in the examples of these chapters, does a woman have the freedom of movement to access transport or the finances to pay for transport (e.g., gas, drivers, food, accommodation, medicines while away). Women also must receive permission from their husbands and their in-laws, who may decide that she is not "sick," and, thus, antenatal care, for them, is a waste of time, minimizing the work she could be doing in her gardens (Yakong and McPherson; Yakong).

Whether or not women are at "risk," they are subjected to ongoing pressure (often couched in terms of obeying government and clinical edicts and a fear of death during childbirth) to attend a clinic and to give birth in the presence of a trained attendant. Probably one of the most egregious failures of the health care facilities in rural areas in the cultures represented here (and often in urban areas as well) is that these same clinics, more often than not, lack equipment, medications, and personnel to actually protect and save women's lives when the birthing process does goes wrong (Wogaing; Hobbis). Our ethnographic studies show that clinics are often closed when needed, nurses and other staff are absent, medication is not available, and technology does not work. A large part of the problem is that health facilities are understaffed, personnel are overworked, and resources are not forthcoming from government ministries of health.

Nonetheless, there are successful examples to report here. Among the Murik in the Lower Sepik region of PNG, Barlow shines a light on the work of a Catholic nursing sister in the 1980s and 1990s. Despite a government health clinic in another village, Mendam villagers preferred the Catholic mission clinic operated and supported for ten years by one nursing sister. Sister Marianna was careful to respect local practices and women's sensibilities and offered women privacy and a means to deal with the placenta, umbilical, and bodily products of the birthing process, thus keeping such "polluting" substances away from the potentially destructive forces of sorcerers. This mission clinic is now defunct due to lack of mission-funded resources, and the government did not step in with financial support.

Gibbs and William also discuss the work of a Catholic mission clinic run by Sister Gaudentia among the Mendi in the Highlands region of PNG. Here, for twenty-eight years, the focus was on women's sensibilities and customary birthing practices. When HIV became an issue in PNG, the mission clinic introduced HIV education for mothers and the community, began testing and providing treatment and counselling for seropositive women, and provided facilities for the women to await their child's birth. Gibbs and William report (chapter two, this volume) that, as of 2014, "113 [HIV-positive] mothers have given birth to 116 healthy babies," no mothers died from complications and "all babies were born without HIV infection." Indeed, "prevention of HIV transmission continues to be one of the bigger challenges in the national response to date" (Thanenthiran 119). Gibbs and William show in chapter two that the Mendi mission is a model of what can be done by respecting local culture, having proper resources and trained and reliable staffing, and developing "a culture of care," which will go "a long way toward reducing maternal mortality in Papua New Guinea." Both these studies of mission clinics in PNG show what can be accomplished when trained and dedicated health workers provide their clientele with a culturally safe environment. But as in the case described by Barlow, when mission funds and personnel become scarce, clinics and schools collapse if national governments are not willing or able to provide the same services.

Often implicit in the studies presented here is that the MDGs are generally oblivious to a notion of "cultural safety," that is, the provision of health care that is not an assault on peoples' cultural identities and well-being (Williams, 213; Brascoupé and Waters). In health care delivery, culturally unsafe practices include "any actions that diminish, demean or disempower the cultural identity and well-being of an individual" (Cooney qtd. Brascoupé and Water 7). Originally developed in New Zealand with regard to the manner by which health care, especially nursing practices, affected Maori people, the concept of "cultural safety" has expanded to encompass health care services and delivery to indigenous peoples in Canada, Australia, and New Zealand who are recovering from their experiences of colonialism. Thus, given the history of colonialism and the trauma associated with assimilation policies, it is "important to locate the concept of cultural safety within the context of cross-cultural relationships, between Aboriginal service-recipients and non-Aboriginal service deliverers, and to consider how the concept affects relationships, power structures and trust" (Brascoupé and Water 7). All the studies in this volume are situated in previously colonized nations. By its very nature, cosmopolitan obstetrics, as ideology and as practice, is unconcerned with a concept of cultural safety, since its mandate is to replace customary health care with a cosmopolitan, biomedical model of illness and disease. Much of what is wrong with health care delivery in postcolonial developing nations is the universal application and implementation of cosmopolitan medicine, which is insensitive to indigenous systems of reproduction and the positive kinds of practices and care that emanate from those models. Cosmopolitan obstetrics has no regard for cultural safety.

These case studies are exemplary of the fine detail that ethnographic research brings to understanding the complexity of women's lived experiences and their everyday realities. The following studies are concerned with highlighting the lived experience of the women who are meant to be the recipients of the changes inferred in the goals and targets described in MDG 1 (eliminate poverty), MDG 3 (women's equity and empowerment), and MDG 5 (improve maternal health). Every study in this volume makes the case that improving women's reproductive health is much more than taking care of the biology of reproduction. As Smith argues (this volume), all development goals should integrate ethnographic research, given that the social determinants of health are "more complex than simple access to a hospital, but include nutrition, bodily stress, gender inequality and other diseases of poverty and patriarchy." Understanding these complex cultural circumstances is a precondition to an even larger imperative: the necessity to embrace a concept of cultural safety within the delivery of health care in non-cosmopolitan postcolonial societies if the intent is truly to alleviate the suffering in the lives of women and girls and men and boys in so-called developing countries.

POSTSCRIPT

As the book goes to press, the 2000-2015 MDG deadline has passed and international attention has already turned to the reconfiguration of the MDGs into a the "Sustainable Development Goals 2015-2030" or SDGs. As noted above, MDGs are goals of human development that are to be "measured at the micro level," the level of individuals and villages (Loewe 1). But results and statistics, however, are reported at the country or regional (macro) level, which tends to obscure what is going on at the micro level. Our ethnographic studies have offered some insight into that grassroots world of women's lived experiences and although there are some good results, too many women continue to suffer. The proposed SDGs "refer to the preservation or establishment of global public goods [e.g., limiting climate change, financial stability, equitable development, etc.] that can thus only be measured through macro indicators" (Loewe 1). In other words, the SDGs will focus on macro-level, global issues of development sustainability. (Here I ignore the fraught nature of what constitutes "development" and "sustainability.") Loewe argues that the difference between MDG and SDG makes a kind of sense, because they have conceptually different goals, although the goals of both are "instrumentally linked" (4). While this may be true enough, it does not preclude the fact that stronger influences have a much better chance of realizing their goals, often at the expense of other goals. The likelihood of macro goals of a global nature to have a "trickle-down effect" or to "enable" achievement of the SDGs is doubtful.

Of the seventeen SDGs, the closest reconfiguration of MDG 5 (improve maternal health) is found in SDG 3, which is to "ensure healthy lives and promote well-being for all at all ages" (*Millennium Development Goals* 25). This goal includes targets for lowering maternal mortality ratios and zero-to five-years-old mortality ratios; raising the rate of contraceptive use; lowering death rates from HIV, TB, and malaria; and other health issues, such as obesity and road traffic deaths. SDG 3 also lists thirty-five other indicators, including birth attended by skilled birth attendants, antenatal and postnatal care, prevention of mother-to-child transmission of HIV, and stillbirth rates. MDG 3 (gender equity and female empowerment) is worked into SDG 5 goal to "achieve gender equality and empower all women and girls" (27), which includes tracking gender and sexual violence against women and children, the number of seats held by women in government and meeting the demand for family planning. While it is surely timely to deal with the global shame of gendered and sexual violence against women and to get more women representatives in their respective parliaments, I am skeptical about the causal links among these targets for achieving the goals of gender equity and female empowerment.

In sum, as I read these goals and indicators—from women's human rights to sexual and reproductive health to gender equity and empowerment—the issues pertaining to women are spread throughout the new SDGs, where they will be just one "indicator" of any number of goals or objectives. This suggests to me that the alleviation of poverty, the achievement of gender equality and women's empowerment, and the improvement of women's maternal and reproductive health, which also affects the health and well-being of their children and communities, will not be high on the various agendas "of technocrats, diplomats and government officials with no experience" any more than they were for the 1979 convention on the *Elimination of All forms of Discrimination Against Women* (Crossette 74). The research and literature cited in these chapters make a strong case that improving maternal and reproductive health clearly depends on women achieving gender equality and empowerment in order to be able to carry out their reproductive health decisions. Those reproductive decisions are multitude, culturally complex and, indeed, the bedrock of any woman's lived reality and must be approached from within a framework of cultural safety.

ENDNOTES

[1] Canada is equally adamant on this matter and, despite promising money to support maternal, newborn, and children's health, the previous government of Canada, under conservative Prime Minister Stephen Harper, refused to allocate funds for condoms, contraception, family planning and abortion. It would also appear that the federal government of that time, did not provide promised aid funds to supply ambulances in Mursi (LaTosky, chapter five, this volume).

[2] PGK is the Papua New Guinea kina. In 2009, one Papua New Guinea kina was worth approximately 42 cents Canadian. Although the sums might seem insignificant, when there are several children to educate and no cash income, these small sums are often impossible

to accumulate. Hence, not everyone gets to go to school.

[3] In 2012, the PNG government initiated free tuition in primary and elementary schools but permitted "project fees" which meant the financial burden remained, especially as project fees were often as much as the tuition fee (Walton).

[4] This teacher was my namesake and adopted daughter. I helped fund her teacher training. She was one of the "new woman" of PNG and was smart, educated, and concerned about the direction of her country and her culture. I was devastated to hear that she died on 5 February 2015 from what I can only assume was complications from endemic malaria. She was thirty-four years old and is survived by her husband and her now two-year-old daughter.

[5] These numbers are hardly straightforward and must be taken with a large grain of salt. According to *The Source for Women's Health*, "Although Canada has one of the lowest reported maternal mortality ratios in the world, it is important to capture the differing rate of maternal mortality in specific subpopulations such as Aboriginal and immigrant women. Reporting in this detail is not currently available" ("Maternal Health"). In other words, MMRs for First Nations, Métis, and Inuit women in Canada are not included in these MMRs.

WORKS CITED

Arnup, Katherine, Andrée Lévesque, Ruth Roach Pierson, with Margaret Brennan. *Delivering Motherhood: Maternal Ideologies and Practices in the 19th and 20th Centuries*. London, New York: Routledge, 1990. Print.

Blanc, Ann K. "The Effect of Power in Sexual Relationships on Sexual and Reproductive Health: An Examination of the Evidence." *Studies in Family Planning* 32.3 (2001): 189-213. Print.

Brascoupé, Simon and Catherine Waters. "Cultural Safety: Exploring the Applicability of the Concept of Cultural Safety to Aboriginal Health and Community Wellness." *Journal of Aboriginal Health* 5.2 (2009): 6-41. Naho. Web. 29 Nov. 2015.

Brewis, Alexandra. "Gender Conflict and Co-operation in Reproductive Decision-Making in Micronesia." *The Journal of the Polynesian Society* 110.4 (2001): 391-400. Print.

Brolan, Claire E. and Peter S. Hill. "Sexual and Reproductive Health and Rights in the Evolving Post-2015 Agenda: Perspectives from Key Players from Multilateral and Related Agencies in 2013." *Reproductive Health Matters* 22.43 (2014): 65-74. Web. 29 Nov. 2015.

Coates, Amy L., Peter S. Hill, Simon Rushton, and Julie Balen. "The Holy See on Sexual and Reproductive Health Rights: Conservative in Position, Dynamic in Response." *Reproductive Health Matters* 22.44 (2014): 114-124. Web. 29 Nov. 2015.

Crichton, Susan and Brown Onguko. "Appropriate Technologies for Challenging Contexts." *On the Move: Mobile Learning for Development*. Eds. S. Marshall and W. Kinuthia. Charlotte, NC: Information Age Publishing, 2013. 25–42. Print.

Crossette, Barbara. "Reproductive Health and the Millennium Development Goals: The Missing Link." *Studies in Family Planning* 36.1 (2005): 71-79. Web. 20 Mar. 2015.

Dawson, A., T. Howes, N. Gray and E. Kennedy. *Human Resources for Health in Maternal, Neonatal and Reproductive Health at Community Level: A Profile of Papua New Guinea*. Sydney, Australia: Human Resources for Health Knowledge Hub and Burnet Institute. 2011. Web. 29. Nov. 2015.

Dunn, Frederick L. "Traditional Asian Medicine and Cosmopolitan Medicine as Adaptive Systems." *Asian Medical Systems: A Comparative Study*. Ed. Charles Leslie. Berkeley: University of California Press, 1976. 133–58. Print.

Ginsberg, Faye D. and Rayna Rapp, eds. *Conceiving the New World Order: The Global Politics of Reproduction*. Berkeley: University of California Press, 1995. Print.

Inhorn, Marcia, C., and Frank Van Balen, eds. *Infertility around the Globe: New Thinking on Childlessness, Gender and Reproductive Technologies*. Berkeley: University of California Press, 2002. Print.

Inter-Parliamentary Union (IPU). "Women in Politics Map: 2014." IPU, 2015. Web. 15 Mar. 2015.

Jordan, Brigitte. *Birth in Four Cultures: A Crosscultural Investigation of Childbirth in Yucatan, Holland, Sweden and the United States*. 4th ed. Revised and expanded by Robbie Davis-Floyd. Prospect Heights, IL: Waveland Press, Inc., 1993. Print.

Kvernflaten, Birgit. "Meeting Targets or Saving Lives: Maternal Health Policy and Millennium Development Goal 5 in Nicaragua." *Reproductive Health Matters* 21.42 (2013): 32-40. Web. 29 Nov.2015.

Leonard, Lori. "Problematizing Fertility: 'Scientific' Accounts and Chadian Women's Narratives." *Infertility around the Globe: New Thinking on Childlessness, Gender and Reproductive Technologies.* Eds. Marcia Inhorn and Frank van Balen. Berkeley: University of California Press, 2002. 193-214. Print.

Loewe, Markus. "Post 2015: How to Reconcile the Millennium Development Goals (MDGs) and the Sustainable Development Goals (SDGs)?" Briefing Paper 18. German Development Institute (DIE), 2012. Web. 29 Nov. 2015.

Luck, L. "Safe Motherhood Intervention Studies in Africa: A Review." *East African Medical Journal* 77.11 (2000): 599-607. Web. 29. Nov. 2015.

"Maternal Mortality" *The Source for Maternal Health.* Women's Health Data Directory, 2013. Web. 29 Nov. 2015.

Merica, Dan. "Clinton Ties 'Broader Human Development' with Women's Reproductive Rights." *Politicalticket.blogs.cnn.com.* Cable News Network, 7 Mar. 2014. Web. 17 Mar. 2015.

Mcintyre, Martha. "Gender Violence in Melanesia and the Problem with Millennium Development Goal No. 3," *Engendering Violence in Papua New Guinea.* Eds. Margaret Jolly, Christine Stewart, and Carolyn Brewer. Canberra: Australia National University E-Press, 2012. 239-266. Print.

McPherson, Naomi M. "Modern Obstetrics in a Rural Setting: Women and Reproduction in Northwest New Britain." *Urban Anthropology and Studies in Cultural Systems and World Economic development. Special Issue: Women in Development in the Pacific* 23.1 (1994): 39-72. Print.

McPherson, Naomi M. "Women, Childbirth and Change in West New Britain, Papua New Guinea." *Reproduction, Childbearing and Motherhood.* Ed. Pranee Liamputtong. New York: Nova Science Publishers, 2007: 127-41. Print.

McPherson, Naomi M. "*SikAids*: Deconstructing the Awareness Campaign in Rural West New Britain, Papua New Guinea." Eds. Leslie Butt and Richard Eves. *Making Sense of AIDS: Culture,*

Sexuality, and Power in Melanesia. Honolulu: University of Hawai'i Press, 2008. 224-45. Print.

McPherson, Naomi M. "Black and Blue: Shades of Violence in West New Britain, Papua New Guinea." *Engendering Violence in Papua New Guinea*. Ed. Margaret Jolly, Christine Stewart and Carolyn Brewer. Canberra: Australia National University E-Press, 2012. 47-72. Print.

Okonofua, Friday E. and Helen Obi. "Specialized Versus Conventional Treatment of Infertility in Africa: Time for a Pragmatic Approach." *African Journal of Reproductive Health* 13.1 (2009): 9-11. Web. 29 Nov. 2015.

Papua New Guinea. National Department of Health. *Ministerial Taskforce on Maternal Health in Papua New Guinea*. Port Moresby: National Department of Health, 2009. Print.

Pollock, Nancy. J., Ed. *These Roots Remain: Food Habits in Islands of the Central and Eastern Pacific since Western Contact*. Honolulu, HI: Institute for Polynesian Studies, 1992. Print.

Rapp, Rayna. "Gender, Body, Biomedicine: How Some Feminist Concerns Dragged Reproduction to the Center of Social Theory." *Medical Anthropology Quarterly* 15.4 (2001): 466-77. Print.

Scaletta (McPherson), Naomi M. "Childbirth: A Case History from West New Britain, Papua New Guinea." *Oceania* 57 (1986): 33-52. Print.

Sustainable Development Solutions Network (SDSN). *Suggested SDG Indicators Sustainable Development Solutions Network. Revised Working Draft*. SDSN, 2015. Web. 27 Mar. 2015.

Thanenthiran, Sivananthi, Sai Jyothir Mai Racherla and Suloshini Jahanath. *Reclaiming and Redefining Rights ICPD+20: Status of Sexual and Reproductive Health and Rights in Asia Pacific*. Resource and Research Centre for Women (Arrow), 2013. Web. 29 Nov. 2015.

United Nations (UN). *The Millennium Development Goals Report 2013*. UN, 2014. Web. 27 Mar. 2015.

United Nations (UN). "Official List of MDG Indicators." *Millennium Development Goals Indicators*. UN, n.d. 7 Feb. 2015.

United Nations (UN). *Overview: the Millennium Development Goals Report*. UN, 2014. Web. 27 Mar. 2015.

United Nations. "Unmet Family Planning Needs." *Millennium*

Development Goals Indicators. The United Nations, n.d. Web. 25 Mar. 2015.

United Nations Development Program (UNDP). "About Papua New Guinea." UNDP, 2012. Web. 3. Feb. 2015.

Van Balen, Frank, and Marcia Inhorn. "Interpreting Infertility: A View from the Social Sciences." Eds. Marcia C. Inhorn and Frank Van Balen. *Infertility around the Globe: New Thinking on Childlessness, Gender and Reproductive Technologies*. Berkeley: University of California Press, 2002: 3-32. Print.

Wardlow, Holly. *Wayward Women: Sexuality and Agency in a New Guinea Society*. Berkeley: University of California Press, 2006. Print.

World Health Organization (WHO). Bulletin. "Mother or Nothing: The Agony of Infertility." WHO, 2015. Web. 25 Mar. 2015.

Walton, Grant. "Eliminating Project Fees in PNG Schools: A Step Too Far?" *Devpolicy Blog*. Development Policy Centre, 20 April. 2015. Web. 11 Nov. 2015.

Williams, T. "Cultural Safety — What Does It Mean for Our Work Practice?" *Australian and New Zealand Journal of Public Health* 23 (1999): 213–214. Print.

World Bank. *Reproductive Health at a Glance: Papua New Guinea*. World Bank, 2011. Web. 20 Mar. 2015.

Yakong, Vida Nyagre. *Ethnographic Perspectives on Rural Women's Reproductive Health Decisions in Ghana: The Cultural influences of Gender Relations, Kinship and Belief System*. Diss. University of British Columbia, 2013. Print.

1.
Integrating Western Medicine and Local Practice

Contributions of a Mission-Based Maternity Clinic to Maternal and Child Health in the Lower Sepik Region of Papua New Guinea

KATHLEEN BARLOW

MILLENIUM DEVELOPMENT GOAL (MDG) 5—to reduce maternal mortality and provide universal access to reproductive health care by 2015—is not being met in parts of the world where women living in remote rural areas have limited access to communication networks, transportation, and health care that could save their lives. Although proposed by the United Nations as a global priority, these goals must be accomplished in diverse local contexts. Examples from developing countries—Liljestrand and Pathmanathan for Malaysia and Sri Lanka (301-7), and Koblinsky for Bolivia, China, Egypt, Honduras, Indonesia, Jamaica and Zimbabwe (viii)—show that government-supported change and step-by-step implementation of appropriate health services eventually do make impressive improvements.

By contrast, for Papua New Guinea (PNG) as a whole, maternal and infant mortality have risen in recent decades ("Papua New Guinea: Tackling Maternal Health 'Crisis'"). The United Nations Development Program (UNDP) in Papua New Guinea reports that "the challenges of distance, isolation, lack of transport and an extreme shortage of skilled birth attendants, highlight the hazards of childbirth in PNG" (UNDP and PNG, "The Future We Want 2013" 13). Investment in needed infrastructure has been underfunded nationally, and maternal health care has been underprioritized at provincial and regional levels (Kiessler and Clark vii). Papua New Guinea ranks 49th from the bottom out of 178 countries on rankings of maternal mortality developed by WHO, UNICEF, UNFPA, and the World Bank ("Maternal Mortality Ratio"). A national survey found that maternal mortality rates in Papua New Guinea doubled between 1996 and 2006. Dame Carol Kidu cites the same 2006 national survey finding that the maternal mortality rate for rural women was as high as 731, with an overall total fertility rate of 4.3, due mainly to lack of access to basic health services ("Papua New Guinea: Tackling Maternal Health 'Crisis'" 180-181). She calls for increased health education and services to enable positive change for women and their families. Also in response to these alarming statistics, *The Report of the Ministerial Taskforce on Maternal Health in Papua New Guinea*, edited by Kiessler and Clark, recommends 1) developing a system of maternal "waiting houses" with trained birth attendants; 2) providing appropriate information on reproductive decision-making; and, 3) enlisting community support to make services culturally "friendly" and respectful (14).

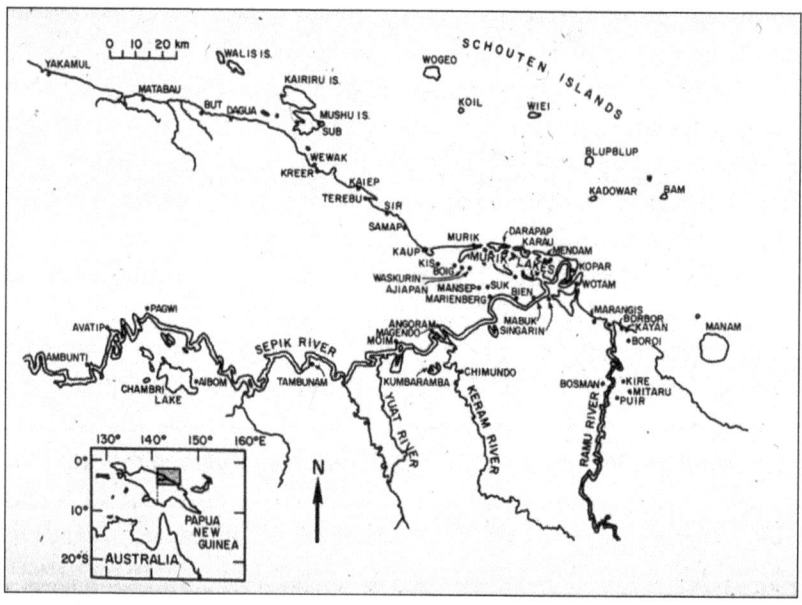

Map 1: Map of Sepik Region with Lower Sepik roughly indicated. ©K. Barlow.

In June 2011, on a recent visit to Manam settlement camps and the Murik Lakes region of Papua New Guinea, I noticed the lack of access to medical care, information, and facilities. Men and women alike expressed dismay at their growing populations and decried the lack of information and support for family planning. In Murik villages, births were taking place unattended, follow-up health care was lacking, and local practices that formerly supported pregnant and postpartum women were no longer practised. Based on historical data from a time when infrastructure was stronger, I explore in this chapter issues involved in improving maternal and reproductive health care in the Lower Sepik in terms of social structural systems and cultural processes. Data come from intensive fieldwork with mothers and young children in Murik villages and shorter term work throughout the Lower Sepik region. I also draw on records and anecdotal accounts of Sister Marianna of the Marienberg Catholic mission station, who developed and maintained a maternity hospital and general clinic for several decades.

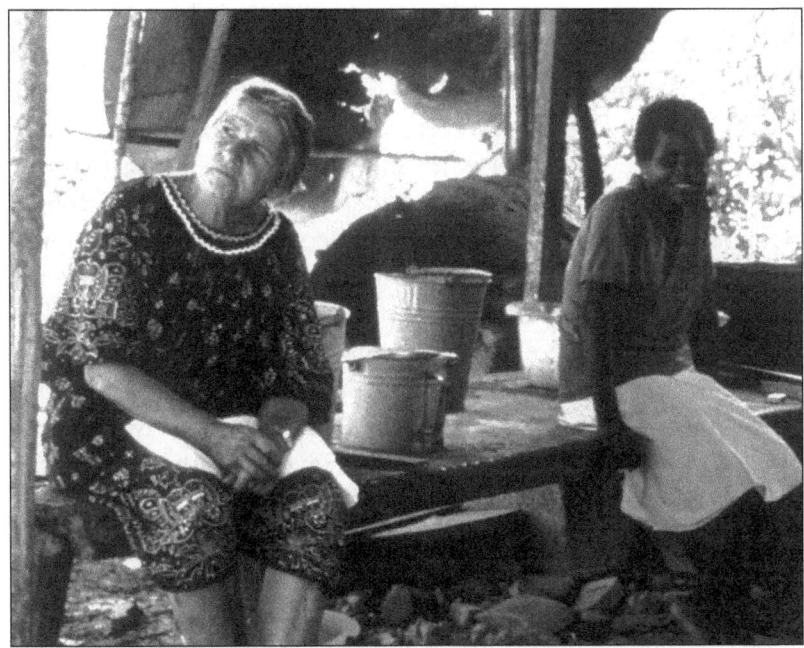

Fig. 1: Sister Marianna in the kitchen area for the maternity clinic with one of her staff of birth attendants. Photo © K. Barlow, 1988.

The *Papua New Guinea—Millennium Development Goals Second National Progress Report 2010* emphasizes that pursuing these goals successfully requires careful attention to local circumstances, priorities and cultures (vi). In the Sepik region of

Papua New Guinea, general and reproductive health services have declined over the past several decades. Although macro factors of funding and infrastructure are beginning to be addressed from national levels (for example, through recent legislation supporting free public health and education in 2013), my concern is with cultural differences at the local level that must be addressed for health care based in cosmopolitan biomedicine[1] to be offered in ways that support mothers and infants in rural villages. Based on field research in rural villages of the Lower Sepik region that had access to a mission-sponsored maternity health clinic, I consider the challenges of delivering reproductive health care from a local cultural perspective.

From approximately 1981 to 1997, Sister Marianna created and ran a maternity clinic at Marienberg Mission station on the lower Sepik River, successfully delivering much needed health care to pregnant, birthing and postpartum women. Comparison of this clinic to recommendations of the UN Task Force on Maternal Health and Child Health (Freedman et al.) and of the Ministerial Taskforce on Maternal Health in Papua New Guinea (Kiessler and Clark) suggests ways that general recommendations might be modified to suit local cultural understandings. For example, understandings about kinship, gender, body, and substance are culturally variable and crucial to the context of human reproduction, perhaps nowhere more so than in Melanesia.[2] Although the focus here is on maternal health, I also address aspects of infant and child health because children's health and survival directly affect women's health and well-being. Having healthy children can contribute to reducing the number of pregnancies and associated risks for an adult woman during her reproductive years. This case study reveals some dimensions of culture to be considered and how mediation between the worldviews that inform local practice and cosmopolitan medical contexts might contribute to better health outcomes for women and children.

Historically, Papua New Guinea health services, particularly mission health services, have prioritized attending to children more readily than to their mothers (Denoon 103), and current statistics on maternal and infant mortality continue to provide evidence for this bias ("About Papua New Guinea"). The clinic at Marienberg was a notable exception, as it focused on caring for expectant, birthing and postpartum women. Nevertheless, it was disadvantaged by a larger institutional framework that did not put women's health first. It served an area along the main river and its tributaries from Kopar to Angoram that included many different language and culture groups with a range of subsistence adaptations. The coastal Murik, among whom I worked, accessed mangrove and ocean resources for fish and shellfish. Groups along the river had extensive gardens and rain forest resources. Cultural differences among groups were marked, including differences in kinship, conceptions of the body, and ideas about pollution and substance. Using examples from Murik culture, I show how being culturally well informed is crucial for effective delivery of reproductive health care services.

For women in Murik villages, Marienberg was the closest place where they could give birth with the assistance of attendants trained in cosmopolitan biomedicine. When I first visited the clinic in 1981, such care was also available at a government clinic upriver in the town of Angoram and at Boram Hospital in Wewak town. A government-run aid post in Mendam village was not regularly staffed or supplied. (See Map 1.) Except for the aid post, services were located outside of Murik villages, among people whose languages and cultures, while related in general, were in many ways quite different. As traders, Murik were used to interpreting other people's ways of doing things, yet this did not reduce the risks of dealing with strangers—an important factor especially around birth and death.

In what follows, I describe how my research experiences relate to this subject and summarize from current literature general recommendations for developing and improving maternal health care. I then compare this framework to the Marienberg clinic and discuss its challenges and accomplishments in relation to understandings about reproduction, pregnancy, and birth in Murik culture. Understanding local cultural perspectives is important for interpreting the behaviour of those who come to a clinic; moreover, such an understanding allows health workers to be sensitive to factors that inhibit people's willingness to use clinic services and helps health workers provide better explanations to patients and their families.

RESEARCH BACKGROUND

My early research (1981–82) concerned how children learn cultural meanings and focused on mothers and children. I conducted field research primarily in the Murik villages of Darapap, Karau, and Mendam in the Lower Sepik region (see Map 1). Early on, I visited the Marienberg mission upriver from my research site, where I met Sister Marianna and learned of the maternity clinic. Several times over the course of my research, she visited Murik villages, including Darapap where I resided, providing immunizations and basic health care. These visits gave me an opportunity to observe her interactions with local people and to talk with her about the relationship of the Marienberg maternity clinic to remote villages. I learned first-hand from villagers what these services meant to them and, from Sister Marianna, how she went about developing relationships of trust and introducing cosmopolitan biomedical services.

In 1986 and 1988, I was part of a team sponsored by the Australian Museum doing research on material culture and exchange in coastal, island, and lower river exchange networks. Travelling throughout the region helped me learn about cultural differences and commonalities. In 1988, my family and I were based in Marienberg and lived in a room adjacent to the maternity clinic. Although we respected the privacy of the women who came there to bear children, and they ours, I learned about aspects of the clinic's challenges and success by observing comings and goings at the clinic and by talking with Sister Marianna and her team of birth attendants.

Because of my research interests and because in 1986 and 1988 my own young children travelled with me, I spent large amounts of time with women and children during each of these research periods. As a result, I was privy to or involved in discussions and activities around pregnancy, birth, postpartum seclusion and care of infants and young children. I learned about changing ideas and practices and sometimes decision making about when and how to access traditional and cosmopolitan health care resources.

In 1997, I gave lectures on the tour boat, *Melanesian Explorer*. As large numbers of children gathered on shore to greet us or wave good-bye, I frequently heard villagers' concerns about too high fertility. Looking at the assembled crowd, adults would remark on the skewed age distribution.[3] These parents were struggling under the tremendous workload of raising many children who were too young to help with subsistence work.

A visit in 2011 to Murik Lakes, Marienberg, and to nearby Manam Island and Bogia gave me another window on how things have changed over several decades with regard to health services for mothers and children, which, unfortunately, were not for the better. Visiting the Marienberg Mission Station to see members of a family from Darapap who were living there, I learned that the maternity and general health clinics were no longer in operation. Following Sister Marianna's retirement, there had been no one to continue her impressive work, and a general retrenchment of mission services had led to the closure of both clinics. The recent call for improving maternal and child health has led me to reflect on Marianna's accomplishments and her attention to the relationship between the medical services that she offered and local cultural norms. Her interpretations and negotiation of local people's concerns about health and illness were crucial to developing the trust and confidence that led to better treatment and outcomes for women. Her example is best considered in the context of current official recommendations about how to improve maternal and child health.

TASK FORCE RECOMMENDATIONS

Two reports on Millennium Development Goals provide a description of the health care infrastructure required to improve maternal and child health outcomes. The first is *"Who's Got the Power? Transforming Health Systems for Women and Children"* by the United Nations Task Force on Child Health and Maternal Health (Freedman et al.), and the second is the *"Report of the Ministerial Taskforce on Maternal Health in Papua New Guinea"* (Kiessler and Clark). Together, they outline what is needed to develop health care systems that meet the needs of mothers and children in rural Papua New Guinea.

At the most general level, certain features of political and economic context are required—foremost among them, national political stability and a strong link between the rural poor and the ruling political establishment (Liljestrand and Pathmanathan 305). Compared to elsewhere in the world, PNG enjoys a relatively high level of political stability, and since independence in 1975, this has been the case generally throughout the East Sepik Province. This provides a context in which health care systems can be established and maintained and services provided as a right of citizenship (Freedman et al., 106). The UN Task Force also advises that policymaking should be inclusive rather than mechanistic and top down. New initiatives in Papua New Guinea need to be based on the needs and wants of local people (Kiessler and Clark 15). In order to know whether changes are effective and to identify inadequacies, political commitment needs to include professionally trained health care workers and well-maintained health care records (Liljestrand and Pathmanathan 308).

The task force reports recommend free, state-supported health care.[4] Research has shown that market-based (fee for service) approaches are not effective because cost is a major barrier to accessing care (Freedman et al. 96). Smoothly functioning health services require adequate financial support for personnel, equipment, facilities (including electricity and running water), drugs, and consumable supplies. To prevent frequent turnover and trained staff leaving the profession, staff must have working conditions, supervision, and incentives that maintain their expertise and morale and the respect of the community (Liljestrand and Pathmanathan 301). Maternity care workers are mainly women who need working conditions that support their staying in the workforce and career paths that work for them and their families (Freedman et al. 126).

Maternity health services operate best as part of a well-functioning general health care system. Maternal and child illness and mortality can be reduced significantly by providing care that treats and reduces major illnesses—such as malaria, TB, HIV, and AIDS—that complicate and compromise the health of pregnant women and their children. For example, Townsend cites the frequency with which anemia associated with malaria leads to women hemorrhaging at birth, a complication that cannot be addressed easily in remote villages (37). Better general health care would reduce the frequency of this dangerous condition.

Both reports cited above emphasize that maternal and child health are best improved in the context of an alliance with public education (Freedman et al. 50; Kiessler and Clark xii, 22). It has been widely demonstrated across the globe that primary education for women enables them to look after their own best interests and to know when and how to access health care for themselves and their family. In Papua New Guinea, education is an important element in reducing violence against women (McIntyre 256). Sex education about reproduction, sexually transmitted infections, and contraception are components of public health that can be taught in schools to help prevent premature pregnancy and those conditions and illnesses related to becoming sexually active at young ages (The National Sex and Reproduction Research Team and Carol Jenkins 135-6).

Four kinds of delay have been identified as critical factors in preventing maternal deaths. These are delays in: 1) identifying problems that require medical intervention; 2) deciding to seek treatment; 3) getting to an appropriate health care facility; and 4) accessing care and treatment once there. The reasons for delays are often complex and linked to cultural differences between local people and cosmopolitan medical personnel, but, along with decision making at all phases, there are also practical considerations of communication, transportation, and effective planning for handling medical emergencies (Yakong and McPherson, this volume). Research shows that an effective health care system for pregnant women must enable immediate access to a health care facility that is fully equipped to deal with emergency obstetric complications (Kiessler and Clark 13-14).

Both reports cited above emphasize the importance of skilled birth attendants. Liljestrand and Pathmanathan (301) and Freedman et al. (15-16) point to the need for these attendants to be supported by a system that provides continuous—every day, all day, 24/7—access to qualified obstetrical care and emergency services. "Skilled birth attendance" includes adequate facilities, equipment, supplies, training, and qualified supervision of medical staff.

Discussing the difference between trained birth attendants and traditional midwives, Townsend concludes that for most of Papua New Guinea, there is no existing local role that easily transitions into trained birth attendant (23). Most women rely on more experienced female family members or other women in their villages, but these women do not have extensive special knowledge and training for dealing with complications of pregnancy and birth, such as breech presentation, hemorrhaging, or retained placenta. In 2007, most women of the East Sepik were reported to have access to antenatal care, but the percentage of supervised births in health centres and hospitals was only about 25 percent (Kiessler and Clark 11). Moreover, women's experiences at government health centres were often deplorable. The Papua New Guinea Millennium Goals report states that many women prefer mission health services to those provided by the government because

> women do not trust the [government] health system to look after them respectfully and safely. Maternity care can be disrespectful and contingent upon the payment of fees. Offensive and demeaning language by health personnel and ridiculing of women's poverty, clothing, parity, smell, hygiene, cries of pain or desire to remain clothed is not only disrespectful but abusive. (Kiessler and Clark 9)

An adequate maternal health care system must be built from the ground up. For the past several decades, few improvements have been made and, in fact, as public expenditure on health care declined over the period from 1995 to 2009 ("Maternal Mortality Ratio"), population growth soared. The combined effect in rural areas has been that many government aid posts are closed or lack staff and supplies (Kiessler and Clark, 16; UNDP PNG, *Comprehensive Report* 23).

Fortunately, in 2013, legislation was passed to provide free health care and public education for the citizens of Papua New Guinea, and the UNDP convened a workshop to find ways to direct wealth from natural resource extraction to these public services (UNDP and PNG, "The Future We Want" 13). If and when the needed infrastructure develops, its success will depend on adjusting services to local contexts in a nation of extreme linguistic and cultural diversity.

THE CLINIC AT MARIENBERG

The clinic at Marienberg is a valuable example of efforts to address the problems of poor maternal health care and the risks of unassisted births. Comparing the success of Sister Marianna's clinic in the period from 1981 to 1988 to the criteria listed above is instructive about the reasons for the clinic's success, challenges, and eventual demise. Marienberg, during this period (only six years following Papua New Guinea's independence from Australia in 1975), was a thriving mission station that included the church itself, a logging operation and sawmill, a general health clinic, and the maternity clinic. The station was part of an independent communication system via radio and a local transportation system on the river. Marienberg was supplied from the much larger Wirui mission station in the coastal town of Wewak. Clergy consisted of one priest who resided in Marienberg and several others working throughout the region and based at Marienberg. In 1981, several Sisters lived at Marienberg and taught at the mission school. By 1988, only Sister Marianna was there, and she maintained her clinics with the help of local staff.

Throughout this time, she travelled to villages on the lower Sepik River and reached most of them at least once and sometimes twice a year. Usually two or three local men accompanied her, who managed transport and the setting up of a local clinic and accommodation in the *haus kiap*.[5] They stayed with others in the village or in another vacant house. Sister Marianna only saw patients who came to her because she wanted to avoid even the appearance of coercion or any action that might arouse suspicion that she had interfered inappropriately or with bad intentions. One of her main goals was to provide immunizations for children (measles, TB, and polio), but she also weighed them and tended to tropical ulcer sores, skin parasites, and other ailments. If she thought that she could offer better care at the clinic in Marienberg (always the case with TB), she would encourage people to go there to stay and receive the treatment that they needed. For those whose health needs exceeded what she could provide in Marienberg—such as, pregnant women whom she judged to be high risk because of health conditions, age, or a history of miscarriages or other complications—she would recommend that they go to the hospital in Wewak.

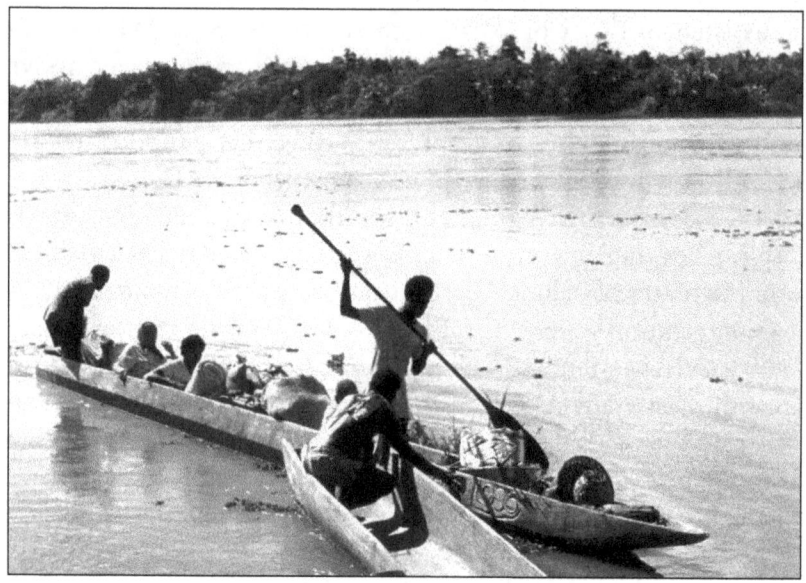

Fig. 2: Caption: Sister Marianna returns to the mission station with a woman coming to the maternity clinic. Photo © K. Barlow, 1988.

At the Marienberg clinic, people received general health care from trained nursing staff on a walk-in basis, including a wide array of services for illness, injury, infections, and chronic conditions. Much of Marianna's attention was devoted to the maternity clinic, where she was assisted by local women whom she had trained. Women came by canoe from throughout the region to give birth there, and she encouraged them to come well before they went into labour. Housing was provided for each woman and one or two women companions, but they were expected to bring their own food. An outdoor kitchen, a bathhouse, and toilet facilities were located nearby. The maternity clinic was located next to the path along the river, removed from housing areas up and down river, in deference to pollution beliefs of the local people.

In 1988, we (my husband and two children, aged one year and four years) lived in one half of the clinic. This space would otherwise have been available for birthing women and their attendants, but

Marianna had been asked by the mission to support the maternity clinic on her own, and we were paying guests who shopped at the outdoor market, bought petrol and other items from the mission and paid for laundry services. Two other members of our research group rented a room in Marianna's house. Although we tried to be considerate guests and the mission staff were friendly and hospitable, I have no doubt that the most important factor in our being able to base ourselves at the clinic and mission station was the income it provided to help maintain the clinic.

Even more critical was Marianna's crocodile farm. In several large ponds near the base of the hill on top of which stood the main mission buildings, Marianna raised crocodiles commercially with the help of a crew of local men. By identifying paid work appropriate for men to do, Marianna enabled men to support women's health in a way that was acceptable to them. The crocodiles were sold for skins and meat and returned enough income to keep the maternity clinic open.[6] During the months we were there, an expensive crisis occurred that caused Sister Marianna much concern. The crocodiles developed conjunctivitis, a potentially fatal infection, and all had to be shipped to Madang for treatment and for premature sale if they could not be cured. This jeopardized her profit margin and threatened not just the health of the crocodiles but potentially that of women and infants in the Lower Sepik.

The activities of the maternity clinic were conducted with a high degree of discretion. During the few months we lived there, women quietly came and went, and their babies were all delivered safely. They arrived, sometimes in the middle of the night, and stayed in seclusion. We rarely saw or heard them. The arrival of an expectant mother was signaled usually by a pile of bananas, yams, coconuts, and garden produce set briefly on the porch as she moved in and by a new flood of sheets and then diapers at the laundry operation by the water tank. Marianna kept records as best she could—she shared with me records for two Murik villages—but she did not voluntarily talk about the goings on at the clinic. Neither she nor the birth attendants talked about their patients to the rest of us and if asked, they gave minimal answers. Only women would come to visit us there and most often people would not call out to us as they walked by. More than just con-

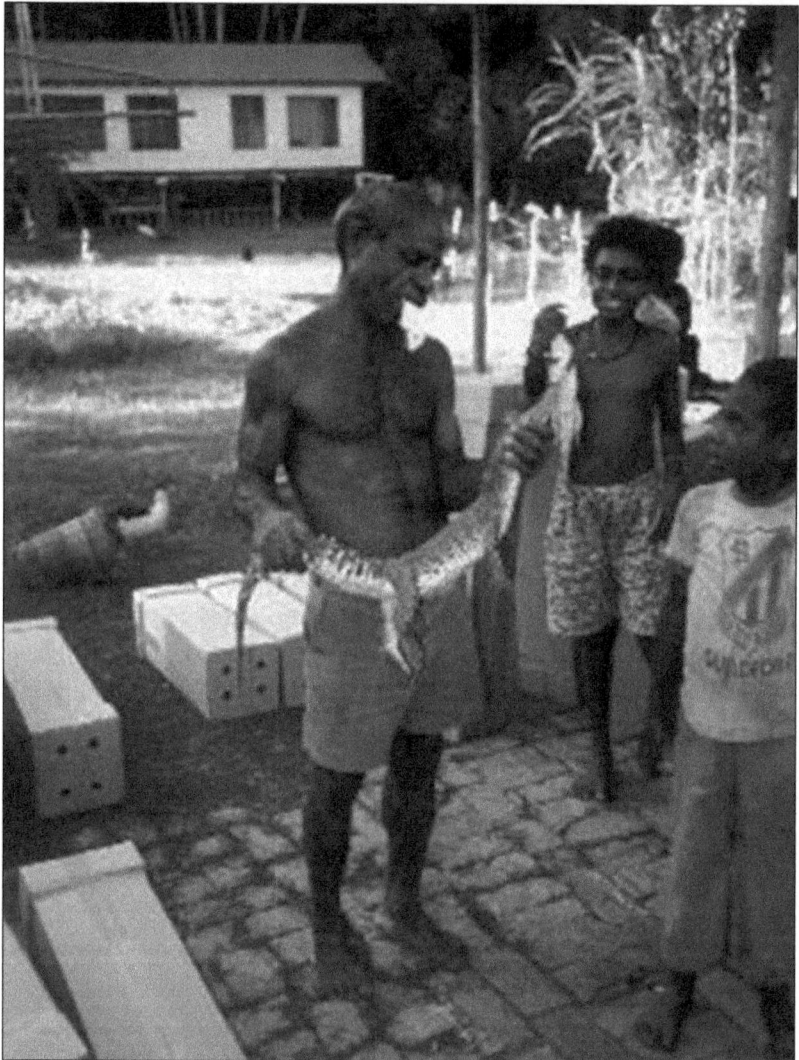

Fig. 3: Sister Marianna's crocodile farm supported the maternity clinic. In 1988, the laundry became a staging area for packing them for shipping to a dealer in Madang for medical treatment. Housing for maternity clinic staff is in the background. Photo ©K. Barlow, 1988.

sideration for the clinic residents, their quiet and distance fit with the importance of separating birth from daily life in general and from masculinity in particular. For much of the time we were there, either we or Marianna travelled away from the station for days at a time. Consequently, I learned less than I would have liked about the actual workings of the maternity clinic.

SISTER MARIANNA'S PERSPECTIVE

From Marianna's perspective, the main issues for birthing women were inadequate nutrition and malaria, which left women susceptible to anemia and sometimes unable to become pregnant or to sustain a pregnancy. She saw them as vulnerable to a cascade of illnesses once they contracted one disease, and she emphasized the importance of suppressing malaria during pregnancy. Other diseases she mentioned that compromised the women's health were TB, diarrhea, pneumonia, scabies, and syphilis. Several times she said to me, "These are fragile people. Once they get sick, they get very sick and go downhill quickly."

In her view, local women were inclined to start feeding infants solid foods too early, which reduced lactation and increased the likelihood of inadequate nutrition.[7] These foods were not always sterile enough for infants, which put them at risk for diarrhea and dehydration. She encouraged mothers to delay solid foods for babies for at least three months and, then, to supplement breastfeeding with overboiled rice or soup with vegetables and fish when their first teeth came in.

Sister Marianna wanted the clinic to have a positive reputation so that women would come there several days prior to giving birth and stay at least until the baby's umbilical cord had become dry and fallen off. In 1981, she worried that women who were at risk or were having difficulties would wait too long to come to the clinic. In 1988, my observation was that women were coming before they went into labour, staying for two weeks and more, and having successful deliveries and healthy babies. As a nurse with only clinic facilities, Sister Marianna was not able to provide a full range of emergency obstetric services. She had limited access via radio to refer patients to hospital services in Angoram or Wewak, but they had to be transported by their own kin. If complications required a Caesarean, then the delay of going first to Marienberg could seriously endanger a woman's life and her child's. It seemed that women who were primaparas or had previously had complications often took her advice to go directly from the village to the hospital in Wewak or Angoram.

Marianna was aware of local beliefs about pollution that influenced men and women to avoid being involved in childbirth. Gradually and by example, she hoped that people would realize that these fears were not necessary and that the clinic and maternity clinic provided safe and effective health care. On the other hand, by situating the maternity clinic away from residences and maintaining clear separation from daily life at the mission station, she respected local practices of seclusion and separation from men.

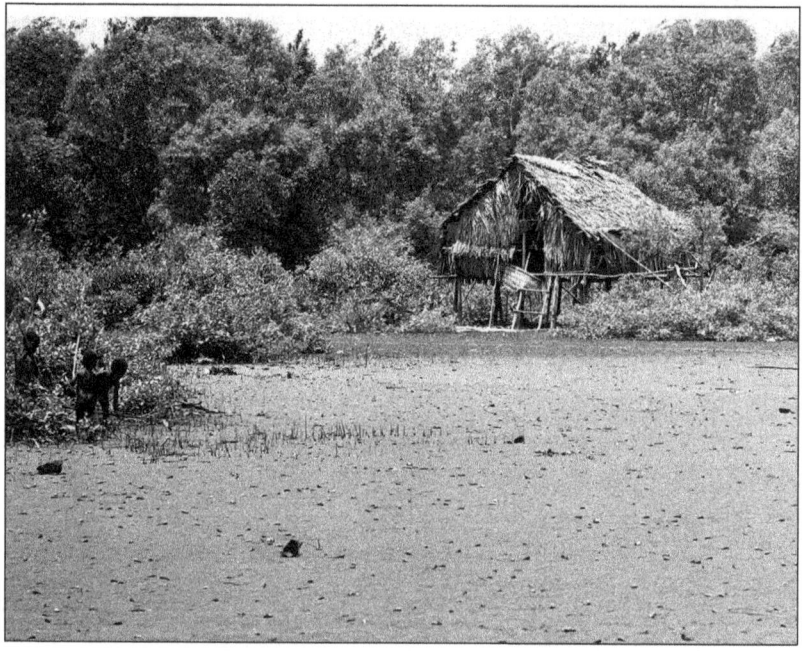

Fig. 4: Birth house in Darapap village, set well away from other houses at the edge of the mangroves. Photo © K. Barlow, 1981.

She also respected women's desire to be assisted by other women and to maintain a high degree of privacy before, during, and after birth. Staff for the maternity clinic was all female—young women from throughout the area who assisted the birthing women, did laundry, and cooked. Her young clinic staff members were paid a salary and had living accommodations there, but turnover tended to occur when they married and began families of their own in their home villages. One benefit was that they were then able to act as village birth attendants in their home communities.

THE CLINIC'S IMPACT ON HEALTH CONDITIONS

Sister Marianna's maternity clinic developed into a facility that people throughout the Lower Sepik region relied on. How does it compare to those aspired to and recommended in the Millennium Development Goal reports? Many features were definitely there, but there were also challenges. Although not government supported, the clinic had access to a larger support infrastructure through the Catholic Mission, which made it possible to maintain facilities, equipment, supplies, communication, and transportation. Marienberg Mission station provided a general health clinic, efforts at health education, infrastructure (buildings, electricity, running water), and systems of provisioning and maintenance that assisted the maternity clinic in delivering care. On the other hand, Sister Marianna had to support the maternity clinic financially mostly on her own. Because of her resourcefulness in developing the crocodile farm, she was able to keep the clinic running but on a tenuous basis. When she was no longer there to contribute her commitment and drive to this work, the maternity clinic was not maintained. Although not fully integrated into a larger, ongoing health care system, the maternity clinic showed what could be accomplished through committed leadership and a small equally committed staff.

Recommendations for effective health care emphasize good recordkeeping not only to maintain patient health histories and provide better care but also to document general health conditions for analysis and improvement. In the case of the Marienberg maternity clinic, financial challenges also meant that there were never enough staff members both to carry out the work and maintain records. Sister Marianna was tireless herself and exacted the same high level of effort from those she employed. Many of them provided exactly what she asked of them and more. Nevertheless, the first priority was to care for people; recordkeeping was secondary. Even though these are, in most cases, the only health record a person has, the records are inconsistent and partial at best. They do not provide a health history that could be used as a basis for ongoing care or as a database for assessing quality of care.

Based on my census and field notes for 1981 and 1982 and Marianna's records for the two villages of Darapap and Karau for 1981-88, the maternity clinic was successful at protecting women's health in childbirth. Marianna recorded birth histories for 95 women, which included 254 pregnancies and no maternal deaths. My field notes from 1986 and 1988 record two deaths of pregnant women—one a suicide and the other a death while en route by boat to the hospital in Wewak following several days of obstructed labour in the village. Based on what I was told about the first death, the young woman's suicide was not related to her physical health or pregnancy. Better maternity care would probably not have prevented her act of despair. The other death was a clear case of delay factors leading to mortality, as described in Millennium Goal reports (Kiessler and Clark 13-14). Had this woman's symptoms been recognized and had she had access to care at an earlier stage, it is likely her death could have been prevented. As with several life and death cases that occurred in 1981 and 1982, a long delay in deciding to go to the hospital or clinic, while other remedies were tried (including going first to an aid post), contributed to patients not surviving a boat ride of several hours or longer to reach a staffed clinic or hospital.

Although maternal survival was high, outcomes (and statistics) for successful pregnancies and healthy babies were not as positive. Of the 254 recorded pregnancies, there were fifty-four that failed: twenty-nine were miscarriages, nine were stillbirths, and sixteen were newborns who died within a few days of birth. This count includes hospital, clinic, and village births reported to Sister Marianna, many of which did not specify where the birth took place. Her records show five premature births (three to the same mother) and five breech births (three to one mother in the village) in which the infants did not survive. Another note specifies that the child was born on the way to the clinic and died there. Skilled birth attendants could change these numbers. Improving health care so that women do not suffer the grief of failed pregnancies or go through many pregnancies to have the children they want would contribute greatly to maternal and child health and well-being.

A related issue comes across clearly in Marianna's records of children weighed at intervals of about six months to a year. They reveal a predictable and serious issue in children's health. From about the age of eighteen months to three years, many children do not gain any weight for one or more (sometimes three or four) of these intervals. These are typically the ages of weaning, when children do not get enough nourishment from either breastfeeding or solid food. Murik children often initially dislike the sour taste and smell of sago, and mothers find it difficult to substitute other foods for this staple, which provides mainly calories. Although fish and shellfish provide good sources of protein and minerals, other vitamins available in garden vegetables and fruit are in short supply. My observation during long-term fieldwork on children was that once young children become undernourished, they are vulnerable to multiple illnesses, most often persistent malaria and/or diarrhea, with very high risks of dehydration. During a prolonged drought in 1982, people resorted to using water from ground holes, and many children developed diarrhea. One child about six months old succumbed within twenty-four hours to dehydration caused by diarrhea. Whole families of women (those of childbearing age and the wider network of female kin who assist them) experience added work, immense stress, and grief when poor health conditions occur and children become gravely ill. Improving general health issues, such as availability of clean water and more diverse food resources, would benefit women of reproductive age and those who support them.

Contraception is an important aspect of maternal health that was not part of the maternity clinic's program as it was not consistent with Catholic sponsorship. Women of the region spaced their children through traditional practices[8] but also freely expressed their desire for access to modern contraception methods that they had heard about, such as birth control pills and IUDs. In 2011, HIV and AIDS informational campaigns were making condoms more available and awareness of their protective and contraceptive benefits more widely known (Bennesch, this volume). Traditionally, Murik women preferred to space their children three years or more apart, but some who belonged to the mission no longer practised postpartum abstinence and had children closer together. Other women tried to induce early miscarriage to avoid having children too close together or more children than they wanted. There was a marked difference in men's and women's point of view on this issue. Women were concerned about the work and physical toll that pregnancy and nursing had on them. Men were concerned about the possibility that a child was not theirs, and senior men averred that a woman should abort a pregnancy if there was doubt about who the father might be. Willingness to control fertility was less of an issue than access to methods of contraception that women themselves could control.

LOCAL CULTURAL PERSPECTIVES ON CLINIC CARE

Optimistic UN Development literature tends to imply that local customs should be tolerated where necessary but, eventually, education will free people of their "superstitious" ways of thinking and lead them into the clean, safe world of cosmopolitan biomedical practice. Mary Douglas has long since shown the extent to which safe and dangerous, clean and unclean emerge from fundamental cultural understandings and are powerful symbolic expressions of social order and disorder (Douglas 3-7). Thus, "customs" associated with reproductive health care are deeply embedded in cultural worldviews and are not simply surface manifestations of "primitive" thinking. Commentators on the Millennium Goals recommend that where traditional practices are unlikely to cause any harm, they should be retained and even encouraged (Kiessler and Clark, 14). In an earlier report on maternal health, Townsend described local practices that make a health facility more familiar and comfortable for birthing women, viz., having a fire, accommodating supportive female kin, giving birth in a standing or squatting position, delaying cutting the umbilical cord, supporting lactation and encouraging birth spacing (51-53). While incorporating these practices into a contemporary health clinic would reduce its strangeness, simply providing for practices deemed non-harmful may seriously miss the point. Through practice, meanings are negotiated. In many ways, local cultural meanings about reproduction and cosmopolitan biomedical care are based in very different meaning systems. Communication and health care practices that respectfully negotiate different systems of meaning should be a priority in creating improved health care systems.

Sister Marianna made many adjustments to local culture and always showed respect for people's choices regarding health care, but she regarded cultural features that influenced reproductive health and early child care as similar throughout the region (Personal interview). She looked forward to a time when many of the "primitive" beliefs that informed people's choices and actions would no longer be relevant (personal communication 1988). From an anthropological point of view, there were not only differences between Western and local worldviews to be acknowledged but there was also substantial cultural variation among groups in the region that affected choices and behaviour related to pregnancy, birth, and infancy. A more thorough and nuanced appreciation of how local practices express a cultural world view would positively affect health care delivery for women and children.

Important understandings at odds with Western medical care but widespread throughout Papua New Guinea are ideas about illness and health as indicators of the state of social relationships within a kin group, among kin groups, and with outsiders. In general, conflicts, rifts, and unfulfilled obligations among relatives are dangerous to those in unstable health conditions, including pregnancy. Non-kin and strangers are potentially dangerous as their intentions may not be benign. How these beliefs are expressed locally may vary greatly. Understanding particular social factors to which people are sensitive is important for improving communication between those providing and those seeking health care. I describe entailments to this basic understanding with regard to pregnancy, birth, and infancy in Murik culture to demonstrate the importance of understanding people's choices and actions in terms of local cultural knowledge.

Among Murik, a pregnant woman should avoid people or spirits who might bear ill will towards her or someone within her kin group. During gestation, important decisions are being made in the spirit world about whether and how to allow a spirit to become a newborn person, and the whole period from conception through about six months of age is one of unstable boundary diffusion between the realms of humans and of spirits (including ancestor spirits—the dead). Therefore, a pregnant woman should stay close to home, behave with circumspection, and especially not eat food from unknown or potentially unreliable sources. She must be careful with whom she associates and talks, as should her husband, whose kin and ancestors also have an interest in the coming child. Careless socializing and failure to follow proscriptions gives hostile others access to harm her or her fetus—the main source of such hostility being unfulfilled social obligations. Those providing health care need to be aware that a hospital or clinic is a dangerous place, as is travel through others' territories to reach health facilities. These factors expose vulnerable people to strangers and other social hazards that could endanger their health (Wogaing this volume; Yakong and McPherson, this volume).

Given the emphasis on the social context of health and illness, there are a range of family and community members associated with each pregnant woman's well-being. A critical factor in effective care is awareness of who is involved in a woman bearing a child—who the appropriate people are in her support network and what their roles are. Differing kinship systems construct these relationships, obligations, and privileges quite differently.

The PNG Millennium Goal Report states that maternal health services should include men as active participants and that husbands or partners should be involved in their wife's care during pregnancy and birth (Kiessler and Clark 15). Murik have a cognatic kinship system, which is different from the patrilineal ones that prevail throughout the Sepik. For them, the main people involved in a woman's pregnancy and childbearing are not she and her husband. Unlike patrilineal groups, the child's father's kin are not immediately welcomed into a pregnant woman's circle of care. Husbands are definitely involved, but perhaps not in the ways modelled by cosmopolitan health care.

Roles, rights, and duties are quite clear, some of which extend throughout the kin group, while others are very specific to individuals. If illness or trouble occurs, healing and curing are not individual choices but family-based decisions of the larger kin group, often its senior members. Those who should be supporting a pregnant woman are her own kin, especially her mother and sisters, but also crucially her father who protects her by providing for her seclusion before, during, and after birth. A woman's father, not her husband, is responsible for preparing the birth house or building an enclosure in or near his home in which she can give birth. He or his senior male or female sibling (their descent group leader) may be the main person(s) deciding what treatment(s), if any, to seek. Her father and brothers are the ones most likely to convey her to a maternity clinic or hospital, and her husband accompanies them if their relationship with him is a positive one.

Expectations of support from a woman's husband could be misplaced if health care workers are unaware that if anything goes wrong, he is likely to be suspected as the cause. For Murik, if something goes wrong with a pregnancy, a woman or her husband is immediately suspected of infidelity, as such actions communicate to the unborn child that it is not wanted by one of its parents, and it may then decide not to be born or not to be born alive. On the other hand, during the birth process, traditionally a husband should go to his own sleeping mat, loosen his clothes, and stay quietly in seclusion so that his activities can in no way jeopardize the delivery. Unless aware that his act of going home to bed was intended to facilitate the birth, one might well misinterpret a man's absence from the clinic where his wife labours as indifference.

The father's kin, especially his sister, may represent a competing maternal influence. Therefore, it is incumbent on the father's sister to support the pregnancy and assure her benign intentions. If the child is a first born, it is crucial that the father's sister not see the baby or encounter the baby and mother before the appropriate ritual "coming out" ceremony at around six months. During this time, the mother and child live at her parents' home while preparations for the ceremony are being made. Her husband (with help from his kin) should help to provide plentiful food. He may visit his wife and baby but only briefly and discreetly, perhaps only at night.

If a woman makes use of a maternity clinic, any or all of these people may be in the vicinity, so awareness of their proper roles and interests would greatly facilitate communication among clinic personnel, the patient, and her family. When there were Murik staff at a hospital or clinic, people often chose to go there because they knew their particular circumstances and practices would be readily understood (Wogaing, this volume).

Beliefs around pregnancy, birth, and infancy are more than just expressions of anxiety or nervousness surrounding the risks of reproduction. They are expressions of a comprehensive worldview in which the boundary between humans and spirits (including ancestors) becomes porous and fragile under certain conditions—birth is one of them, but also dreaming, illness, loss of consciousness, death, and ritually empowered moments. Such conditions must be treated with utmost care to effect necessary transitions and restore firm separation between the living and the dead. Certain actions and substances (especially water) are intimately bound up with such moments and safe passage through them.

The moment of birth is a moment of transition, not just for the newborn but also for a woman as mother, especially one who is giving birth for the first time. Here, there is a drastic split between ideology and practice that creates serious tension between ideal circumstances for claiming the power of motherhood and "safe" medical practice. In Murik culture, mothers represent the power of giving to indebt and control others and are the epitome of those on whom others depend. For a woman to give birth unassisted and alone is an idealized expression of her complete sufficiency in this role, and is an accomplishment that many women desire to claim. I often heard birth stories recounted with pride about giving birth alone in a secluded spot at the beach or in the mangroves. Even in 2011, these accounts were not uncommon. The practice of going off alone to deliver a baby is, of course, the antithesis of "birth attendance" and is understood by cosmopolitan medicine to maximize risks for women and their babies.

Other factors also are conducive to women avoiding clinic and hospital settings to give birth. Murik women are modest and stoic. Many of them abhor the thought of being seen entering the birth house (on the margins of the village) and of having other women come to see how they are doing or hear them cry out. They are horrified if their labour goes on for long enough that others become aware of it, so they wait until the absolute last moment to go to the birth house and take a circuitous route or go under the cover of darkness. Most births are attended by only one or two female kin, although afterward their larger network of female kin is expected to provide food and companionship throughout the seclusion period. As mentioned, the baby's father may come to visit, but he most often comes at night and stays outside. Anyone who has visited the birth house is required to bathe before rejoining others and especially before eating with others, in order to avoid polluting them with the unstable condition of being in or near a transition between human and spirit worlds.

From the birth house, a woman and her new baby go to her parents' house until all of the birth fluids have "dried up" and the child is able to "laugh and recognize a person at a distance" (in Tok Pisin: *lap na lukim man longwe*). At this point in time, the baby is able to see his or her joking partners coming and the mother is expected to begin to resume her normal activities around the village. Thus seclusion and separation are crucial to everyone's well-being with respect to birth. Postpartum recovery is an aspect of maternity care that allows for a sense of security and rightness in the world. Although not all Murik subscribe to this full set of beliefs, local interpretations often draw from them, and feelings of appropriate and inappropriate behaviour throughout the community are based on them.

Gender roles are, of course, central to maternal and child health considerations and play a very important role in the personnel and actions related to birth. Men's participation takes place at a distance and has mainly to do with material support, but a husband's actions also sympathetically affect the progress and success of pregnancy and birth. A woman's male kin, and especially her father, are the guardians of her health and security. Nevertheless, I observed that pollution beliefs about women's sexual and reproductive fluids deterred nearly all men from supportive activities that might have exposed them to contact with birth even indirectly. In 1981 and 1982 in Darapap, the birth house, already in bad repair, sat on the tide flat away from village residences and disintegrated over the course of a year and a half. No men were willing to repair it, even though their female kin harangued and pleaded with them as each birth neared. Women gave birth there but complained bitterly about the leaking roof, poorly built ladder, and holes in the floor. Most of them left it within a day of giving birth. By 1986, it was gone. Women had to give birth either in their father's house or somewhere on the margins of the village. Under these conditions, some of them went to Wewak, Angoram or Marienberg in advance of going into labour.

The importance of bodily substances (blood, semen, breast milk, vaginal secretions) in Melanesian gender ideology has been written about extensively (M. Strathern; Jolly et al. 8). Carsten describes the symbolic importance and multivalent meanings of blood, which range from vitality and life to injury and death (20). In Murik life cycle rituals, all of these substances have heightened power and meaning in multiple contexts, both secret and widely known. They are often the main symbol and medium of transformation in life cycle rituals. These substances and their power to effect changes were the focus of quiet attention at even the most mundane of times. Occasional outbursts about someone's lack of care in disposal, contact, washing or toileting reminded everyone that bodily substances have great impact on the ongoing life cycle and well-being of everyone and had to be dealt with properly. At village meetings, through casual remarks and sometimes sharp reprimands, vital substances were monitored, controlled, and deployed with purpose—but they were not ignored.

Practices surrounding food are crucial to women's status as mothers and can ensure their own and others' health and well-being or expose them to illness conveyed through pollution or sorcery. For Murik, giving food establishes kinship and can even surpass biological relatedness as a claim on a person's identity and loyalty to specific kin groups. In order to claim a newborn child as a member of one's kin group, mother's kin have first priority and primary responsibility for providing good food, but the father's kin also have some responsibility. Not infrequently, adoptive parents must shoulder responsibility for feeding a child's birth mother before, during, and after the child's birth. If the firstborn of a sibling group has no children, he or she may ask a younger sister for a child, a request that may not be refused. Other relatives may also ask and be given a child but must show their good intentions by feeding the birth mother. These practices involve a specific set of kin and near kin in the support group of those who feed and care for a pregnant woman.

Finally, there is a repertoire of beliefs and practices having to do with bathing and health that are significant factors in maintaining the connection of a person's soul to his or her body through the medium of water. Murik routinely bathe in the early morning and near dusk whenever possible, as bathing strengthens the connection of the soul with the physical body at transitional times of day when it is thought possible to slip between realms of spirits and humans. At other times as well— when a person is asleep, ill, or unconscious—the body and soul are tenuously connected and bathing first in salt water and then in fresh water is important to restore a strong connection. Birth itself constitutes a transition of this kind and at each birth I attended, women poured seawater over a labouring woman's belly and genitals to both cool and protect her. Once a child was delivered and its air passages cleared, the vernix was rubbed into its skin and the child was wrapped firmly in a cloth to be bathed morning and evening in warm water. The mother is also expected to bathe immediately after the placenta has been delivered. At one birth I attended, where the labour was overlong and obstructed, fear for the first-time mother's life ran high. Not only was she scolded for not going to the hospital to give birth, but her mother and grandmother yelled at her to hurry up and wash immediately after delivering the child, as she shivered with cold. When she hesitated, one of them ran to where she huddled over an opening in the floor and dumped a full bucket of water over her. Such a dramatic gesture in the context of a health clinic would arouse strong negative responses from anyone unfamiliar with local cultural meanings, yet an appreciation for the significance of culturally embedded concepts of health, well-being, and concern in a life and death situation is absolutely necessary for a maternal health clinic to succeed in rural Papua New Guinea.

DELIVERING LOCALLY APPROPRIATE HEALTH CARE

The Marienberg maternity clinic was unique in the Lower Sepik Region as a health care facility that exclusively cared for women. While it thrived, its circumstances conformed to MDG recommendations that maternity health care be subsumed within larger, operational systems of education, general health care, communication and provisioning. In this case, maternal health care was provided by Catholic Mission infrastructure rather than the government's, and providing maternal health care was a secondary priority within this structure. No doubt many women's and children's lives were saved and improved by supervised births. That no maternal deaths at the maternity clinic were recorded over more than seven years for women from the two villages of Darapap and Karau testifies to the value of such a health resource. The success of this local maternity clinic suggests important factors to keep in mind when developing a new government-supported system of maternal health care.

The (now defunct) mission-based health service was not staffed to provide frequent care at the village level. Then and now, large numbers of births happen in villages where no other resources are available, and obstetrical emergencies are unsupported. These risks were substantially reduced by the kind of clinic that Sister Marianna developed, where women and their kin could come in advance of a birth and remain in relative seclusion throughout the birth and postpartum period. Their needs in terms of personnel, food, privacy and hygiene were provided for and respected. Sister Marianna's willingness to respect women's need for privacy and seclusion did much to develop the sense of trust that made the clinic effective. Had she disregarded these concerns by allowing the women to be exposed unnecessarily to people who were not kin and to strangers, male or female, the feeling that the clinic was a safe and reliable place to give birth would have been much weaker.

A problem of condescension and disrespect has been identified among health care workers in Papua New Guinea who are not from rural backgrounds (Wentworth, this volume). The staff at the Marienberg clinics came from the region. Sister Marianna relied on and respected the advice of local staff about separating birth from mundane activities and maintaining a maternity clinic that did not challenge local pollution beliefs. Health practitioners who are selected from the region and redeployed there following training are better equipped to operate from the basis of a shared worldview and local level experience. Such personnel can fine tune adaptations in health care to local understandings and communicate appropriately about health care services to people of different ages and backgrounds.[9]

Reservations about pollution that lead to the lack of any appropriate facility in the village for giving birth might actually encourage women and their kin to come to a maternity clinic if they are confident about receiving conscientious treatment, concerning not only cleanliness and the handling and disposal of bodily substances but also the implications for others of proximity to the birth process. However a maternity clinic deals with them, such matters will be closely observed and interpreted. Careful attention should be paid to this entire domain of maternal and reproductive health care, not only for its importance to hygiene and health safety but also for how it will be understood by those who use the health services.

Health practices proceed from larger worldviews, and meanings and practices surrounding birth are highly attuned to them. In order to improve health care, safety and survival for rural women, health care workers should be trained, not just in the practical aspects of healthy birthing but also in how to develop respectful communication across cultural differences within the region they serve and in relation to cosmopolitan biomedicine. The maternity clinic at Marienberg was staffed mainly by local people. In general, the operations of the clinic were consistent with and respectful of important local practices having to do with birth. Local people became ever more confident that its services were safe and supportive (Wogaing, this volume). Due to the intention that health care services would contribute to culture change—that is, help to convert people to Catholicism—the maternity clinic did not provide one of the most essential and hoped for reproductive services: family planning and contraception. The Marienberg clinic was not fully prepared to deal with obstetrical emergencies and would have required much better communication and transportation systems to cope with such emergencies and to get women to hospitals in the region. Its ongoing existence depended on the strength of the larger system in which it was embedded (See Freedman et al.; Kiessler and Clark; Wentworth, this volume on the importance of a holistic approach to improving maternal health care).

Equally as important was the leadership of Sister Marianna, without which the clinic did not continue. Because of her high level of commitment, skill and energy, Sister Marianna inspired those around her and provided strong leadership in a crucial and challenging area of health care. She often dealt with turnover among her staff because many of the young girls she trained eventually married and moved back to their villages. With the knowledge that they had gained, their ongoing presence in rural villages improved the outlook for women who gave birth there. The crucial role that Sister Marianna played was more difficult to replace, but planning for transitions in leadership as well as staff is an essential part of developing and maintaining effective maternal health services.

A successful government-run system to improve maternal and child health must provide reliable infrastructure and appropriately trained staff and leadership. Perhaps the greatest strength of the Marienberg clinic was that in major ways it was well attuned to local needs and understandings. New facilities intending to provide such crucial health care would do well to follow this lead and to develop not just practices but also communication strategies and understandings that take into account local worldviews in the service of improved health and survival for women and their babies.

Funding for the research presented here came from Sepik Documentation Project, The Australian Museum, Sydney; University of Minnesota; University of California, San Diego; Department of Anthropology, Central Washington University; and the Wenner-Gren Foundation and Institute for Inter-cultural Studies. Many thanks go to Naomi McPherson for proposing the idea for this book and for her leadership on the project and to Sister Marianna and the women of the Lower Sepik region.

ENDNOTES

[1] "Cosmopolitan medicine" as used here refers to the dominant health care beliefs and practices of industrialized countries. This category often implies hierarchical decision making under the aegis of medico-technical specialists in an overall male-dominated power structure.

[2] Melanesia commonly refers to island nations of the southwest Pacific, principally Papua New Guinea, Solomon Islands, and Vanuatu.

[3] UN statistics confirm that 75 percent of the population in Papua New Guinea is under thirty-five years of age, and 40 percent is under fifteen years of age ("About Papua New Guinea").

⁴Basic statistics for Papua New Guinea provided by the UNDP show the importance of free health care: 85 percent of the population lives in rural areas; 75 percent of the population is dependent on subsistence agriculture; and 40 percent live on less than one dollar a day ("About Papua New Guinea").

⁵Under Australian administration, each village was required to build and maintain an empty house where a visiting Australian patrol office could stay. Many villages continued to have such a house for visitors, especially official ones.

⁶She was able to diagnose many illnesses and told me of several different conditions people suffered from based on others describing the symptoms to her. Her hard and fast rule was that she would treat those who came to see her. She did not go to people's homes, even if they requested it. She wanted to avoid even the appearance of imposing diagnosis or treatment on people who did not want it, whether it be others in the household or the patients themselves. If she had done so, it would have left her open to interpretations of her actions as making someone more ill or even causing their death. She was very sensitive to local people's belief that the causes of illness were social. Likewise, at the clinic, if she knew someone was fatally ill, she would do all she could to alleviate their suffering but would then send them home to die. She recognized both the importance of the clinic not developing a reputation as a place where people died and the local preference for finishing life in one's own home territory.

⁷Among Murik, nursing mothers commonly complained that they were becoming too thin as a result of prolonged nursing, but this was also a sign of good mothering of which they were proud.

⁸Postpartum abstinence from sex was most frequently mentioned. But women who thought they might be pregnant and did not want to bear a child sometimes worked very hard to try to induce a miscarriage through hard physical work; some women were said to know how to use mangrove pods to prepare a medicinal concoction that would induce miscarriage.

⁹In 1982 and 1986, Murik villagers personally knew several Murik health care workers (one doctor and several nurses) at Boram Hospital, which vastly increased their willingness to go there and to trust that they would be given reliable and respectful treatment.

WORKS CITED

Carsten, Janet. "Substance and Relationality: Blood in Contexts." *Annual Review of Anthropology* 40 (2011):19-35. Print.

Denoon, Donald. "Medical Care and Gender in Papua New Guinea." *Family and Gender in the Pacific: Domestic Contradictions and the Colonial Impact.* Eds. Margaret Jolly and Martha MacIntyre. Cambridge: Cambridge University Press, 1989. 95-107. Print.

Freedman, Lynn P., Ronald J. Waldman, Helen de Pinho, Me E. Wirth, A. Mushtaque R. Chowdhury, and Allan Rosenfield. *Who's Got the Power? Transforming Health Systems for Women and Children. United Nations Millennium Project: Task Force on Child Health and Maternal Health. United Millennium Project.* United Nations, 2005. Web. 8 October 2015.

Integrated Regional Information Networks (IRIN). "Papua New Guinea: Tackling Maternal Health 'Crisis.'" *IRIN Humanitarian News and Analysis.* IRIN, 30 Nov. 2011. Web. 8 Oct. 2015.

Jolly, Margaret, Christine Stewart, and Carolyn Brewer. *Engendering Violence in Papua New Guinea.* Canberra: Australian National University Press, 2012. Print.

Kiessler, Tony and Geoff Clark, Ed. *National Department of Health Report. Ministerial Taskforce on Maternal Health in Papua New Guinea 2009. Soroptimist International.* Soroptimist International, 2012. Web. 8 Oct. 2015.

Koblinsky, Marjorie, Ed. *Reducing Maternal Mortality: Learning from Bolivia, China, Egypt, Honduras, Indonesia, Jamaica and Zimbabwe.* Human Development Network, Health, Nutrition and Population Series. Washington, DC: World Bank, 2003. Print.

Liljestrand, Jerker and Indra Pathmanathan. "Reducing Maternal Mortality: Can We Derive Policy Guidance from Developing Country Experiences? Critical Elements in Reducing Maternal Mortality." *Journal of Public Health Policy* 25.3/4 (2004): 299-314. Web. 8 Oct. 2015

"Maternal Mortality Ratio (Modeled Estimate, Per 100,000 Live Births)—Country Ranking" N.p., n.d. Web. 24 June 2015.

McIntyre, Martha. "Gender Violence in Melanesia and the Problem of Millennium Development Goal No. 3." *Engendering Violence in Papua New Guinea*. Eds. Margaret Jolly, Christine Stewart and Carolyn Brewer. Canberra: Australian National University, 2012. 239-266. Print.

National Sex and Reproduction Research Team and Carol Jenkins. *National Study of Sexual and Reproductive Knowledge and Behaviour in Papua New Guinea*. Goroka: Papua New Guinea Institute of Medical Research, 1994. Print.

Sister Marianna. Personal interview. 1981, 1988.

Strathern, Marilyn. *The Gender of the Gift: Problems with Women and Problems with Society in Melanesia*. Berkeley: University of California Press, 1988. Print.

Townsend, Patricia K. "Traditional birth Attendants in Papua New Guinea: An Interim Report." IASER Discussion Paper No. 52. Prepared by the Papua New Guinea Institute of Applied Social and Economic Research for UNICEF. Boroko: IASER, 1986. Print.

United Nations. "Papua New Guinea" *Millennium Development Goals Second National Progress Comprehensive Report for Papua New Guinea 2010.*" United Nations Development Project, 2010. Print.

United Nations Development Program (UNDP). "About Papua New Guinea." UNDP, 2012. Web. 8. Jan. 2014.

United Nations Development Program and Papua New Guinea. *Papua New Guinea— Millennium Development Goals Second National Progress Comprehensive Report for Papua New Guinea 2010*. UNDP, 2010. Web. 8 Jan. 2014.

United Nations Development Program and Papua New Guinea. "The Future We Want." UNDP, 2013. Web. 8 Jan. 2014

2.
Second Chance

Caring for HIV-Infected Mothers and Their Children in Mendi, Papua New Guinea

PHILIP GIBBS AND WINNIE WILLIAM

CHILDBEARING IN PAPUA NEW GUINEA (PNG) is a risky business: reports over the last twenty-five years have made this clear. It is estimated that 1500 PNG women and girls die each year in relation to pregnancy and childbirth (*Ministerial Taskforce on Maternal Health* v). Demographic Health Survey data for PNG estimate the maternal mortality rate (MMR) to be 773/1000 in 2006 (*Papua New Guinea Demographic and Health Survey*). Estimates based on mathematical models give a figure of 250 in 2008. In a study based on facility-based survey data and Health Ministry Information System Records from 2009, Drs. Glen Mola and Barry Kirby estimate the national MMR to be 450 (Mola and Kirby). Despite their variance, all these figures indicate a serious health situation for mothers in PNG and an urgent need to improve maternal health outcomes.

This paper is about maternal health and how care for pregnant mothers can ensure healthy children. The focus is not on all mothers but rather on mothers whose health has already been compromised by the HIV virus and whose health is further stressed by pregnancy. Among the concerns of pregnant women infected with HIV is whether they will survive to carry their pregnancy to term and if their child will be born infected with HIV. In the Papua New Guinea Highlands, Catholic Health Services in the diocese of Mendi has taken these concerns seriously and has sought ways to ensure that infected mothers can remain healthy, that they can have supervised delivery, and that their child will not be infected with HIV. Our paper focuses on efforts by Catholic Health Services and their partners to improve maternal and child health outcomes in the Southern Highlands (SHP) of Papua New Guinea. This paper tells the story of an attempt to take seriously MDG 5 (improving maternal health) in the context of implementing MDG 6 (combatting of HIV and AIDS).

The Southern Highlands Province is situated in the interior of the mainland of Papua New Guinea. In 2011, the former Southern Highlands Province was divided into two parts: one part retained the name Southern Highlands, and the second, western part was named Hela Province. The 2011 census recorded populations of 510, 245 in Southern Highlands Province and 249,449 in Hela Province (*Papua New Guinea Demographic and Health Survey*). The majority of the population in both provinces lives in scattered hamlets and supports itself with subsistence horticulture.

SERVICES FOR MATERNAL CARE

Care for mothers and newborn babies is inadequate throughout much of PNG. Demographic and Health Survey data (*Papua New Guinea Demographic and Health Survey*) show that although about 71 percent of women make one antenatal care visit, only 50 percent complete four or more antenatal visits. Similarly, only about 50 percent of women deliver at a health facility or with a skilled provider.

Compared with national data, the situation in SHP and Hela is even more limited. The Southern Highlands has the lowest antenatal coverage and lowest supervision of births in health centres and hospitals in the whole of Papua New Guinea (*Ministerial Taskforce on Maternal Health* 10-11). This is mostly due to geographic and infrastructural barriers, limited availability of health services, shortage of human resources, and lack of equipment. Mendi Hospital is the only hospital in the SHP with qualified doctors and facilities for dealing with severe birth complications requiring surgery or transfusion. There are only fifteen registered midwives in the province, most working out of Mendi Hospital—some of these are not working now as midwives but in administrative positions as matrons and supervisors.

Most rural women continue to give birth at home where only a small fraction of maternal deaths are reported. The most common reason for giving birth at home is due to lack of money and (transport) infrastructure, which makes it difficult for them to come to an operating health facility. About half of all rural health services in Papua New Guinea are provided by church-based groups. Southern Highlands is typical in this regard. Catholic Health Services from the Catholic Diocese of Mendi, which covers both Southern Highlands and Hela provinces, provides services with six health centres and seven aid posts.[1] There is a day clinic at Tari secondary school, a community health worker training school, stand-alone voluntary counselling and testing (VCT) centres at Tari and Lake Kopiago, and an urban clinic in Mendi that also serves as a VCT centre. This study focuses on the services at the Mendi urban clinic, better known as the Epeanda clinic at Kumin Catholic Mission in Mendi.

TRADITIONAL PRACTICES ASSOCIATED WITH CHILDBEARING

The Southern Highlands is one of the few provinces in Papua New Guinea where in some cultures, a woman is expected to deliver alone (Townsend).[2] Custom allows another woman to call out to the labouring woman from outside the delivery hut, but another woman is not allowed to enter (Alto et al. 613). The practice is hazardous because it does not allow women assistance while giving birth, which means that women only get experience about childbearing through their own deliveries. The reason for this is that woman's blood is considered dangerous to both men and women and that contact with blood is believed to result in illness or death.

Sister Gaudentia Meier, a trained midwife from Switzerland, first came to Mendi in 1969. She describes the practice when she first arrived at Det, near Mendi.

> *The standard practice was that there was a house behind the women's house, which she also used [for seclusion] when she had her period. The mother would go in there when she started labour and no other women were allowed to go in. They just could tell her ... the grandmother or someone ... tell her what to do ... that was the way it was here. In Tari, they had birth attendants, usually the hus-*

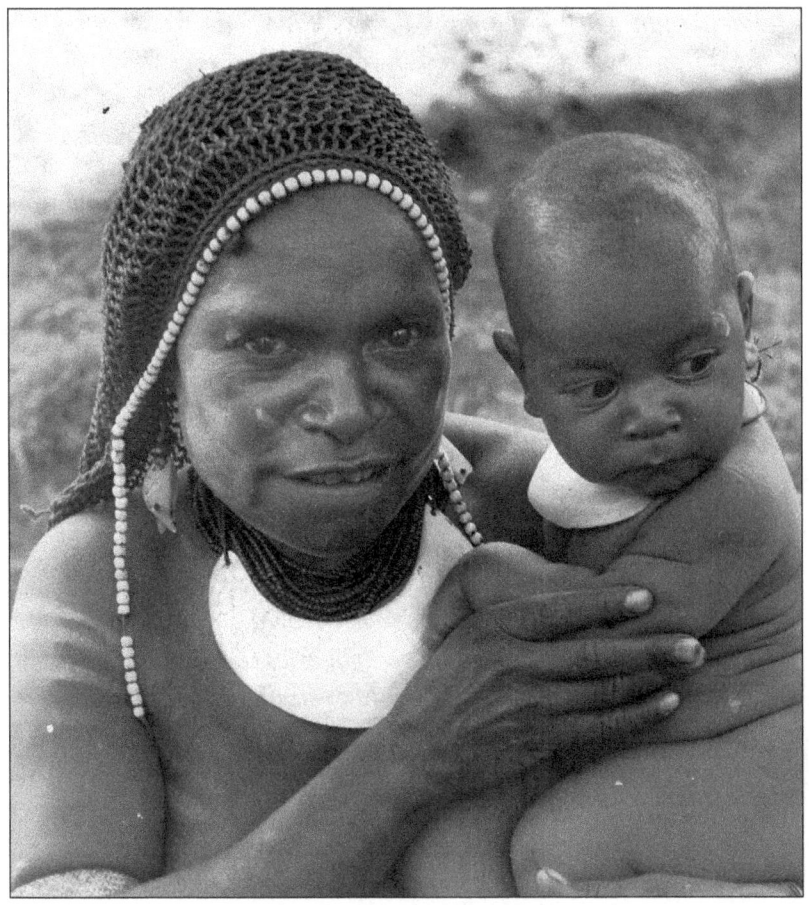

Mother and child at Nipa in late 1960s.
Photo from collection of Olddenbank Sisters. Used with permission.

band's mother. What they did here at Det was the way it was in the lower Mendi area. (Meier, Personal interview)

As a midwife, Sister Gaudentia thought that supervised delivery would be beneficial, and she invited women to come to the aid post for childbirth. She tells of the first mother she assisted to deliver in 1969.

Father Ben was here, and he knew the language, and he told them that there is someone here, so you don't have to deliver by yourself. When the mothers came for clinic,

> *we would learn how many babies had died or that some children would be adopted because the mother died. We started in a bush house to "fix sores" [medicate tropical ulcers] or whatever. Then the catechist's wife was the first one that I assisted to deliver. She sent a message down, so I went to her village and walked to where she was. She was quite in labour. I walked back to the car with her. We had to stop because of strong contractions. I was rubbing her back and everybody was watching me. A lot of women came along, and they were talking to each other. I brought her to the car, got to Det [the mission aid post], and she delivered. The husband was happy, but then I asked what the women had been talking about … it seems they were saying, "How does she know where the pain is when she has never had a baby herself. She says she has no baby." When I heard that, we got the mothers around, and we talked about it. I told them that I learned it, and that is how I know. I had three more deliveries the same month. By the end of the year, I had fifty-six deliveries.* (Meier, Personal interview)

At the same time, Sister Gaudentia engaged with local practices associated with birth. Customarily, women give birth in a kneeling position. The mission health centre provided a bed, but women were free to choose their own position.

> *I asked them, "which would you prefer," and they said, "we prefer our way and position." So I would let her because that's the way she feels better. She would kneel with her head against a post and her feet against something firm so she could really get some pressure. We would put a towel or a piece of plastic on the floor for hygiene purposes.* (Meier, Personal interview)

Mothers wanted to take home a piece of umbilical cord, which they would hide in the roof of their house in the belief that this would prevent them getting pregnant again quickly.[3] Traditionally, after some weeks, when there was no more discharge, a woman

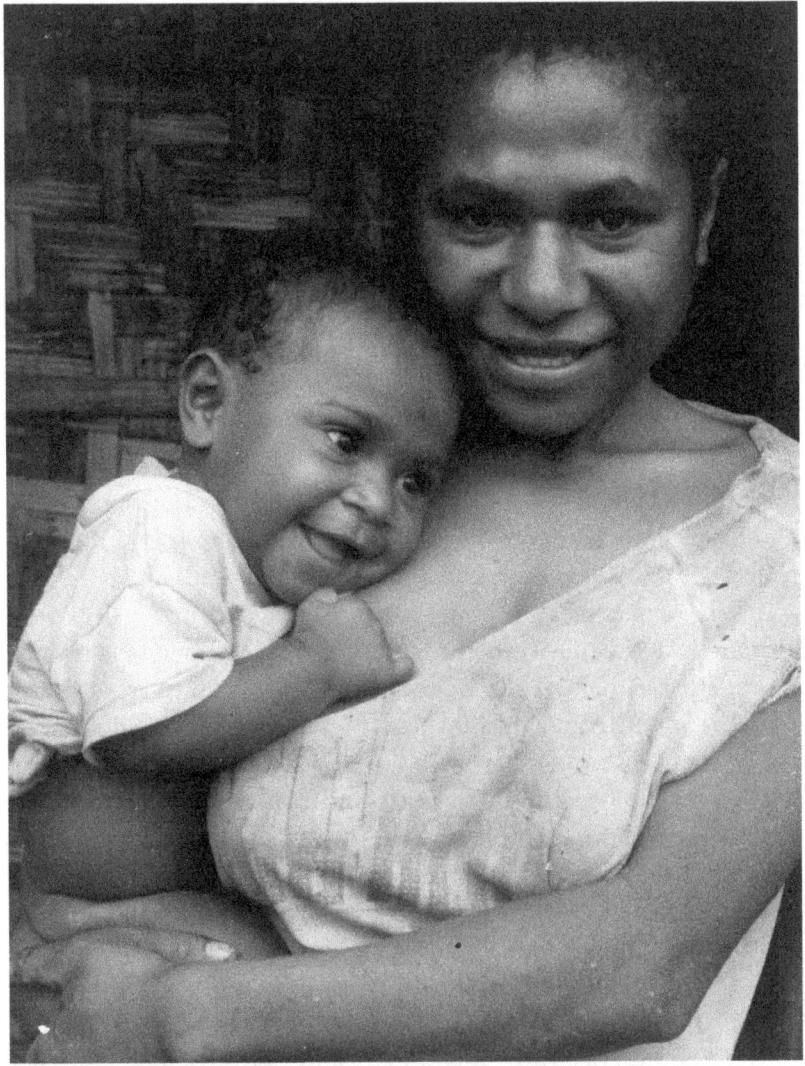

Mother and child at Margarima in the late 1970s.
Photo from Oldenbank Sisters collection. Used with permission.

was required to jump over burning leaves in order to "dry the blood" and, thus, be allowed to be seen with her baby in public. When asked if they should have a similar practice on leaving the mission aid post, the people said that was not necessary, and the mother could simply return home. Word went around and soon, in the early 1970s, there were over two hundred births a year at the small Det aid post. In one month, there were thirty-nine births.

In the twenty-eight years Sister Gaudentia was at Det, she assisted several thousand mothers and none died. "We had to send a few mothers for Caesarean section in Mendi, but none died" (Meier, Personal interview).[4]

Two decades later, health workers were alarmed to hear that HIV had arrived in PNG.[5] In 1994, after (Lady) Margaret Anjo from Ialibu in the Southern Highlands went public over her seropositive status, Sister Gaudentia started providing awareness training in high schools and through community health workers (CHW). The module on HIV that she developed for the CHW training curriculum was adopted for home-based care throughout the country by the National AIDS Council in PNG. The first case of HIV was recognized in Mendi in 1998, and Sister Gaudentia moved to Mendi that year to work with hospital staff at Mendi Hospital.[6] Stigma ran high, and Sister Gaudentia recalls how the first woman found to be infected with HIV was hiding in a shelter for pigs.

At that time, there was no antiretroviral therapy (ART) and, although ART drugs were available by 2002, nobody was trained to administer them. The "Born to Live" program to train health workers on ART began in 2003 at Mingende Hospital in Simbu with the help of Dr. Ann Doherty who previously had been working in Kenya. In 2003 and 2004, Sister Gaudentia went for Prevention of Parent to Child Transmission (PPTCT) training. By Easter 2006, with the help of Dr. Arun Menon of the Australasian Society for HIV Medicine (ASHM), they started HIV rapid testing, and Dr. Menon put four people on treatment, including one pregnant mother.

The Epeanda urban clinic at Kumin Mission in Mendi started in 2005.[7] In 2006, Sister Gaudentia, along with the Epeanda staff, started the practice of having all HIV-infected "friends" together for some days at Kumin Mission twice a year.[8] Infected people would support one another (for example, giving advice about what to do when rats chew the teat on a feeding bottle!). Now some of these people have become "mentor mothers," sharing their own experience as infected mothers with other infected women.

HIV AND MATERNITY

The risk of pregnancy-related death is six to eight times higher for

HIV positive women than their HIV negative counterparts (Gathigah). Studies in Africa reveal that pregnant women with HIV die at much higher rates than women who do not have HIV. Indeed, HIV increases maternal mortality directly, from the progression of the HIV disease itself and indirectly through higher rates of sepsis, anemia, and other pregnancy-related conditions (Gathigah).[9] Hence, the health workers in Mendi were very concerned about how the spread of HIV would affect the mothers they were caring for.

HIV in Papua New Guinea

HIV spread exponentially in PNG during the 1990s, and by 2003, the prevalence of HIV among women attending the Port Moresby General Hospital antenatal care clinic surpassed one per cent (UNGASS, *Country Progress Report 2010* 4). The recorded increase began to level off in recent years, partly due to more accurate ways of recording data in different parts of the country. Recognizing the varying sources of data, figures are now given as ranges. According to the most recent United Nations Global Report in 2013 (UNAIDS):

- In 2013, there were between 20,000 and 31,000 people living with HIV in PNG (UNAIDS 123);
- The estimated prevalence in 2012 was 0.4–0.7 percent (120);
- Estimated AIDS deaths in 2012 was <1,000–1,600 (128);
- HIV-infected female adults in 2012 estimated at 10,000–16,000 (183);
- The coverage of antiretroviral prevention services for pregnant women living with HIV in PNG in 2012 is less than 50 percent. (40)

Data from the Southern Highlands in 2009 gives an estimated HIV prevalence rate of 4.7 percent through VCT centres, 0.1 percent from blood bank tests, and 0.4 percent from antenatal testing (*Ministerial Taskforce on Maternal Health* 34). Table 1 below gives prevalence rates of those tested from Epeanda. Mothers testing seropositive have the choice of going to Epeanda or to the Nina clinic at Mendi Hospital for follow-up visits.

Table 1: Antenatal Catholic Health Services Mendi

Year	Reactive HIV	Total Tested	% Reactive	Comment
2006	5	365	1.37	3 repeat test
2007	6	1603	0.37	1 tested twice
2008	6	336	1.79	
2009	9	1418	0.64	
2010	4	1069	0.37	
2011	9	1470	0.61	
2012	8	1777	0.45	
2013	7	737[10]	0.95	

COMPREHENSIVE STRATEGY FOR ENSURING HEALTH OF MOTHERS AND BABIES

With the growing danger of HIV (and other STIs), Catholic Health Services Mendi developed a comprehensive strategy for improving the health of mothers and babies. This included special training of health workers, education for mothers about STIs (including HIV) and treatments available, antenatal clinic with testing, provision for those testing seropositive to receive prompt treatment, facilities for mothers close to term to come and wait near health facilities, and a follow-up program for infected mothers to ensure that their children remained healthy.

Training of Health Workers

All Catholic Health Services (CHS) health workers were trained in STI syndromic management, voluntary confidential counselling and testing (VCCT), provider initiated counselling and testing (PICT) and home-based care (HBC). Hence, the task of identifying and caring for affected people was not left to a few specialists but was expected of all health workers within the Mendi Catholic Health Services.

Other health workers were selected for specialist training, including rural laboratory assistants (RLA), the use of CD4 count equipment, and antiretroviral therapy (ART) prescribers. Since

2010, working with the CHW school at the mission and supervision from Sister Gaudentia, some Community Health Workers have been trained as ART prescribers resulting in more health workers qualified to prescribe ART treatment. In other parts of PNG, this service is reserved only for registered nurses. Feedback from health workers whom we interviewed spoke of how the most important outcome of the training was a reduction in fear associated with HIV and a reduction in stigma and discrimination on the part of the health workers. There was also the realization that the essential ingredient in care is just that, care.

Education for Mothers

Antenatal clinics offer an important opportunity to educate mothers (and the few fathers who attend) on STIs, including HIV and clinics, which were organized so that this educational component was not missed. Education information also dealt with healthy attitudes and practices. For example, previously there was a practice for mothers in the Southern Highlands to under-eat during pregnancy thinking that this would mean a smaller baby and a smaller baby would be easier to deliver. Health workers spoke about the importance of healthy foods that would assist both mother and baby. Attitudes are important too, and in Papua New Guinea, where pigs represent wealth and status, some mothers needed convincing that their own health is more important than that of their pigs. Mothers in polygamous marriages who perceive that their husband is giving more attention to another wife might think, "Who cares [about me], the father [of my child] is looking out for another woman" (Meier, Personal interview). Sister Gaudentia has impressed on health workers the importance of health worker's attitudes, since to ensure mothers return for care, depends very much on their first therapeutic communication. A mother who trusts a health worker will return to that health worker.

GREATER COVERAGE OF ANC CLINICS AND TESTING

In 2011, of the estimated 210,000 pregnancies for the whole of PNG, 125,892 pregnant women had at least one antenatal care visit (60 percent) and HIV testing was offered to less than 50,000 of them (National AIDS Council Secretariat, *Global AIDS Report 2012* 75; UNAIDS). There is less coverage in the Southern Highlands according to the Southern Highlands Health Department, as only 39.6 percent of pregnant women made at least one antenatal clinic visit for 2012 and only 1,927 women between 15 to 49 years of age were tested for HIV at these clinics. This is because HIV testing is normally available only to those attending town (as opposed to rural) clinics and when test strips are available, only a minority of pregnant women in the province attending ANC clinics are offered tests for HIV.[11] The majority of those tested were at clinics run through CHS Mendi or at outreach clinics also run by CHS Mendi.[12]

Provision for Mothers Who Test HIV+

Clinical examination and CD4 count results can help the health worker to assess the health of the person infected with HIV. However, with mothers, CHS Mendi has a policy of "test and treat," so all pregnant women who test seropositive are put immediately on antiretroviral therapy. This has required considerable management work to ensure that medication is available. The program involves more than medication, however, as it also includes confidential counselling and clean daycare facilities. The program is designed to help mothers physically, mentally, and spiritually.

Due to geographical distance and poor or non-existent roads, many mothers are not able to reach a health facility once they feel the signs of labour. CHS Mendi thus offers facilities for infected expectant mothers to stay at the Epeanda clinic when they come close to full term or when they feel the need for medical care. When labour begins, they are provided with free transport to the maternity ward at Mendi Hospital for a supervised birth. After they have recovered, the mothers return with their baby to the Epeanda clinic.

Follow-Up Program

Mothers are advised to give exclusive breastfeeding for four to six months (depending on when the child would start putting things in its mouth). Then they were given solids with Lactogen for three weeks with sweet potato water and other soft foods, which ensured that babies would not be infected with HIV. Previously, mothers were instructed to wean the child as soon as the child started on other foods, but, now, those mothers on ART treatment can continue mixed feeding with breast milk and other food.

RESULTS

As of July 2015, 133 HIV positive mothers have given birth to 144 healthy babies (one had twins and another triplets).[13] No mothers coming through the Epeanda clinic have died from childbirth complications and all babies were born without HIV infection.[14] This is a better result than the national figure for healthy mothers.[15] Without interventions such as PPTCT, transmission rates range from 15 percent to 45 percent (WHO, "Mother-to-Child"). One mother did die months after giving birth to a healthy baby but this was due to her joining a Revival church that convinced her to stop taking ART medication.[16]

Some of the mothers coming to the Epeanda clinic have had to travel very long distances. Those coming from the Kopiago area have to walk two days and then travel a full day on a bus. Some have survived very traumatic experiences. For example, one of the first to attend at Epeanda was a young woman who had been gang-raped, infected with HIV, and was made pregnant at the same time. She came for help three weeks after the incident, which was too late to start post exposure prophylaxis (PEP). A health worker recalls her saying, "How will I cope? I did not plan to have a child. Besides, I am HIV positive." When this occurred in 2005, ART was not widely available; however, with the help of Sister Tarcisia of the National Catholic HIV-AIDS Services in Port Moresby, the young woman started ART at thirty-two weeks gestation. She was helped to deliver a healthy baby girl and she remains HIV-positive but continues with treatment; she is now married with a second child.

A sixteen-year-old girl was carried to the Epeanda clinic. She had been ill for a long time, and her legs were contracted from being left in a sitting position. She tested positive for HIV. With care and treatment, she was able to able to walk and even to play basketball within two months. On returning to the village, she became pregnant by the same person who had infected her. She came back to the Epeanda clinic for help during her pregnancy, and her son was not infected. However, he was hydrocephalic and died after a year. She has since remarried. She would surely have died if she had remained in the village.

Another woman was brought from her home village to the Epeanda clinic gravely ill with a serious skin infection and TB. Upon testing, she was found to be HIV infected. With treatment she recovered, married, and became pregnant, at which point her husband rejected her and sent her away. She returned to clinic for help during her pregnancy and had a healthy baby. But then her husband's sisters came and took the baby from her, and she was left to return childless to her home village where she remains.

Dealing with some cases can be traumatic for the staff at the Epeanda. Occasionally infected mothers become aggressive due to HIV psychosis (toxoplasma). After punching and threatening health workers, one infected woman had to be locked in a room for a week. With treatment and care, she recovered and gave birth to a healthy daughter. Since then, the woman developed TB of the spine and could walk only with the help of crutches. She was convinced that her illness was caused by sorcery or witchcraft, defaulted in taking her medication, and subsequently died. There is little that the health workers can do when a person refuses to believe that they are infected with HIV.

LESSONS LEARNED

There have been a number of lessons learned through the PPTCT program at the Epeanda clinic. Training for health workers is very important. It is through the health workers that mothers and their partners receive sound counselling on how to live healthily despite HIV infection. They are prescribed medication to reduce the viral load, and this is followed up with the help of "mentor mothers." These women, also infected with HIV, have volunteered to help other HIV+ women and mothers. If someone fails to come to the clinic for new ART supplies, a mentor mother will go to their homes to check on them and to encourage them to come to the Epeanda clinic for their medicines.

Reliable staff personnel are also important. Sister Gaudentia has worked out of Mendi since 1969 and her co-worker Clare

Kopipi has been with CHS Mendi since 1981. Clare seldom needs to consult records, as she knows all returning mothers personally and remembers their case history and personal information. The long-term commitment of other locals in the small group of health workers attached to the Epeanda clinic, such as Maria Koke and Clare Andawa, all contribute to a sense of teamwork, which carries over in service to their clients. CHS Mendi has been fortunate to have assistance from the Oil Search Company, which is part of the oil and gas extraction industry in the area. When reagents run short or the CD4 count machine is out of action, Oil Search has come to their aid. "They are doing CD4 cell count, so now we send our blood samples directly to Kutubu, to Oil Search. They do the full blood count. They do even hepatitis B, they do everything. So we are really fortunate" (Meier, Personal interview).

Perhaps the most important lesson learned concerns the attitudes of mothers. For a woman who comes to the antenatal clinic and finds out that she is HIV positive, it seems to her like the end of everything. "Once the PPTCT program is introduced into her life, she sees that she has chances of living positively and having another child, and she participates in the program with all her heart" (Meier, Personal interview). For positive mothers, being healthy and having a healthy child becomes a priority in their lives. When they have trouble, they know where they can go to get caring assistance. After giving birth at Mendi Hospital, mothers call the Epeanda staff to help make sure that the baby receives the right medicine. Co-author Winnie William notes that "we have over a hundred committed mothers. They have a second chance to have a child and they are one hundred percent committed."

This second chance makes a big difference to a marriage. N[17] was infected with HIV through her first husband. She remarried and with the program for discordant couples run through the Epeanda, they were able to have children and her husband remains HIV negative. "My husband takes care of me and our daughter so that we may not get other infections. Last week after getting the DBS [dry blood spot] result from the Epeanda clinic, for our last daughter, my husband was so happy with the result that he suggested we should have another child again, this time, a son."

P and L commenced ART treatment in 2007. P now serves at the Epeanda as a mentor to others who test seropositive. P and L had a healthy child in 2009, who is now four years old, and L is expecting again. P says, "We are happy and confident that by following the program at the Epeanda, our child will be born HIV free."

DIFFICULTIES

There have been difficulties, too. During a medication supply crisis for several months in 2012, staff had to change the treatment for clients who had been on regular ART. Some patients went onto oral suspension, a medication meant for children. Fortunately, Dr. Menon from the Australasian Society for HIV Medicine (ASHM) could give advice.

Confidentiality is a big issue. Because of the fear of stigma and discrimination, there are people on treatment who do not want to be seen coming to get their supply of medicine. Some ask to meet in a quiet place in town; they open their bag to allow the Epeanda health worker or mentor mother to discretely drop the medicine in the bag. There have been crises over confidentiality. For example, on one occasion after a man died, his wives were accused of practicing witchcraft [*sanguma*] to cause his death, leading others to call for burning them them alive (Gibbs, "Engendered Violence"). Fortunately, the health workers were able to convince the infected person to disclose, so as to save the lives of the accused women. Stigma and discrimination appear to be lessening, and some people reveal their status to their community; as a result, most now often get support in that community.

APPLICATION

The "Second Chance" PPTCT program is running successfully with high-risk mothers in a high-risk rural province. Since 2005, of the 133 mothers participating in the program, there have been no maternal deaths for those who stay with the program. This is an example of what can be done to reduce maternal mortality in PNG. What is to prevent similar measures being offered to all pregnant women? A report from the National Department of Health (*Ministerial Taskforce on Maternal Health*) lists the first four characteristics of a successful public health program:

1. A package of evidence-based and cost-effective interventions contextualized for PNG;
2. An adequate supply of trained, competent, and willing workforce who have
3. A functional, supplied, enabling environment that is
4. Supportively supervised and managed (*Ministerial Taskforce on Maternal Health* 9).

The PPTCT program run by CHS Mendi through the Epeanda goes a long way to fulfilling these characteristics.

Staff running the PPTCT program tell how they have MDG 5 and MDG 6 in mind when doing annual performance reviews based on the National Health Plan 2011–2020. Key Result Area 5 of that plan is to improve maternal health, with objective 5.2 being "increase the capacity of the health sector to provide safe and supervised deliveries." Health workers say that numbers and percentages do not mean a great deal to them; rather, human behaviour, such as women coming for antenatal clinics or delivering in a health facility, means a lot. Health workers do all they can to encourage such practices and to provide safe deliveries and, in this way, contribute to implementing MDG 5.

Aside from interventions specifically for HIV infected mothers, such as ART treatment, other aspects of the Mendi program—in-service training for staff, education programs for mothers, access to facilities, adequate supply of functioning equipment and necessary medicines—which have worked through CHS Mendi, could be made more widely available with sufficient political and managerial resolve. Increased funding would surely help. Papua New Guinea spends 0.6 percent of GDP on health expenditure, compared to 4.1 percent in Fiji and 8.8 percent in Australia (*Ministerial Taskforce on Maternal Health* 25). In fact, the PNG government funding on health decreased 9.4 percent in real terms between 1997 and 2004 (*Ministerial Taskforce on Maternal Health* xii).

A 2011 report recommends the establishment of family and community health care (FCC) with village health volunteers (VHVs) (Byrne and Morgan). Village birth attendants were being trained and were working in the SHP in the 1980s but this stopped in 1989 during a tribal fight in Nipa (Townsend; Alto et al.). This program, begun by the Tiliba Mission, was taken over by the government but has not resumed in the years since 1989. If the government were to restart the program, it would be wise for the National Department of Health to learn why the VHV program stopped and the PPTCT program continues.

The most important lesson from the CHS Mendi program is the culture of care that continues to sustain the program. It is hard to imagine how any program can function effectively without it. The culture of care obviously applies to dedicated and long-serving health workers and mentor mothers. One HIV infected mother noted, with a tone of admiration, *marasin ol i save holim long han na givim mipela* [they give us the medicine (personally) with their (bare) hands]. As Sister Gaudentia notes, "if a mother has a good experience the news spreads and she will tell the other mothers, that 'we have to go'" (Meier, Personal interview). However, as noted by the health workers, the culture of care also applies to the mothers themselves. Forty-five years ago, the mothers at Det were concerned enough to break with cultural tradition to deliver their babies at the mission aid post because they considered it safer for themselves and their child. Now, mothers who discover they are infected with HIV and, thus, are faced with the prospect of a grave threat to their child respond by making their own health care and the health care of their child a priority. Apart from finance, facilities, and political will, the development of a culture of care with all health workers and those who assist them will go a long way towards implementing MDG 5 and to reducing maternal mortality in Papua New Guinea.

ENDNOTES

[1] The six health centres are at Det, Wiliame, Tamenda, Yepi, Purani and Hiwanda. The seven aid posts are at Karanda, Mapenda,

Kema, Waip, Tiri, Tugiri/Lake Kopiago and Topani.

[2] Bryant Allen recorded the following description of village birthing:

> We had children by ourselves, and we cleaned and cared for them after the birth.... In childbirth, we got on our knees and hands to have the baby. The other women made magic for me. We fasted before birth. We had the child by ourselves in a small house. Nobody else stayed with us. Other women who had had babies told us what to expect and how to have the baby. Some women died. One every now and again. We stayed in the small house for eight days. Other women brought food only. We were afraid of the new child in those days. Those that died, died because the child became stuck inside them. We had our babies using our own strength and if we were not strong enough we died. (Allen, Personal interview)

[3] Sister Gaudentia refutes the account by Leanne Merrett-Balkos of a protest in 1970 over placentas taken from mothers, with the compromise of them being given a few inches of umbilical cord (Merrett-Balkos). Sister Gaudentia, who was there at the time, says that a problem arose from mothers rubbing ground on the umbilical cord stump with the intention of having it dry and detach more quickly. She discouraged that practice after one baby developed tetanus and encouraged the mothers to wait three or four days for the umbilical cord to detach naturally before they took the child home.

[4] Sister Gaudentia gives an example of the challenges some women face:

> I identified a woman who was to have twins—her first babies. She said, "I have so many pigs I have to look after." One afternoon, a truck comes and that woman comes off from the truck holding a baby. And I said, "why did you not come early?" And she laughed, and said, "one is still inside." She told me that as soon as the pain started she began to walk and she must have walked about three hours. And then her pain got so strong, she went into the bush and somebody helped her to deliver the first baby and then the other didn't come. So still connected with the chord she got to the road and stopped a truck and they brought

> *her here. So then, we delivered the next baby—the other twin.* (Meier, Personal interview)

[5] HIV was first detected in Papua New Guinea in 1987 (UNGASS, *Country Progress Report 2008* 17).

[6] In 2001, a massive tribal fight erupted in Mendi. In one month, there were seventeen cases of rape. Concerned about HIV infection for the rape victims, Sr Gaudentia tried to send blood serum to Mt. Hagen for testing but bandits on the road stole it, and she had to try to follow up and get the blood samples all over again.

[7] The name means "good house." There are seven positions at the Epeanda clinic. One position is paid by the government. The other positions are supported through the National Catholic HIV and AIDS office.

[8] The "friends" gathering is shown in the film directed by Philip Gibbs, "World AIDS Day in Mendi 2010."

[9] A study in Zambia showed that rates of maternal mortality increased eightfold over the past two decades, despite better obstetric services. Indirect causes of maternal mortality were responsible for 58 per cent of deaths, with malaria and AIDS-related tuberculosis the most common of these. In the Rakai district of Uganda, maternal mortality was five times higher in HIV-positive women than in HIV-negative women, reaching rates of over 1,600 per 100,000 live births in the infected group. In Malawi and Zimbabwe, pregnancy-related mortality has increased 1.9 and 2.5 times in parallel with the increasing AIDS epidemic (McIntyre).

[10] The record of numbers tested in 2013 is lower because testing at the Mendi town clinic was done by staff from the Clinton Foundation during part of that year.

[11] According to the Health Department records, in Mendi, four women (0.2 percent) of those tested in 2012 were confirmed seropositive. I note the difference between the Health Department records and those records from the Epeanda clinic in Table 1 above. Sister Gaudentia estimates that, at clinics offering testing, after pretest awareness talks, 90 percent of mothers agree to be tested for HIV (Meier, Personal interview).

[12] Catholic Health Services Mendi runs between four and six outreach clinics each quarter to rural areas.

[13] Of these mothers, six are returning to give birth to a second child,

and one is returning to give birth to her third child supervised through the PPTCT program.

[14] The result is similar to that from Mingende Rural Hospital run by CHS Kundiawa (Prasanna).

[15] Subsequently, three babies died, two from pneumonia and one due to gross deformity (hydrocephalic and downs syndrome).

[16] The Revival Church convinces people to stop taking medication and to rely solely on faith for their continued health. Unfortunately, many HIV-infected people die after trying to follow this policy.

[17] Letters were given to all participants to protect their identity.

WORKS CITED

Allen, Bryant. Personal interview. 29 June 2014.

Alto, William A., Ruth E. Albu, and Garabinu Iraho. "An Alternative to Unattended Delivery. A Training Program for Village Midwives in Papua New Guinea." *Social Science and Medicine*. 35.5 (1991): 613-618. Print.

Byrne, Abbey and Chris Morgan. *Improving Maternal, Newborn and Child health in Papua New Guinea through Family and Community Health Care. Compass Women's and Children's Health Knowledge Hub.* Australian Agency for International Development, Oct. 2011. Web. June 2014.

Gathigah, Miriam. "Maternal Deaths Due to HIV a Grim Reality." *ipsnews.net*. Inter Press Service News Agency, n.d. Web. June 2014.

Gibbs, Philip. "World AIDS Day in Mendi 2010." *Vimeo*. Vimeo, 9 Aug 2010. Web. June 2014.

Gibbs, Philip. "Engendered Violence and Witch-killing in Simbu." *Engendering Violence in Papua New Guinea*. Eds. Margaret Jolly, Christine Stewart, Carolyn Brewer. Canberra: Australian National University E-Press, 2012. 107-136. Print.

Meier, Gaudentia. Personal interview. May 2014.

Merrett-Balkos, Leanne. "Just Add Water: Remaking Women Through Childbirth, Anganen, Southern Highlands, Papua New Guinea." *Maternities and Modernities: Colonial and Postcolonial Experiences in Asia and the Pacific*. Eds. Kaipana Ram and Margaret Jolly. Cambridge: Cambridge University Press, 1998. 213-238. Print.

McIntyre, James. "Mothers Infected with HIV." *British Medical Bulletin* 67 (2003): 127-135. Web. June 2014.

Mola, Glen and Barry Kirby. "Discrepancies between National Maternal Mortality Data and International Estimates: the Papua New Guinea Experience." *Reproductive Health Matters* 21.42 (2013): 191-202. Web. June 2014.

National AIDS Council Secretariat. *Global AIDS Report 2012. Country Progress Report, Papua New Guinea.* UNAIDS. United Nations, 2012. Web. June 2014.

Papua New Guinea. National Department of Health. *Ministerial Taskforce on Maternal Health in Papua New Guinea.* Port Moresby: National Department of Health, 2009. Print.

Papua New Guinea. Department of Health. *National Health Plan 2011–2020 Volume I Policies and Strategies. WHO Representative Office Papua New Guinea.* World Health Organization, June 2010 Web. June 2014.

Papua New Guinea. National Department of Health STI, HIV and AIDS Surveillance Unit. *The 2009 STI, HIV and AIDS Annual Surveillance Report. East-West Centre: Communicating with Policymakers about Population and Health.* N.p., 2012. Web. June 2014.

Papua New Guinea. National Statistics Office. *Papua New Guinea Demographic and Health Survey 2006.* Port Moresby: National Statistics Office, 2009. Print.

Prasanna Sumithra. *Together We Can: The Success of the Mingende Practice Model for Preventing Parent-to-Child Transmission of HIV in Papua New Guinea.* Geneva: UNICEF, 2011.Print.

Townsend, Patricia K. *Traditional Birth Attendants in Papua New Guinea: An Interim Report.* Port Moresby: Papua New Guinea Institute of Applied Social and Economic Research, 1986. Print.

UNAIDS. *Report on the Global AIDS Epidemic.* UNAIDS. United Nations, 2013. Web. June 2014.

United Nations General Assembly Special Session (UNGASS). *Country Progress Report: Papua New Guinea.* Port Moresby: PNG National AIDS Council Secretariat and Partners, 2008. Print

United Nations General Assembly Special Session (UNGASS). *Country Progress Report. Papua New Guinea.* Port Moresby:

PNG National AIDS Council Secretariat and Partners, 2010. Print.
World Health Organization (WHO). "Mother-to-Child Transmission of HIV." WHO, n.d. Web. June 2014.

3.
Faith, Hope, and Charity

Barriers to Condom Use Among Women and Girls in Southern Malawi

NICOLE C. HAYES

UNITED NATIONS (UN) MILLENNIUM DEVELOPMENT Goal (MDG) 5 aims to improve women's maternal health by reducing maternal mortality rates, as they stood in 1990, by three quarters and by ensuring universal access to reproductive health by 2015. The UN identifies access to contraceptives as an important component of this overarching goal. Dissemination of one of the cheapest and most widely available forms of contraception, the condom, is critical across sub-Saharan Africa because condoms are one of the most effective ways of reducing HIV transmission during sexual intercourse. Nevertheless, condom use throughout sub-Saharan Africa is low and inconsistent, despite constant promotion of condoms through AIDS education programs. Studies have shown that across the continent, women face more barriers to condom use than men (Benefo; Prata et al; Sinding; Schoepf; Zellner). In this chapter, I examine some of the reasons behind the unpopularity of condoms in Malawi, with a particular focus on obstacles faced by women and girls in acquiring and using condoms. First, I consider the moral crisis created by a recent perceived rise in "promiscuity," particularly among women who engage in transactional sex, leading to the stigmatization of condoms by the population at large and faith groups in particular. Second, I examine how gender roles in Malawi encourage women's sexual submissiveness and make it difficult for girls and women to negotiate safer sex with their partners. This is compounded by the fact that condoms are also contraceptives, and fertility is a key component of adult status among women. Third, I explore widespread mistrust of initiatives promoted by the government and the international donor community, including condom promotion. This mistrust has led to a flourishing body of conspiracy theories regarding the perceived fallibility and even danger of using condoms. Unfortunately, barriers to condom use are reinforced by the efforts of non-governmental organizations (NGOs) to market condoms in Malawi, as social marketing campaigns persistently link condoms with sex work and foreign sexual practices. The majority of girls and women in Malawi, therefore, find it extremely difficult to access or use condoms, which has obvious negative implications for their ability to prevent HIV and to control fertility, both key components of their overall reproductive health.

CONTEXT

Research on condom use in sub-Saharan Africa has repeatedly shown that usage is both uncommon and inconsistent. In Zambia, although condom sales have clearly increased, they remain unpopular. According to a Zambian survey on sexual behaviour, condoms were only used in 32 percent of reported relationships, and they were used consistently in only eight percent of relationships. At the same time, more than two-thirds negatively evaluated condoms as promoting promiscuity, and over half of respondents reported barriers to accessing them (Benefo 23). Similar results were obtained across the continent in Côte d'Ivoire, where only 23 percent of men and 7 percent of women admitted to ever using a condom. These low figures were obtained despite the fact that 92 percent of men and 80 percent of women mentioned at least one sexual mode of transmission when asked how HIV was acquired (Zellner 41). As was the case among Zambians, Ivoirians associated condoms with infidelity and, therefore, avoided them for psychological reasons. A similar profile of condom use prevails in Malawi. According to a sample of 3,386 people in three districts, only 22 percent of those interviewed had used a condom with any of their last three sexual partners, and only 1 percent of respondents reported consistent condom use (Doskoch 207).

There is no consistent evidence to suggest that condom use is increased by knowledge of AIDS, including personal knowledge of someone who has died of AIDS (Zellner 42; Kayiki and Forste 58). Although Kofi Benefo's (24) multilevel analysis of the determinants of condom use in Zambia concluded that condom use went up with increased exposure to HIV and AIDS education and knowledge that condoms prevent HIV, Sara Zellner's (45) study of condom use in Côte d'Ivoire found only a slight association between knowledge of AIDS and condom use. Also, on the positive side, a comparison study of data from Zambia, Kenya, and Uganda showed that knowing someone with AIDS and having correct knowledge about AIDS were both associated with adopting safer sex practices (Prata et al. 192). On the other hand, a survey of fifteen hundred Rwandan women revealed that although the vast majority had correct knowledge about HIV and AIDS, only a very small number had adopted protective sexual behaviour within the past year. And in Tanzania, university students who were aware that condoms prevent HIV were actually *less* likely to use them. In Ethiopia, a study of factory workers with high rates of HIV prevalence showed high risk sexual behaviour and low rates of condom use, despite the fact that the majority of those interviewed cited condoms as the best way of preventing HIV (Prata et al.v193).

Barriers to condom use are also gendered. Note the consistent discrepancies between reported male and female condom use in the studies cited above. In many sub-Saharan African contexts, men make decisions related to sex, and women are expected to ask male partners' permission to use contraceptives, which would naturally include condoms (Zellner 41). Therefore, even when a woman is aware of how to protect herself from HIV, she may not be able to do so if she cannot gain the approval of her partner. Women who exchange sex for access to cash or commodities may also find that they are not in a position to insist on condom use. The resources of poor, single women are often so limited that they are not able to avoid these types of encounters (Schoepf 374). Increasingly, however, being married is seen as a risk factor for AIDS among women. Health care workers in sub-Saharan Africa report that "married, monogamous women are highly vulnerable to HIV infection due to their lack of rights within marriage, difficulties negotiating safer sex, extended partner absence and domestic violence" (Sinding 38). In fact, the majority of recently HIV positive women in sub-Saharan

Africa contracted the virus from their husbands. In Rwanda, for instance, 25 percent of HIV positive women interviewed reported having only one sexual partner ever (Sinding 38). This situation is not unique to sub-Saharan Africa. In this volume, Sarah Smith notes marriage is also the greatest source of vulnerability to sexually transmitted infections (STIs) in Chuuk, Micronesia (for Papua New Guinea, see also Hammar; McPherson). Yet married women are not typically the target of condom social marketing. Instead, they are encouraged by AIDS educators to remain strictly faithful. The problem is that "emphasis on fidelity often means *women's* fidelity and falsely reassures faithful women that they are not at risk [emphasis in the original]" (Schoepf 374). The unpopularity of condoms in sub-Saharan Africa, and their association with promiscuity and sex work is very troubling.

METHODS

Malawi is a small county in sub-Saharan Africa sharing a border with its much larger neighbours, Zambia, Mozambique, and Tanzania. This paper focuses on Malawi's Southern Region. The majority of my research is based in Blantyre and Chiradzulu Districts at the western edge of the Shire highlands, an area known for population pressure, soil erosion, land degradation, and deforestation. Another notable feature of this part of Malawi is that it is both matrilineal and matrilocal: descent is traced through women, and couples are expected to live in the wife's village after marriage (although this latter expectation is changing). This area is also recognized within Malawi for the highest rates of HIV infection. Recent studies estimate more than 17 percent of women and 11 percent of men are HIV positive in the Southern Region. Among the Lomwe and Yao ethnic groups with whom I principally worked, rates are 17 and 13 percent respectively (NSO and ICF Macro 198).

This chapter is based on eighteen months of participant observation, focus groups, and interviews.[1] The first period of research occurred in 2000 and 2001 when I was acting as Human Rights Education Officer in the Canadian International Development Agency Youth Internship program. During this eight month placement, I conducted focus groups on gender roles and human rights among secondary school students in Blantyre, Chiradzulu, Mangochi, and Zomba Districts. The second stint was my dissertation fieldwork conducted in 2006 and 2007. This fieldwork was roughly divided into two phases. Throughout the first phase, I maintained a base in the home of a village headman in rural Chiradzulu District, where I interviewed extensively. While in Chiradzulu, I taught several days a week at the Catholic University of Malawi, where I also interviewed among the student body and maintained another home with a family of teachers. During the second phase, I relocated to urban Blantyre District to conduct interviews among the employees of NGOs doing work on HIV and AIDS. However, I travelled back to rural Chiradzulu several days a week for follow up interviews and focus groups. In my interviews and focus groups, I obtained relationship histories and asked about sexual behaviour in Malawi, including condom use, abstinence, and fidelity. I also asked about attitudes towards AIDS and AIDS social marketing campaigns. I conducted interviews and focus groups in English among university students and NGO workers and in the villages, I used Chichewa, except where individuals asked to speak English. For my rural research I employed three research assistants, two men and a woman, from the local community who also acted as translators when needed.

FAITH

Transactional Sex

Despite recent strides in reducing the rate of maternal and under-five mortality in response to the Millennium Development Goals as well as seeing a substantial increase in overall life expectancy to 55 years, Malawi is still one of the poorest countries in the world ("Data: Malawi"). The United Nations Development Programme's Human Development Index places Malawi 174th on a list of 187 countries. It should not be surprising that poor socioeconomic indicators in Malawi have affected sexual relationships between women and men by increasing opportunities for transactional sex. Transactional sex is generally conceived of as sex that occurs outside of marriage, often involving multiple concurrent partners, in which money or commodities are exchanged for sex (Hunter

100). It is, however, unlike prostitution because the individuals involved consider one another as "boyfriends" or "girlfriends" rather than as sex workers and clients.

Although the overt mingling of sex and money is considered immoral by most North Americans and Europeans, this is not the case everywhere. Certainly, there is ample evidence to suggest that money and affection are linked in a number of quite different cultures (Bloch; Mills and Ssewakiryanga; Sobo, "One Blood"; Van den Borne). Despite the fact that money *can* be linked to sexual behaviour in morally neutral ways, linkages between the two have been accelerated and altered by the neoliberal principles associated with rapid economic globalization. In developing economies such as Malawi, neoliberalism has typically worn the face of structural adjustment programs and conditional loans implemented by International Financial Institutions (IFIs) such as the World Bank or the International Monetary Fund (IMF). I will go into further detail about Malawi's relationship with IFIs below, but it is necessary to state here that one unanticipated result of these types of loan has been an increasing gap between rich and poor in adjusting countries (Altman 22). For instance, by 2001, after two decades of "successful" structural adjustment, Malawi's levels of income inequality were the third most extreme in the world (Harrigan 315). Such income disparities, which are frequently gendered, have opened the door for new kinds of connections between sex and money.

Moral Crisis

A perceived increase in "promiscuity" and transactional sex, particularly among youth, is widely discussed in southern Malawi, and most people feel that this seismic shift in the Malawian sexual landscape has been a very recent occurrence. When I asked my informants whether they thought sexual behaviour had changed within the last one hundred years, most of them were derisive of my deliberately naïve time scale and gave answers similar to that of Gertrude, a program officer for a church-based NGO in Blantyre, who replied: "Don't even talk of one hundred years! Or even fifteen! It has tremendously changed." Perception of a rapid shift in Malawian sexual mores, particularly among young people, has created a kind of a moral crisis in Malawi in which elders increasingly denounce youth for "promiscuous" behaviour, whereas youth judge each other and readily accuse young women of being *mahule* (singular, *hule*) or "prostitutes."

Intergenerational tensions focused on "sexuality, specifically sexual misdemeanors and the sexual irresponsibility of young adults" in Malawi have also been observed by sociologist Amy Kaler ("Many Divorces" 533). She notes that elders characterized youthful sexual encounters as indiscriminate and increasingly transactional in nature and blamed these developments on rapid modernization.[2] A similar moral panic focused on perceived increase in transactional sex is explored by James Pfeiffer in neighbouring Mozambique. Although the Mozambican economy has grown considerably since the end of the civil war in 1992, the improved GDP masks rising levels of income disparity. The end of the decades-long civil war was characterized by a rapid roll out of massive development project loans, similar to what happened in Malawi after the implementation of multiparty democracy in 1994. In Mozambique, one of the unintended consequences of economic transition and adjustment was a rapid "commoditization of social life" (Pfeiffer 86). The sudden demand for cash among the poor majority undermined previous social obligations and safety nets. Predictably, a heightened demand for cash in an environment of increasing income inequality led to a rise in transactional sex. Pfeiffer describes an "ensuing moral panic" focused on sexual behaviour and characterized by frequent accusations of adultery (87). It was in the midst of this toxic atmosphere of economic disparity, increased sex work, and lack of trust that condoms as a method of preventing HIV were introduced to Mozambique, leading to widespread suspicion and disapproval.

The situation in Malawi was disturbingly similar. In Malawi, condoms very early developed such a bad reputation that most women and many men have not wanted to be associated with them. Population policy had never been high on Malawi's agenda, and it was not until the early 1990s that a fairly low-key family planning initiative was introduced, in which condoms were offered as one of several contraceptive alternatives. The introduction of condoms unfortunately coincided with the first official recognition of the AIDS epidemic within the borders of Malawi (Kaler, "The Moral

Lens " 110). The timing could not have been worse. According to Kaler (112), "Because of the temporal association of the first large-scale condom promotion in Malawi with the emergence of AIDS there, condoms are virtually synonymous with sexually transmitted diseases, despite efforts of family planning associations to position them as alternative contraceptive methods" (112). So unfamiliar were Malawians with condoms prior to the days of HIV and AIDS that many no longer recall that condoms were first introduced as a family planning method.

When I spoke with George Macheka—director of Banja la Mtsogolo [Family of the Future], one of Malawi's premier family planning NGOs and also a distributor of the Manyuchi condom—he was not aware that condoms were available as a family planning method prior to the advent of HIV and AIDS. He first encountered condoms in the early 1990s when Population Services International (PSI) marketed their Chishango condoms as a method of HIV prevention. This campaign primarily targeted sex workers, a marketing decision with disastrous and lasting consequences. For this reason, according to Mr. Macheka and several others with whom I spoke, Malawians associate condoms with prostitution. Certainly this was the impression I received when I talked about condom use with my research participants. When I asked Agnes Zalimba, a thirty-five-year-old woman living in rural Chiradzulu, about condoms, she informed me that very few women are brave enough to ask a man to use a condom because people say that a woman who uses condoms is a *hule* or a "prostitute." Similarly, Christine, a radio DJ, told me that although it is "everyone's responsibility to have condoms," people say that a woman who has condoms must be "promiscuous." Young people in particular were clear that a girl or young woman who insists that her partner use a condom probably has more than one partner.

Religion

Given the moral crisis surrounding infidelity and the association of condoms with promiscuity, it should not be surprising that in Malawi, many religious leaders oppose or at least do not support condom use. Both times I was in Malawi, I attended church services frequently, both in English and Chichewa. I attended church services in two different denominations: Presbyterian and Catholic.[3] A sizable portion of the sermons that I attended dwelt heavily on themes of sin, especially with reference to AIDS. Congregants were exhorted to stop promiscuous behaviour, to be faithful to their partners, and to abstain from sex before marriage. The underlying message was that the AIDS epidemic was a direct consequence of sinful behaviour. I did not hear any religious leaders encouraging condom use in any of the public sermons that I attended and by my calculations, I attended over forty church services in five different congregations over the course of eighteen months of fieldwork. My impressions are borne out by the findings of the 2004 Malawi Religion Project, which interviewed the religious leaders of 187 congregations (Doskoch 207). Of the religious leaders interviewed, eighty-eight percent said they frequently preached on topics of morality, 73 percent said they frequently discussed sexual morality in their sermons, and 72 percent said they frequently gave sermons touching on AIDS. In their private lives, 95 percent enjoined congregants to avoid promiscuity, but only 27 percent said they encouraged congregants to use condoms (Doskoch). The relatively small number of religious leaders who promoted condoms is due to the close association between AIDS, condoms, and promiscuity, which is characterized as a sin. Of course, in the case of Catholicism, condom use is explicitly forbidden by church doctrine.

In his illuminating study of the conflict between condom social marketing and Pentecostal and African Independent Churches (AICs) in neighbouring Mozambique, James Pfeiffer noted similar trends. In Mozambique, as elsewhere in sub-Saharan Africa, including Malawi, Zionist AICs and Pentecostalism have recently gained large followings. The movement away from traditional mission Christianity to Pentecostalism has almost entirely overlapped the period of the AIDS epidemic and subsequent widespread condom social marketing campaigns throughout sub-Saharan Africa. Pfeiffer found that Pentecostal churches and AICs were very good at addressing the "moral panic" about "promiscuous" behaviour and HIV infection (79). Zionist churches in Mozambique overwhelmingly oppose condom use, which they associate with promiscuity. Pastors and congregants of these churches were deeply offended by the efforts of PSI to market condoms using slogans and images which were perceived by the general population as encouraging licentious behaviour (Pfeiffer 79).

In her work on condom discourse in Malawi, Amy Kaler ("The Moral Lens") analyzed the informal journals of six trained Malawian research assistants who were asked to record everything that they heard people say about AIDS over the course of a five-year period. She noted that "condoms were overwhelmingly described in disparaging tones" (108). Religious objections to condoms were the second most common type of negative condom discourse after complaints about technical failure (108). This is significant because the data are based on journals kept by research assistants in Balaka, a district with a relatively high percentage of Muslim residents. In Malawi, the Muslim faith has proved less resistant to condom use than most Christian denominations. So even in a district with a higher than average number of Muslims, condoms are still seen to be objectionable from a moral and religious standpoint.

Women in Malawi, therefore, face a variety of moral and religious barriers to condom use. Although it is true that men face similar barriers, the threat posed by condoms to a woman's reputation is much greater. Men and women whom I interviewed objected more or less equally to condom use, but I never heard of a man being referred to as a "prostitute" simply for being found in possession of condoms. The potential damage that known condom use can do to a woman's reputation will be discussed in greater detail below.

HOPE

Gender Roles

For most rural southern Malawians, an important source of information about gender roles is pre-puberty initiation ceremonies, which are segregated by gender. These ceremonies have a long history of promoting sexual intercourse as life-affirming behaviour (Phiri 268). In fact, according to traditional notions of sexuality, completely abstaining from sex is unnatural and unhealthy, and desire for sex is likened to desire for food and drink (Morris, *Animals and Ancestors* 70). Initiation ceremonies, therefore, generally celebrate sex within the context of marriage, especially in girls' initiations (Fiedler). Sex positive messages appear to be less context dependent in boys' initiations (Bonongwe). A key element of girls' initiation ceremonies is to provide instruction on sexually pleasing future husbands (Fiedler; Kalalo 84; Morris, *Animals and Ancestors* 94). Girls are also warned that sex is part of marriage, and they, therefore, should not refuse to have sex, even when they are ill or tired (Kalalo 84). Messages of respect and obedience to elders and men, particularly husbands, are driven home in psychologically distressing and sometimes physically painful dramas involving masked dancers (animated by men) and simulated injury and death (Fiedler 37; Minton 78; Morris, *Animals and Ancestors* 101). Boys' initiations are similarly sex positive but less focused on sexual instruction *per se*. In these initiations, boys are tutored in traditionally male activities and offered moral instruction that focuses on respecting elders and becoming an adult member of the community (Bonongwe; Morris, *Animals and Ancestors* 120; Stannus and Davey). Crucially, boy initiands make the costumes used by the masked dancers to frighten and torment the girls in *their* initiations (Morris, *Animals and Ancestors* 128).

As conveyed through initiation ceremonies, then, Malawian gender roles encourage socially sanctioned sexual activity while undermining women's sexual autonomy. They also promote the idea that the husband is the head of the family. This may strike some as surprising given that the vast majority of southern Malawians are matrilineal. One would expect to see a situation in which women enjoy a reasonable amount of autonomy, and maternal uncles rather than husbands are regarded as the head of the family. Some historical background is, therefore, necessary. Prior to colonization late in the nineteenth century, it seems that, in general, women did hold considerable ritual and political power. Malawian historian Elias Mandala writes that the earliest accounts of this region suggest that prior to the ravages of the slave trade and subsequent colonization, age rather than gender was the best indicator of social rank (25).

Although there are economic causes for women's loss of status, here I would like to further explore the influence of Christianity on sexual behaviour and gender roles. The first Malawian mission was established by the Scottish Presbyterians in 1876, quickly followed by the Dutch Reformed Church in 1889, the Anglicans in 1895, and the Catholics in 1901. By the 1920s, the country had essentially been divided up by these four pioneering groups (Morris, *The Power of Animals* 44). Missionaries did not approve of male or female initiations, the power of maternal uncles or, indeed, matriliny itself (Mair 107; Morris, *The Power of Animals* 44). From a missionary perspective, matrilineal institutions were un-Christian, so the churches set about undermining them in every way they could: banning initiations among congregation members, emphasizing conjugal bonds over solidarity between siblings, and preaching the authority of the father over that of the matrilineage (Morris, *The Power of Animals* 44; Phiri 268).

Although the opposition of Christian missionaries did not succeed in eradicating matrilineal institutions, their teachings certainly had an influence (Morris, *The Power of Animals* 44). At first, missionaries faced an uphill battle. Missionaries' attempts to convince families to send boys to mission schools ran counter to the participation of youth in initiation rites prior to marriage, and they incurred the steady resistance of powerful matrilineage elders (Phiri 268). It was not until the 1920s that some missionaries grasped the potential of initiations as a teaching tool (268). This realization was followed by attempts to co-opt the rituals by offering Christianized versions in which missionaries emphasized the Pauline view that the husband, not the wife or her uncle, is the head of the family.

The effects of Christian initiations on matrilineal institutions have continued to the present day because of their lasting popularity as either an alternative or an adjunct to traditional initiation ceremonies. In fact, research suggests that there is now little to choose between the two different types of initiation in contemporary Malawi, except that Christian initiations do not encourage initiates to have ritual sex at the conclusion of the rite (Fiedler; Minton; Morris, *Animals and Ancestors*). Despite missionaries' early objections to the erotic overtones of traditional initiations, contemporary church-sponsored initiations graphically emphasize that it is a woman's duty to please her husband sexually (Fiedler 34). Many of the songs and dramas incorporated in Christian initiations are also used in traditional initiation ceremonies, and they teach girls that they should be submissive to their husbands, they should neither refuse nor request sex, and they should not ask for too many material goods or too much money (Fiedler 37; Minton 78). As no accounts of girls' initiations exist prior to the introduction of Christian initiation ceremonies, it is difficult to say how much the Christian initiations affected traditional rites. However, given the very un-matrilineal emphasis on the husband as head of family in *both* types of contemporary initiation, it is fair to say that the influence has most likely been substantial. One result has been the emergence of a kinship system similar to the one described by Smith in this volume: contemporary Malawi is at once matrilineal and patriarchal. Some of the effects of Christian activities on gender hierarchies in a patrilineal society are described by Stephanie Hobbis in her article about maternal health in the Solomon Islands, also in this volume.

Contraceptives

In an atmosphere in which sex is highly valued but women are told to subordinate their desires to those of men, the marketing of condoms to women has proved problematic because women have limited ability to negotiate sexual encounters. Moreover, people are aware that, in addition to preventing HIV transmission, condoms also prevent pregnancy. Although this is a desirable outcome for many people at least some of the time, it is not a desirable outcome for everyone all or even most of the time. Fertility is highly valued by most Malawians and is linked to full adult status, particularly for women. According to my informants, a single Malawian career girl without children, be she only in her early twenties, often finds herself an object of derision for insolent youth:

> *When a girl hits twenty or twenty-one, she's a big person here in Malawi. And now she receives words of mockery frequently ... like sometimes they use Chichewa words* amayi kwa wiyalesi. *That means "mother of radio." Maybe a girl has a radio in her home, in her house, but she's a little bit old to get married, maybe. She has been late a little bit. So they mock her, saying, "Mother of radio, mother of pots, doesn't have children."*

The single career woman is reminded that although she may have a decent job that has allowed her to purchase desirable goods for herself, she is not a real woman because she is not a mother. It is preferable that a woman marry before she starts having children, but the stigma of childlessness is greater than the stigma of single parenthood. Similarly, men desire children as proof of their virility. I frequently heard stories of men beating their wives upon discovering that they were secretly taking birth control pills or receiving injections to prevent or delay pregnancy.

Pleasure

When one takes into account the strong emphasis on male sexual pleasure in initiation rites, described above, widespread resistance to condom use is not surprising. When I queried informants' statements that condoms were not very popular in Malawi, people often responded humorously: "You don't eat a sweet in the wrapper." I heard this saying again and again, in English and Chichewa, until it became a background refrain to my interviews. As Laxton, the self-appointed spokesperson for a focus group of young people I spoke with in rural Chiradzulu, explained, "You don't feel sweet when you are doing that sex with a condom." I asked Laxton whether using a condom made sex feel bad, and he seemed puzzled and said, "No, it's not *bad*" but then he grinned knowingly and reiterated that sex *without* a condom felt *"very, very* sweet" [emphasis in original]. Additionally, I was told on a number of occasions that men did not enjoy having to stop their activities in order to put on a condom and found the pause annoying. In the heat of the moment, men reasoned that putting on a condom was a "waste" of time. Although the decision to use a condom is far more often in the hands of the man than the woman in Malawi, both men and women told me that they prefer "plain" sex, or sex without a condom. Men and women feel that sex is "sweeter" this way because it allows the man to express and the woman to truly feel his *mphamvu*, or "power."

Trust

Despite the moral crisis of perceived promiscuity and the very real incidence of infidelity and transactional sex, people informed me that one of the most important barriers to condom use among women is that they are expected to display trust in their partners. It is only through willingness to have unprotected sex with her partner that a woman demonstrates that she is also worthy of trust. Men are also subject to the need to preserve the fiction of trust, but this does not constrain their activities to the same degree. Martha, an employee in a peri-urban NGO working with AIDS education, explained to me that when a person asks his or her partner to use a condom it is taken to mean either that he or she does not trust the partner or that he or she has been unfaithful. Therefore, women are too "shy" to insist on condom use because they do not want to be accused of infidelity. As Smith (this volume) describes in Chuuk, asking a partner to use a condom is a shameful behaviour for women. Men do not worry about partners' adverse reactions to the same extent because women are instructed to be attentive to men's sexual needs and, therefore, typically accept a man's request to use a condom without comment. Men often use the association between condoms and infidelity to pressure their partners into forgoing condoms. According to Brown, a young actor:

> *If it is women, especially village women and girls, because of tradition, culture, most Malawians are generally more withdrawn, and the women will always not want to show that they know a lot about sexuality and sex issues. And so oftentimes they will not ask for a man to use a condom. In fact, some people would refuse to use a condom because by using a condom it's as if you are giving a message to each other that you are not faithful to each other. So people want to pretend, especially women that, they are alright, they are okay, they are [HIV] negative and they will go ahead without using a condom and will not ask the men ... for fear. Because the men will say [menacingly], "You think ... you are suggesting I use a condom? Is it ... maybe it is you that is [HIV] positive. Or do you think I'm positive?"*

As George Macheka, director of Banja la Mtsogolo, accurately but chillingly noted in his interview with me, the "principle of trust has really killed a lot of Malawians."[4]

Afraid of giving the impression that they are promiscuous and not wanting their partners to know that they do not trust them, women are reluctant to broach the topic of safer sex, and even when they do, they are easily overruled. In order to fulfill gender norms of sexual submissiveness and high fertility, then, women must simply hope that their partners take the initiative in remaining HIV negative.

CHARITY

Given that sexual encounters are typically engineered and controlled by men, women's feelings about condoms would probably not seriously affect rates of condom use if men themselves were interested in using them. Most are not, however, and not only because they feel that condoms negatively affect their sexual pleasure. Kaler ("The Moral Lens" 105) writes that Malawians are deeply suspicious of condoms because their dissemination is sponsored by the government and funded by the international donor community, the two groups most often blamed by locals for the introduction and spread of HIV. Many people suspect that HIV was invented by Western scientists and deliberately introduced to African nations to control population.

There are two different kinds of complaints about condoms that illustrate widespread suspicion of their efficacy and safety: complaints that condoms do not work properly and complaints that they are harmful to users. Technical objections to condoms vary, but all concern the various physical reasons that a condom might fail. Kaler ("The Moral Lens" 108) records people's fears or complaints of condoms breaking, slipping or having holes in them as examples of this theme. When I asked people if they had heard any stories about condoms, focus groups of young men and women, university students of both genders as well as married men and women had all heard that condoms can break or burst. In fact, male university students had heard that not only *can* condoms break but that they *usually* do break. I was also frequently told that condoms fall off and get lost inside the woman, causing infertility or even death.[5] Most people said that they heard that condoms have "tiny holes" in them or are "porous," meaning that although they may be effective at blocking a man's sperm from impregnating his partner, they cannot stop the spread of the microscopic human immunodeficiency virus. This particular complaint probably stems from deliberate misinformation to this effect spread by the Vatican in an attempt to dissuade people from condom use. Although the impermeability of condoms to both sperm and HIV has been conclusively proven by the World Health Organization, the International Planned Parenthood Federation and the U.S. National Institute of Health, this appears to be much less widely known than the earlier statements made by the Vatican (Sinding 39).

The other type of condom objection that I will outline in this section is more political than technical in nature. Concerns about the safety of condom use communicate people's deep suspicions of government and donor interventions. Suspicions of government and donor initiatives that affect fertility are also reported in the Marshall Islands by Nancy Pollock in this volume. In Malawi, these persistent rumors take several forms. Kaler ("The Moral Lens" 112-113) describes how her research assistants recorded conversations about people's fears that condom lubricants cause sores, infertility, cancer or HIV. When I was in Malawi several years after Kaler, only a few people spoke to me about the possibility of condoms transmitting HIV (although this was a common trope among the secondary school students I interviewed when I was in Malawi in 2000 and 2001). However, Malawian NGO workers who worked in AIDS prevention continued to encounter this belief. Perhaps my informants were too polite to tell me that they believed condoms were deliberately introduced by my compatriots to spread HIV, but Billy Mayaya, a long-time colleague of mine from my volunteer days, told me that these stories are still common: "I see it a lot. You know, people saying, 'Condoms are laced with some kind of virus.' Conspiracy theories, you know ... I think [people say that] it's like a conspiracy from the West to reduce the birth rate in Africa—a genocidal thing."

As with Kaler, I mainly heard that condom lubricants cause cancer, infertility, impotence, rashes, or sores. Fear of lubricants may also tie into the contemporary cultural preference for dry sex, a practice that involves women treating their vaginas with various substances to reduce secretions. Indeed, I was told by someone who worked for a manufacturer of condoms that marketing research had led the company to reduce the amount of lubricant on condoms sold in Malawi for precisely this reason. One common theory is that exposure to condom lubricant causes cancer. This rumor came up in focus groups among both young men and young women at Catholic University, and several students commented on it during individual interviews as well. Young men and women I spoke with in the rural areas were also familiar with this rumour, and I was informed that both men and women will refuse to use condoms on these grounds.

Mike Magola from the Youth Ambassadors Organization informed me that in the rural areas, it is also believed that condom lubricants cause infertility. This was a rumour I had often heard from secondary school students during focus groups in my first trip to Malawi. More frequently, I was informed that regular condom use can cause impotence or can affect a man's libido. Male students at Catholic University had heard that repeated use of condoms leads to a "loss of interest in sexual intercourse." Nor was this simply a rumour that boys repeated among themselves. First year student, Raphael Chitete informed me that when representatives of an NGO came to his secondary school to speak about HIV, they confirmed this rumour when students asked about it. Less seriously, many people claimed that condom lubricants cause men to develop penile sores. This rumour was also reported to me by secondary school students in 2000 and 2001, and it was repeated during more recent fieldwork by urbanized university students, rural villagers of all ages and both genders, and by NGO workers. When a rural youth group informed me that condoms caused sores, I asked them whether this was true or just a rumour, and they shouted back, *"Zoona!"* or "It's true!"[6]

Why are people so deeply suspicious of a government and NGO intervention ostensibly geared to the preservation of their health? People in Malawi have good reason for expressing serious misgivings about the intentions of their government, as there has been a long history of the government not having their best interests at heart. From independence in 1964 to the advent of multiparty democracy in 1994, Malawi was under the oppressive rule of self-declared President-for-life, Hastings Kamuzu Banda. In the

Banda days, censorship was draconian, and a country-wide dress code was in effect. Banda openly encouraged people to spy on their neighbours, and any dissent met with swift and brutal repression.

Banda's reign was ended by the suspension of donor aid in 1992, which triggered a referendum on multiparty democracy in 1993, followed by the first multiparty election in 1994. Banda's Malawi Congress Party (MCP) was defeated when Bakili Muluzi's United Democratic Front (UDF) won the election. The UDF also won the subsequent election in 1999, and Muluzi served as president of Malawi until 2004. Multiparty politics under Muluzi "quickly became an ever-changing mosaic of alliances and intrigues, often pursued by party leaders with woeful disregard for their electorate's opinions" (Englund 17). The cynicism of Malawi's newly elected officials was reflected in public attitudes toward the government. Realizing that former expectations of multiparty democracy had been overly optimistic, Malawians coined the phrase "multiparty, multi problems" to express their disenchantment with the new democratic system (van den Borne 35).

After attempting unsuccessfully to change the constitution in order to allow him to run for president a third time, Muluzi turned the UDF over to his handpicked successor, Bingu wa Mutharika. After winning the subsequent election, Mutharika lost no time in breaking with the UDF and forming his own party, the Democratic Progressive Party (DPP). Although conditions initially improved under Mutharika, the latter years of his second term in office were characterized by increasingly autocratic and, in some cases, bizarre behaviour, such as the expulsion of the British high commissioner for criticizing him, as well as highly publicized crackdowns on protestors, activists, human rights lawyers, and journalists. This turbulent period of Malawi's history ended abruptly with Mutharika's unexpected heart attack in early April, 2012. After two days of secrecy and confusion, his vice-president, long time women's rights activist Joyce Banda, was sworn in as president.[7]

Joyce Banda's succession to office was by no means assured. Mutharika had previously thrown her out of the party for refusing to endorse his brother, Peter Mutharika, as his successor. On Mutharika's death, while the Malawian cabinet sought a court order to stop her from becoming the new President, Joyce Banda enlisted the support of Malawi's army commander, who surrounded her house with troops as she was sworn in. Responses to her short tenure in office were mixed. International observers were pleased by her attempts to restore diplomatic ties with the United States and the European Union and by her capitulation to IMF demands that she devalue the Malawian kwacha by 33 percent against the U.S. dollar, something Mutharika had refused to do. However, Malawians were disgusted by the "Cashgate" scandal associated with her administration, in which a number of highly placed civil servants and politicians associated with Joyce Banda's government were suddenly found in possession of huge sums of cash. Additionally, it seemed that Banda herself had inexplicably acquired over USD 75,000. Many Malawians believe that Banda embezzled money obtained from the sale of the presidential jet and fleet of luxury cars, which was supposedly done as a cost-cutting measure. At the same time, thousands protested the inflation that followed her decision to devalue the kwacha. Joyce Banda and her People's Party were resoundingly defeated by Peter Mutharika, still leading the DPP, in the May 2014 elections. Although it is too early to say what lasting effects Peter Mutharika's government will have on Malawi, he has already drawn criticism from human rights observers for his failure to tackle critical economic issues and the fact that his public appointments have heightened regional and ethnic tensions.

People have equally good reason to question interventions promoted by the international donor community. When Malawi's economy collapsed in the wake of the 1979 oil crisis, Malawi became the first country in the Southern African Development Community (SADC) to adopt a structural adjustment program (SAP) through the World Bank (Englund, 17). Malawi implemented three SAPs and various sectoral loans throughout the 1980s, 1990s, and early 2000s through the World Bank as well as stabilization programs through the IMF (Chinsinga 30; Harrigan). These loans came with conditions similar to those of SAPs implemented elsewhere:

> liberalization of marketing of smallholder agricultural produce; liberalization of prices controlled by Ministry of Trade and Industry; introduction of increased user

charges for some social and departmental services; debt management; tax reform and [reform of] government expenditure; elimination of subsidy on smallholder fertilizer and flotation of the Malawian kwacha against other currencies. (WLSART 102-3)

In Malawi, the express goal of SAPs and other loans was to increase Malawi's balance of payments to donor institutions and stabilize the economy. It is now widely conceded that the loans not only failed to stabilize the Malawian economy but they also made things worse for the majority of Malawians (Chinsinga 30; Englund 17; Harrigan 315; WLSART 103). Almost all social indicators declined throughout the 1980s, 1990s, and into the 2000s. The resulting widespread malnutrition worsened AIDS and tuberculosis, and life expectancy dropped from 48 years to 40 years between 1990 and 1999 (Englund, 17). At the turn of the millennium, Malawi had some of the highest rates of infant, child, and maternal mortality in the world (Harrigan 315). Malawi's debt servicing burden more than doubled during this time while government cuts to social services disproportionately affected the poorest sectors of the population, particularly women and children (Chinsinga; Harrigan; WLSART). Although conditions have improved somewhat since then, Malawians remain extremely mistrustful of the motivations of the international donor community.

CONDOM SOCIAL MARKETING

Given that decisions about whether to use a condom are generally in men's rather than women's hands in Malawi, it is not surprising that condom promotion has shifted from targeting women (as sex workers) to targeting men. But even though women are no longer directly targeted by condom marketing in Malawi, their ability to use condoms is still hampered by the messages promoted by condom social marketers. Despite the long-lasting and negative consequences of the early marketing of condoms to sex workers, condom advertisements in Malawi continue to link condoms with promiscuity.

In Malawi, there are two main players involved in condom social marketing: Banja la Mtsogolo and PSI. During my research, Banja la Mtsogolo was responsible for large billboards in prominent urban locations advertising two somewhat racy lines of their Manyuchi condoms. One of these billboards featured an attractive woman in a red dress and sunglasses, holding back her long braided hair extensions. Her head was tilted to one side, and she smiled at the viewer, arms held back and chest thrust slightly forward. Below the photograph of the woman there were two lines of text, in English: "Manyuchi. Studded for extra pleasure." In North America, it is commonly understood that textured condoms are designed to enhance the pleasure of the partner of the condom user. This does not appear to be the case in Malawi. Everyone whom I spoke to about it was surprised to find out that (heteronormatively speaking) studded condoms were supposed to increase women's rather than men's sexual enjoyment. Moreover, the provocative dress of the woman, according to Malawian standards, as well as her direct gaze, suggested to the majority of people with whom I spoke that the woman featured in the billboard was a sex worker.

Their other line of condoms was advertised in a similar style of billboards, but I did not come across them until the end of my dissertation fieldwork. In these billboards, a woman wearing a tight fitting black dress with hair extensions piled on top of her head was posed over an English slogan promoting chocolate condoms. Now, it is possible that this marketing strategy was supposed to address widespread critiques that in addition to being highly suspicious, condom lubricants were also "smelly." Perhaps, also, the reference to chocolate was supposed to reinforce the semiotic link between sex and sweetness already exploited by the fact that Manyuchi means *honey* and is a slang term referring to sex in Chichewa. But to me, and I'm sure many others, the marketing of chocolate condoms connoted oral sex, a practice which is explicitly condemned in initiation ceremonies (Fiedler 69). I well recall that, while working as an intern in 2000, one day when the boss had left the room a group of young male colleagues questioned me closely on what they had heard of the Euro-American predilection for oral sex. Equally fascinated and horrified, they repeatedly asked me why a person would want to engage in such a practice and confidently asserted that no Malawian would ever consider doing something so "disgusting." Given that the Manyuchi condom billboards were located in an urban centre and made use of English rather than Chichewa slogans, it is likely that they were aimed at an educated urban audience—exactly the sort of people who a few years earlier had condemned oral sex to me as revolting.

PSI advertisements for their Chishango or, shield, condoms, were entirely different. Near the end of my fieldwork, I saw posters for PSI's new condom campaign. Both posters that I will describe here pictured a box of Chishango condoms in the corner. Formerly, the condoms were packaged in a box with a picture of a shield on the front. However, over the course of my fieldwork, PSI switched to new packaging that showcased the body of a scantily clad woman from chest to thigh. The anonymous woman was wearing a red brassiere or bikini top and a white sarong that left one of her thighs bare. Keep in mind that a dress code banning trousers and above-the-knee skirts for women was in effect in Malawi until 1994. As late as 2012, there were mass protests in Blantyre and Lilongwe due to a rash of incidents in which market vendors had stripped and beaten passing women for wearing trousers or miniskirts. Thigh-baring sarongs and bikini tops should therefore *not* be construed as normal attire for Malawian women.

The first poster depicted a middle-aged man locking the door of his red vehicle in the parking lot of a guesthouse. In the middle distance, many men and women were seated under a thatched pavilion. The man, with his laptop case and note books, was undoubtedly supposed to represent a travelling business man. Above this image ran the text: "*Kokalima sapita opanda khasu,*" which means "When you go to the gardens, do not go without your hoe." As the farmer should not forget his hoe when he goes to the gardens, so a man should not forget his condoms when he stays at a guesthouse. Guesthouses, which are like small motels, were synonymous with sex work when I was in Malawi.

The second poster displayed a broadly smiling man about to step out of a transport truck at a truck stop. He was looking down at a woman fashionably clad in tight jeans and a pink blouse. Shopping bag in her left hand, the woman pointed to a row of shops in the background. In the middle distance, a woman in a fitted blouse and trousers was talking to another man with his back to the camera against a backdrop of large trucks, a car, and the aforementioned shops. Above the image was the message: "*Ulendo ndi wautali.... Tengani katundu yense,*" which means, "The journey is long.... Bring all your luggage." That the woman greeting him was supposed to be a sex worker was indicated by both the location and the man's profession. Truck stops are notorious haunts for sex workers and truckers' predilection for sex workers is proverbial.

Both of these posters were troubling in that they portrayed respectable men without female companions who could reasonably be construed as wives. Yet the age of the men depicted in the posters makes it unlikely that they were supposed to be single. Widespread male infidelity was, thus, tacitly acknowledged and even condoned so long as condoms were used. The only women in these posters were sex workers. The Manyuchi billboards were also problematic due to their use of provocative, therefore not respectable, women and references to salacious foreign sexual preferences in order to sell condoms. Although these advertisements targeted men rather than women, they were in the public domain, communicating to one and all that the only women who use condoms are promiscuous, and that people who use condoms are more likely to engage in unusual sexual practices. Where women are fearful for their reputations and lacking in negotiating power and where the motivations of the powerful foreigners promoting condoms are treated as suspect, the semiotics of condom social marketing in Malawi are surprisingly insensitive.

One of the major obstacles standing in the way of achieving MDG 5 in Malawi is that women do not have universal access to reproductive health, which includes access to contraceptives such as condoms. As I have discussed in this chapter, women face many barriers to condom use. In Malawi, as elsewhere, condoms are critically important because when used correctly and consistently, not only are they a contraceptive but they also prevent transmission of HIV. As noted by Kathleen Barlow, Shauna LaTosky, and Philip Gibbs and Winnie William in this volume, HIV itself is an important aspect of a woman's reproductive health, particularly during pregnancy and parturition. Condom social marketing in Malawi predates the formation of the MDGs, and dissemination of condoms targets not only MDG 5 but also MDG 6, which is devoted to combatting HIV/AIDS, malaria, and other diseases. People who work in a development capacity in Malawi are well aware of the role condoms play in preventing AIDS and achieving the MDGs in Malawi. Unfortunately, their efforts to market condoms are not paying off as well as they would like and, in some cases, are actually reinforcing pre-existing barriers to condom use, particularly among women and girls. The government and the international donor community have much work to do to repair the trust of the Malawian people, and until this happens, it is unlikely that many initiatives promoted by either of these two groups will be fully accepted. In the meantime, NGOs and civil servants who work in AIDS prevention need to be more aware of the cultural context of condoms in Malawi, or they risk further alienation of the sector of the population that they often most wish to help: girls and women.

CONCLUSION

In Malawi, as elsewhere in sub-Saharan Africa, women face more barriers to condom use than men. The recent history of neoliberal economic adjustment and attendant economic disparities have increased connections between sex and money and have led to a moral panic focused on perceived promiscuity and transactional sex. The association between condoms and promiscuity, particularly but not exclusively among faith communities, makes it very difficult for women to access condoms without inviting negative assessments of their sexual probity. Additionally, Malawian gender roles have evolved to emphasize the need for women to be sexually submissive and attentive to men's needs. Women therefore lack negotiating power when it comes to safer sex, especially when men object to condoms on the grounds that they curtail male sexual pleasure. Finally, both women *and* men are highly suspicious of condoms because they are promoted by the government and the international donor community, institutions that many Malawians find highly suspect. The result is a complex network of rumours calling into question the efficacy and safety of condom use. Despite a legacy of early missteps when it came to condom social marketing in Malawi, NGOs in Malawi remain surprisingly insensitive to these nuances when it comes to promoting condoms, reinforcing beliefs that condoms encourage promiscuity. It is time to move beyond social marketing when it comes to tackling the MDGs in Malawi. The principles of rational free choice that social marketing is based on ignore the structural factors that prevent women, but also men, from using condoms consistently and effectively. Community participation in defining as well as addressing health risks is likely to lead to healthier communities than marketing strategies that exclude and stereotype women.

ENDNOTES

[1] In this chapter, I have adopted a mixed policy toward divulging the identities of my research participants. Prior to each interview or focus group, I asked all participants whether they wanted to be identified by name in any writing that might result from my research. A number of individuals with whom I spoke asked me to use their real names and where this is the case I give their names in full. Where I do not have a person's permission to use their name, I have assigned a pseudonym and do not offer a surname.
[2] Kaler ("Many Divorces" 544) traces complaints of sexual irresponsibility among youth back to the 1940s and 1950s. She argues that ongoing tropes of youthful disobedience indicate that the sexual morality of the past often appealed to by elders is actually an invented tradition. I have argued elsewhere that the elders of the 1940s and 1950s had legitimate grounds for their complaints, as an emerging cash economy, in which they had no role, increasingly sidelined them from the sexual decision making of young people. Although the conservative views of today's elders are not accorded much respect in the modern sexual economy, they are not entirely blameless in this behavioural shift (Hayes).
[3] My affiliation with these two denominations was largely serendipitous. When I applied to the Canadian International Development Agency youth internship program in 2000, I was placed with Presbyterian World Services and Development in Malawi. Then in 2006, at the commencement of my dissertation fieldwork, I was asked by a friend if I would join the first anthropology department in Malawi at the new Catholic University because they

were short of instructors. Presbyterianism and Catholicism were recognized as the two largest single Christian denominations in Malawi at the time.

[4]Elisa Sobo in *Choosing Unsafe Sex: AIDS-Risk Denial among Disadvantaged Women* reports similar associations between trust and condom use among inner-city Black women in Ohio (110-111).

[5]Elisa Sobo (*One Blood* 139) records similar fears about condoms among Jamaican women in the late 1980s and early 1990s.

[6]Possibly this is a description of contact dermatitis due to latex allergy, but latex allergy is not likely widespread. I cannot find any information about rates of latex allergy in African populations but more than 50 percent of individuals who are allergic to latex experience cross-reactions when eating bananas, papaya, passion fruit, pineapple, avocado or tomato, all widely consumed in Malawi. It seems likely that if latex allergy was widespread, I would have heard about or met people with food allergies.

[7]Joyce Banda is no relation to former President Hastings Banda. Banda is an extremely common surname in Malawi.

WORKS CITED

Altman, Dennis. *Global Sex*. Chicago: University of Chicago Press, 2001. Print.

Benefo, Kofi D. "Determinants of Condom Use in Zambia: A Multilevel Analysis." *Studies in Family Planning* 41.1 (2010):19-30. Print.

Bloch, Maurice. "The Symbolism of Money in Imerina." *Money and the Morality of Exchange*. Eds. Jonathan Parry and Maurice Bloch. New York: Cambridge University Press, 1989. 165-190. Print.

Bonongwe, Francis Joseph Mary. "Initiation Rites for Boys in Lomwe Society: A Dying Cultural Practice?" *Research in African Traditional Religion: Initiation Rites for Boys in Lomwe Society and Other Essays*. Ed. J. C. Chakanza. Zomba, Malawi: Kachere Series, 2004. 5-22. Print.

Chinsinga, Blessings. "The Politics of Poverty Alleviation in Malawi." *A Democracy of Chameleons: Politics and Culture in the New Malawi*. Ed. Harri Englund. Sweden: Nordiska Afrikainstitutet, 2002. 25-42. Print.

"Data: Malawi." *World Bank*. World Bank, n.d. Web. 11 Feb. 2015.

Doskoch, P. "In Malawi, Condom Use and Fidelity Are Linked with Religious Leaders' Discussion of These Behaviours." *International Perspectives on Sexual and Reproductive Health* 35.4 (2009): 207-208. Print.

Englund, Harri. *Prisoners of Freedom: Human Rights and the African Poor*. Berkeley: University of California Press, 2006. Print.

Fiedler, Rachel Nyagondwe. *Coming of Age: A Christianized Initiation for Women in Southern Malawi*. Zomba, Malawi: Kachere Series, 2005. Print.

Hammar, Lawrence, J. "Fear and Loathing in Papua New Guinea: Sexual Health in a Nation Under Siege." *Making Sense of Aids: Culture, Sexuality and Power in Melanesia*. Eds. Leslie Butt and Richard Eves. Honolulu: University of Hawai'i Press, 2008. 60-79. Print

Harrigan, Jane. *From Dictatorship to Democracy: Economic Policy in Malawi 1964-2000*. Farnham, Surrey, United Kingdom: Ashgate, 2001. Print.

Hayes, Nicole C. "Human Rights Discourse, Gender, and HIV and AIDS in Southern Malawi." *Anthropologica* 55.2 (2013): 349-358. Print.

Hunter, Mark. "The Materiality of Everyday Sex: Thinking Beyond 'Prostitution.'" *African Studies* 61.1 (2002): 99-120. Print.

Kalalo, Chimwemwe Umboni. "Improving Women's Sexual and Reproductive Health in the Context of HIV/Aids [sic]: The Involvement of the Anglican Church in the Upper Shire Diocese in Southern Malawi." Thesis, Master of Arts. University of Malawi, Chancellor College, 2005. Print.

Kaler, Amy. "Many Divorces and Many Spinsters: Marriage as an Invented Tradition in Southern Malawi, 1946-1999." *Journal of Family History* 26.4 (2001): 529-556. Print.

Kaler, Amy. "The Moral Lens of Population Control: Condoms and Controversies in Southern Malawi." *Studies in Family Planning* 35.2 (2004): 105-115. Print.

Kayiki, Simon P. and Ranata Forste. "HIV/AIDS Related Knowledge and Perceived Risk Associated with Condom Use among Adolescents in Uganda." *American Journal of Reproductive Health*

15.1 (2011): 57-63. Print.

Mair, Lucy P. "Marriage and Family in Dedza District of Nyasaland." *The Journal of the Royal Anthropological Institute of Great Britain and Ireland* 81.1/2 (1951): 103-119. Print.

Malawi. National Statistics Office (NSO) and ICF Macro. *Malawi Demographic and Health Survey.* Zomba, Malawi and Calverton, Maryland: NSO and ICF Macro, 2011. Print.

Mandala, Elias. *Work and Control in a Peasant Economy: A History of the Lower Tchiri Valley in Malawi, 1859-1960.* Madison, Wisconsin: University of Wisconsin Press, 1990. Print.

McPherson, Naomi M. "*Sik*Aids: Deconstructing the Awareness Campaign in Rural West New Britain. Papua New Guinea." *Making Sense of Aids: Culture, Sexuality and Power in Melanesia.* Eds. Leslie Butt and Richard Eves. Honolulu: University of Hawai'i Press, 2008. 224-245. Print.

Mills, David and Richard Ssewakiryanga. "No Romance without Finance: Commodities, Masculinities & Relationships among Kampalan Students." *Readings in Gender in Africa.* Ed. Andrea Cornwall. Bloomington, Indiana: Indiana University Press, 2005. 90-95. Print.

Minton, Carol. *The Social Construction of Gender Inequality in Central Malawi.* Saarbrücken, Germany: VDM Verlag Dr. Müller, 2008. Print.

Morris, Brian. *The Power of Animals: An Ethnography.* New York, New York: Bloomsbury Academic, 1998. Print.

Morris, Brian. *Animals and Ancestors: An Ethnography.* Oxford: Berg, 2000. Print.

Pfeiffer, James. "Condom Social Marketing, Pentecostalism and Structural Adjustment in Mozambique: A Clash of AIDS Prevention Methods." *Medical Anthropology Quarterly* 8.1 (2004): 77-103. Print.

Phiri, Kings M. "Some Changes in the Matrilineal Family System among the Chewa of Malawi Since the Nineteenth Century." *The Journal of African History* 24.2 (1983): 257-274. Print.

Prata, Ndola, Leo Morris, Elizio Mazive, Farnaz Vahidnia and Mark Stehr. "Relationship between HIV Risk Perception and Condom Use: Evidence from a Population-Based Survey in Mozambique." *International Family Planning Perspectives* 32.4

(2006): 192-200. Print.

Schoepf, Brooke Grundfest "Museveni's Other War: Condoms in Uganda." *Review of African Political Economy* 31.100 (2004): 372-376. Print.

Sinding, Steven W. "Does 'CNN' (Condoms, Needles and Negotiation) Work Better than 'ABC' (Abstinence, Being Faithful and Condom Use) in Attacking the AIDS Epidemic?" *International Family Planning Perspectives* 31.1 (2005): 38-40. Print.

Sobo, Elisa J. *One Blood: The Jamaican Body.* New York: State University of New York Press, 1993. Print.

Sobo, Elisa J. *Choosing Unsafe Sex: AIDS-Risk Denial among Disadvantaged Women.* Philadelphia: University of Pennsylvania Press, 1995. Print.

Stannus, H. S. and J. B. Davey. "The Initiation Ceremony for Boys among the Yao of Nyasaland." *The Journal of the Royal Anthropological Institute of Great Britain and Ireland* 43.1 (1913): 119-123. Print.

United Nations Development Programme (UNDP). *Human Development Report 2014.* New York: UNDP, 2014. Print.

Van den Borne, Francine. *Trying to Survive in Time of Poverty and AIDS: Women and Multiple Partner Sex in Malawi.* Amsterdam: Het Spinhuis, 2005. Print.

Women and Law in Southern Africa Research Trust (WLSART). *In Search of Justice: Women and the Administration of Justice in Malawi.* Blantyre, Malawi: Dzuka Publishing Company Limited, 2000. Print.

Zellner, Sara L. "Condom Use and the Accuracy of AIDS Knowledge in Côte d'Ivoire." *International Family Planning Perspectives* 29.1 (2003): 41-47. Print.

4.
Shortages, Priorities, and Maternal Health

Muddled *Kastom* and the Changing Status of Women in Malaita, Solomon Islands

STEPHANIE HOBBIS

SOLOMON ISLANDS HAS BEEN STRUGGLING with Millennium Development Goal 5, which pertains to maternal health, but is especially struggling with MDG 3 concerning gender equality and women's empowerment. In terms of raw numbers, Strategic Asia (commissioned by the United Nations Development Program (UNDP) to prepare the official progress report for Solomon Islands in 2010) has described the country's progress towards MDG 5 as "encouraging" and on track (87). From 1990 to 2010, the Maternal Mortality Ratio (MMR) fell from 150 to 93, with an average annual change in MMR of 2.2 percent (WHO). Ninety-five percent of women who had live births between 2004 and 2009 had received prenatal care from a skilled health care professional at least once. Major remaining problem areas are identified as access to medicinal drugs, the availability of female health providers, and the affordability of medical care. Also concerning is the number of women not using contraceptives (69 percent), despite an almost universal knowledge of family planning options (Strategic Asia). There was a near complete absence of postnatal care until February 2015, when a postnatal ward was opened at the National Referral Hospital in the capital city of Honiara.

The statistical outlook for MDG 3, on the other hand, is mostly grim. Solomon Islands is close to achieving gender parity in primary school enrolment, but significant gaps remain in access to secondary and tertiary education. Women are overrepresented in the non-waged labour market and underrepresented in skilled employment sectors, and they are barely represented in national and provincial governments. Violence against women remains widespread, and efforts to curb it have had only limited success. Statistics concerning domestic violence, insofar as they exist, likely underestimate the problem as well. Gender disparities worsened in Solomon Islands during the 1998–2003 civil unrest which is commonly referred to as "The Tensions." During this period, violence against women and the exploitation of women were particularly underreported, and the continuing effects of the social breakdown that occurred (e.g., family breakdowns, traumas, setbacks in economic development) have not been fully acknowledged or adequately addressed (Strategic Asia).

There does appear to be an increasing commitment among urban elites, from government to civil society actors, to improve the status and rights of women, at least legally and through policy outreach. However, significant shortcomings persist and it remains questionable if centralized policy initiatives are sufficient to challenge gender disparities across Solomon Islands. Over the course of 2014, the Family Protection Act was passed, which, for the first time, systematically criminalized domestic violence. *Seif Ples* or "safe place," a comprehensive first response service for victims of sexual violence, was opened in Honiara. At the same time, a country-wide awareness campaign was rolled out to support female candidates for the November 2014 national election. However, only one woman was elected. Similarly, the extent to which the Family Protection Act will and can be enforced among the country's largely rural population (80 percent) remains questionable. The ability of the Royal Solomon Islands Police Force (RSIPF) to effectively operate outside of urban areas (and in some places even within them) is under ongoing scrutiny and the reach, impact, and enforcement capacities of any state and non-state initiatives outside the urban core remain peripheral.

In other words, MDG 3 is very unlikely to be achieved, whereas MDG 5 may likely be, at least numerically. In this regard, the situation in Solomon Islands differs from several of the other case studies in this volume. Rather than addressing a failure in progress towards MDG 5, I explore challenges to the sustainability of Solomon Islands' achievements, and how failures in the implementation of MDG 3 are linked to continued shortcomings and long-term gains

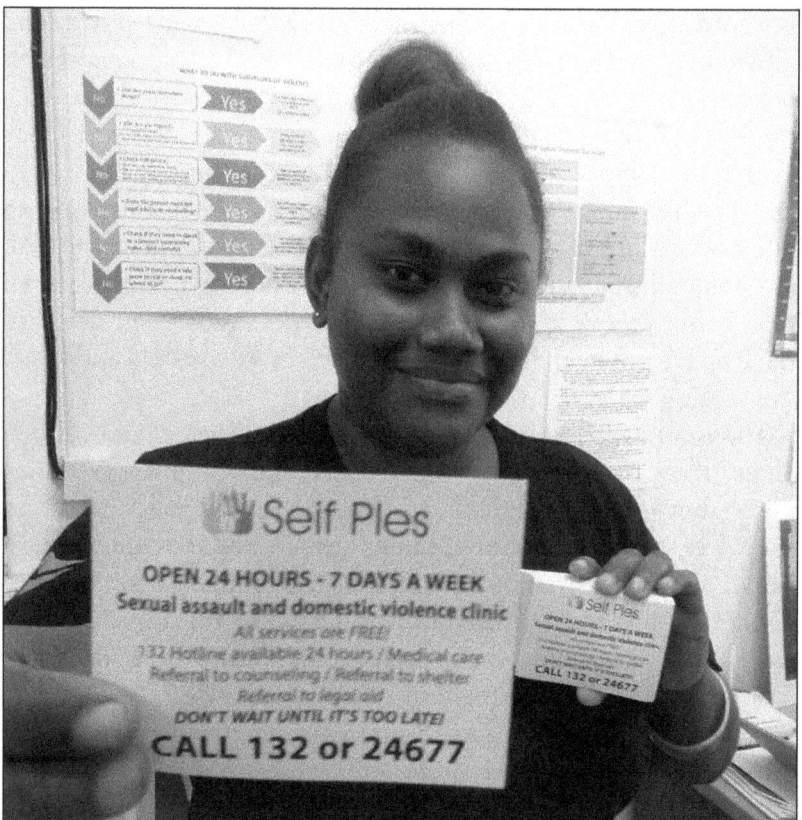

Fig.1: *Seif Ples* Gender-based Violence Crisis and Referral Centre

in regard to MDG 5. I focus above all on the everyday experiences of predominantly rural women and on how they negotiate access to health services, both public (biomedical) and customary, with their roles as women, daughters, sisters, wives, and mothers in the particular context of Malaita, the province that many refer to as the most "conservative" in Solomon Islands.

Ethnographically, my argument is based on twelve months of field research (2014–2015) among the coastal Lau people of North Malaita in the rural Lau Lagoon and their peri-urban settlements around Honiara. As such, I cannot claim to provide a comprehensive answer to my questions. A concentration on Malaita as analytical category is itself artificial, at least in part, given the strong historical and ongoing links with neighbouring provinces and islands. At the same time, Malaita is too broad a category in view of Malaitan heterogeneity in life experiences and local expressions of *kastom* or "ancestral ways," Christianity, and their hybrid iterations. Yet Malaita is also deeply interconnected, increasingly so, as historical events have been creating the narrative foundations for a "Malaitan identity," from the anticolonial Malaita-centered Maasina [Marching] Rule movement—and its attempts to develop a codified canon of Malaitan customary laws (Akin, "Colonialism, Maasina Rule")—to shared socioeconomic challenges[1] and pan-Malaitan responses to them.

With this in mind, this chapter is situated in relation to research on *kastom* or ancestral ways and on Christianity, their hybrids, and their implications for the status of women across Malaita. I begin by exploring cosmological-biological transformations and changes in the everyday life experiences of women in response to ideological and pragmatic developments concerning gender divisions. Then, I examine the impact of these transformations on women's maternal and reproductive health. I argue that the remaining obstacles to achieving MDG 5, comprehensively and sustainably, are located not solely in institutional-structural weaknesses of the public health system but more explicitly in the interaction of those weaknesses with ongoing changes in the status of women towards further devaluation. This is manifested in the intensified physical exploitation of women as labour and, metaphysically, as spiritually "impure" beings susceptible to demonic possession.

MUDDLED *KASTOM*: RE-POSITIONING WOMEN

Recognition of a symbiosis between pre-Christian and precolonial customs, missionary and, more recently, charismatic evangelical Christianity and accompanying organizational political forms is nothing new (Burt). With the continued strengthening of Christian influences in Malaita over the last century, hybrid forms of *kastom* and Christianity have emerged from transnational theocratic movements that link pre-Christian and Judeo-Christian traditions in shared ancestors—Malaitans as descendants of a lost tribe of Israel (Timmer)—to a continued centrality of gender relations and divisions in social life and cosmological or ideological imagination (Burt; Maranda, "Mapping Historical Transformation"). This symbiosis and its various iterations represent local struggles in making sense of a rapidly shifting world and the challenges these changes pose to traditional values and ways of being. As such, they offer ample opportunities for reinterpretations, manipulations, and confusions.

GENDERED SPHERES OF SEPARATION: METAPHYSICAL TRANSFORMATIONS

In the context of gender relations, Christian influence has provided a means by which men have reinforced their claim to power and authority over women. At a symbolic level, Christianity has offered men the potential to continue control on a physical or everyday level while weakening the cosmological structures that traditionally nurtured fear of and a "devilish" superiority of women on a metaphysical level. This is especially so because pre-Christian ways centred on the metaphysical separation of the female realm from the male and particular ancestral realms, including distinct roles in ritualistic practices as well as partial but not radical physical separation. For example, Kwaio men and women would work together in gardens and share family houses, but there were important ritualistic times of separation. For women, these were particularly significant while menstruating and after giving birth and for priestly men, after high sacrifice (Akin, "Kwaio Women's Taboos").

In the context of this (partial) separation, Keesing argues that the power of women and the power of men can be understood on an abstract, symbolic level as mirror images of each other, with both being connected to the powers of ancestors in different ways. This division did create the foundation for male control over female bodies, but it also allowed for women to assume, at least in their own conceptualizations, a position of moral superiority (reflected in their careful following and respect for taboos surrounding their bodily fluids). "In some ways reproductive power, mystified as dangerous and potentially antisocial, represents women's victory, not women's subjugation" (Keesing 222). Herein, Keesing finds evidence that the customary male-female dialectic is not necessarily one of inherent inequality and oppression, even though it certainly allows for it. Instead, symbolic (and partially spatial) separation is, on an everyday basis, said to be a complex struggle and negotiation that, nevertheless, is fixed within the perceived possible and that follows the particular cosmological status of women and men and their respective role in communicating with ancestors (Keesing).

However, one should not overemphasize symbolic analysis of gender relations. Akin demonstrates how, in practice, these taboos, their enforcement and consequences are enmeshed in the particular lives of those involved, and how their roles have changed over time ("Kwaio Women's Taboos"). He identifies an important shift, specifically a notable increase in women's reporting of taboo violations, from the 1940s. Because menstrual taboo violations come with rampant costs to the community at large, "in pigs, houses, gardens, and its good health" creative responses had to be found to both acknowledge the violation and to decrease the costs (Akin, "Kwaio Women's Taboos" 393). One such solution is an increase in *gwari* magic to "'cool down' ancestral spirits so those users can violate their taboos with lesser or no repercussions" (Akin, "Kwaio Women's Taboos" 397-8).

I observed similar flexibilities and recent developments among Lau, especially in usages of Christian magic, to appease or even chase away ancestral spirits. On the other hand, I also found that these very processes strengthen gender differentiation, metaphysically as well as in lived practice. This was visible less in the direct punishment of women for taboo violations than in privately uttered reminders—or threats—to women about the great harm their behaviour could bring onto themselves and, even more so, to their families and communities.

In this context, it is important to note that, only since the introduction of Christianity, has it become cosmologically feasible to maintain the exclusion of women while weakening the metaphysical fears that provided at least partial counterbalance to male dominance over the female body. Specifically, in a comparative examination of the non-Christian and the Christian ontological status of women among the Lau, Maranda argues that men have actively used Christian teachings to "neutralize female power.... With Woman becoming Eve, they [men] can put her in an evil category that suits their purpose and frees them from their ontological paradigm of female radical and unequivocal power. God will subdue women, and—an innovation—his sons can base male supremacy on Adamic 'metaphysical' grounds" ("Mapping Historical Transformation" 106).

Pragmatically, this means that Christianity has allowed the tearing down of the spheres of separation between men's and women's everyday life worlds. Traditionally based on a cosmological-biological fear of menstrual blood, birthing, and women's bodily wastes, Lau men were afraid of ritual poisoning and subsequent death should women, for example, prepare food for them. With conversion, at least in theory, men were able to move beyond this division. Following the missionary example of the nuclear family, men and women can live together during menstruation and even birthing. The woman assumes the role of the primary caretaker. Foods and gardens can be shared at all times.

Among Lau, at least,[2] only a complete rejection of everything *kastom* seemed to allow for safety from the potentially deadly consequences of men's violations. When Ellie K. and Pierre Maranda conducted their field research between 1966 and 1989, Christian men complained about "pain in their guts" in response to ongoing violations of customary gender rules and the subsequent required forgetting of their own genealogies in the learning of new Judeo-Christian ones, those of Jesus and David (Maranda, "Mapping Historical Transformation"). This pain indicates that customary fears persisted, despite what may at first appear to be a cosmologically "liberated" practice.

Twenty-five years later, I find this continuity in discontinuity to be ongoing and even further muddled. This has especially been the case in response to the strengthening of *kastom* as a political ideology that, nevertheless, remains deeply rooted and, at times, conflicted in particular local iterations of pre-Christian cultural practice (Akin, "Ancestral Vigilance"; "*Kastom* as Hegemony?"). Classified as customary in new and different ways, women's disenfranchisement has become more pronounced. Akin notes that, among the Kwaio, contemporary ancestral fears centre, above all, on governing female bodily fluids and mitigating the dangers of a seemingly increasing violation of women's taboos ("Ancestral Vigilance"). Despite the previously noted "new" and creative ways of responding to this shift, with this increase in the violations of women's taboos, women have become "socially indebted to men" to a degree that was previously unknown—"women's violations damage relations with ancestors, and men provide most of the pigs, labor and rituals to repair that damage" (Akin, "Ancestral Vigilance" 310). As a result, women's positions are undermined, and they are more vulnerable to oppression and exploitation on both societal and individual levels.

Among the Lau, the perceived dangers of female bodily fluids have become less prominent. Menstruation and birth have shifted from the public (as community ritual, see Keesing) to the private domain. Typically, women are no longer required to follow menstrual taboos or report their violations of them. In many villages, all spatial and architectural features related to this have disappeared. Menstrual taboos are usually talked about only within intimate family relations or in the abstract, as remembrance of past practices that have limited, if any, relevance today. Among many young men, fear of menstrual blood and birthing has not only vanished but for some, the former has even become sexually desirable. On the other hand, birthing at home is often merely described as "too messy." It is for this reason rather than a fear of spiritual pollution that some men (across all ages and plural social positions) have suggested a return to a house dedicated for birthing for women who, for any given reason, do not go to clinics or hospitals.

WITCHCRAFT ACCUSATIONS: WOMEN AS "LIABILITIES"

At the same time, release of female bodily fluids in the immediate surroundings of a house continues to bring stigmatization and a subsequent indebtedness to men, especially husbands and their families. For example, if a woman admits to defecating in the vicinity of any house, or is caught or suspected of doing so, she can be accused of being a "witch"—a woman possessed by a spirit with malevolent intent. Christian rites, in the form of an exorcism performed by a spiritually powerful priest, may offer some relief. This response silences the spirit and its "evil" effects, but it has limited temporal reach and overarching effect. The spirit is thought to be located in the woman's "blood" and Christian exorcism is thought to be unable to permanently remove it. In other words, the woman's female offspring are certain to inherit a susceptibility to spirit possession and witchcraft. In this, a woman's subordination or obligation to her husband and by extension to his family (repaid in her labour and in unquestioned obedience to her husband) can be intensified, since she remains a "liability" in childbirth, motherhood, and to future generations beyond.

This is not to say that increased exploitation of women's labour is necessarily always and directly linked to witchcraft accusations, or that it primarily focuses on "lazy" women. I witnessed several instances of witchcraft accusations that were directed at women who were known for their willingness to work particularly hard. Also, these accusations were uttered not just by men but also as often, and in some cases especially, by other women (often of the same age group and of comparable social status). Several of the women who were suspected of witchcraft simply shook their heads in response, not in disbelief but in reaction to what many thought to be an indicator of jealousy. Hard work had allowed many of the accused women to accumulate more power than other women and also some, or even many, men. For instance, they had increased access to and control of cash earned (e.g., from betel nut sales or other market activities) and stronger voices in at least some family decisions. These women were often thought to be among the savviest in "modern" financial matters and management.

This elevated status and access to power indicates why accused women suspected jealousy to be the root cause of witchcraft accusations. None of the women I talked to admitted to having used witchcraft, at least not intentionally, but many agreed that there had been an increase in sorcery or black magic in recent history. Several also knew of women who had been found guilty of witchcraft and had been punished for it, most commonly by being exiled from their villages at significant (social) costs to their families. This was most common among women who married into and had settled in their husband's village. Their husbands were given the choice of joining their wives and leaving their house, gardens, and other belongings behind or remaining in their villages—usually together with their children and at least their sons—and divorcing their wives.

The women who had so far only been suspected of witchcraft and who had brushed it away as jealousy, worried about this. They had not intentionally been spiritually impure. However, many believed that there had been witches in their families, and, therefore, they had witchcraft in their blood. Such inherited witchcraft was not associated with intentionality. For example, they would not have any memory of defecating in the vicinity of their houses, but, nonetheless, they were (or felt) responsible for polluting and bringing evil spirits to their houses, families, and community (Akin "Kwaio Women's Taboos"). In this possibility, women who were otherwise successful and comparatively powerful felt disempowered, and I witnessed several occasions at which this insecurity was used as means of control by their husbands and by their husbands' male and female relatives. Family members regularly reminded these women of their place in family hierarchies, of how "lucky" they were for being allowed to stay (that their husbands did not send them away), and of how their success (also in market or financial activities) was always derived from and dependent upon decisions made by the men in her family. These reminders were often uttered in semi-public spaces.

In other words, the female, per se, is no longer feared. Instead, women's perceived predisposition to malevolent spirit possession has become a burden that can be controlled "for free." The expensive labour and sacrifice that were required by pagan rituals is absent in Christian rites. At the same time, spirit possession remains an aggravation in everyday life and in intergenerational transmission. The transformation into Eve is complete, and as Eve is hierarchically lower than Adam and more sinful, she becomes indebted to her husband and family in a different way. Following the example of early missionaries, this debt can be best repaid in her exclusion from decision making, especially in the public domain and in her primary delegation to extended work in the domestic sphere—the distinction itself is, to the degree that it exists today, a legacy of colonial and missionary efforts (Mowbray).

DEVALUING WOMEN'S LABOUR

In this context of cosmological-biological repositioning I find that similar to Mowbray's observations among the Halia- and Haku-speaking people of Buka Island, Papua New Guinea, women's work in Lau has been devalued. Today, women are the primary source of manual labour. They take care of children. They are responsible for most of the work in gardens, both for subsistence and markets, and for any work that is required around the house (cooking, weeding, laundry, cleaning etc.). At the same time, their influence outside the home has been reduced significantly. For example, during the national and provincial election campaigns, (male) candidates often encouraged questions from women, seemingly following urban attempts to increase female participation in the political process. The few times a woman dared to speak, however, the audience, men and women alike, started giggling, sometimes even breaking out in laughter, while close family members often expressed embarrassment. What can a woman ask that could be relevant and substantial? Herein, a woman's labour in the domestic sphere becomes the sole means by which she can repay her husband's family for the troubles that she incurs as a descendant of Eve, perhaps even as witch, as well as for the labour sacrificed to "purchase" her in the first place.

Despite ongoing efforts to reduce payments for brides or even stop the practice, especially by Christian churches (to varying degrees), the bride wealth system persists or rather it has shifted towards increased commodification. Even though a woman's labour and the transferal of rights over it were always key factors in marriage exchanges, bride wealth also used to signify the transition of a girl from child-daughter to woman-wife, and it served as means by which her family was compensated for losing her affections as well as her labour. Today, many feel that these ritual meanings have been lost and that the practice has been transformed into a mere economic transaction, similar to buying a bag of rice—a transformation that is best understood in a conceptual shift from bride wealth to bride price (Wardlow). Indeed, in Lau, costs are soaring and with this a woman's indebtedness to her husband and in-laws is increasing as well. In the words of a non-Malaitan woman married to a Malaitan man and living on Malaita:

I will insist on the smallest possible bride price for my

daughter should she choose to marry a Malaitan man. If the payment is too high, she will be treated like a slave, and her husband's family will say it is only fair because she was expensive. She has to be able to repay her debt in her labour and childbearing, as soon as possible. Then she can retain her ability to make own choices. She is willing to work, and she works hard. I am so worried about what will happen to her.

CODIFICATION, PATRILINEAL RIGHTS AND "DEVELOPMENT"

On a different level, with the strengthening of *kastom* as political tool, gender divisions have become more pronounced in the codification (legalization) of men's patrilineal rights and women's exclusion from land ownership in particular. For political and economic gains, lineages are retraced, and as far as possible, knowledge of ancestors is revived. At times, the ancestors are intertwined with Judeo-Christian roots, which were previously thought of as competing with or unrelated to the indigenous system (Timmer).

Across Malaita, primary land ownership was for generations linked to male lines, but cognatic (secondary) lines, as affinal connections, were often granted access to land for residence and gardening (Guo). In fact, land use requests by members of cognatic lines could often not be refused easily, especially in the southern half of Malaita. Cognatic access to and use of land (though not ownership) is then best understood as a right and not as a mere favour (Ross). Today, this system remains, but lineages linked through only females or a combination of female and male ancestors have become more vulnerable as prospects for development projects increase land values and as fixed landownership becomes a perceived necessity to participate in "development" and the global economic system.

At the same time, the veracity of genealogical claims is often questionable in view of breaks in knowledge transmission that followed Christian conversion (Guo). Nevertheless, following a path first paved by the colonial administration, Solomon Islands is pushing forward with court orders and plans for a land registry. These are based on "simplified" patrilineal land rights that allow "secondary" or cognatic residents to be expelled more easily—often in the name of or in accordance with human and/or indigenous rights provisions—or, at very least, they can be charged rent.

The binary distinction between men and women, and by extension their respective access to "rights" in a muddled *kastom*-Western legal framework, is becoming more visible and also more permanently solidified. The older indigenous system put emphasis on both blood relations *and* "action."[3] Legal codification, on the other hand, prioritizes blood relation as unquestionably the most significant marker of legitimate land ownership (Guo). That said, court decisions are frequently contested and rarely enforced, yet the increasing significance of the legal process has altered understanding of genealogies and the role of female ancestors therein. Among the Langalanga (Guo) and among, I contend, the Lau as well, knowledge of kinship ties has shifted accordingly. Detailed knowledge of ancestral lines and of customary practice with its greater complexity and flexibility has disappeared. It has been replaced with a stronger awareness of who was born into a male or female line at any given place to allow for asserting or "straightening" patrilineal hierarchical systems and subsequent entitlements to power. As such, further disenfranchisement of women and cognatic lines is closely intertwined with the demands of "economic development" and desired integration into the global (capitalist and legal) system.

WOMEN'S SUPPORT NETWORKS

In addition, customary support networks, especially those of wives (and mothers) beyond their husbands' families, have been affected by these broader trends. In some ways, women have always been dependent on their husbands and his family, especially so as marriage has constituted[4] displacement in most cases, with women moving from one family and village to another (Köngäs Maranda). However, mothers were also frequently involved in finding suitable wives for their sons. They would explicitly search in their own natal villages, which meant that, in practice, only women from a few villages would marry into any given village. With shared family histories, these women built mutual support networks that offset the instability of displacement (Maranda, "Mapping Historical Transformation"). Today, women and men (mothers and fathers) often have little to say regarding who their sons (and daughters) marry, and although this weakens both parents' control, it most directly influences women's networks, which continue to be particularly significant for responding to and preventing domestic violence.

Spanning the physical, metaphysical, and legal status of women, these recent developments have repositioned women in such a way that their dependence on men has grown, despite simultaneous urban efforts directed at empowering women and codifying equal rights and despite continued and, at times, even amplified access to and control of financial means. Women are indebted to men and their extended families in an entanglement of "new and old" ways that are, above all, signified by a cosmological depreciation, the increased exploitation of women as labour, and the demands of "development," which build on the patrilineal biases of colonialism in land use, ownership, and reform. In other words, high degrees of contextual flexibility in daily life and religious practice are increasingly curbed by the inflexibilities of codification and the survival of "Western" male-centric missionary and colonial hierarchies in the very rules that are being enshrined today.

WOMEN'S ACCESS TO HEALTH SERVICES

The above described positioning of women and its entanglement with legal codification, "development," and Christianization have had a significant impact on reliable access to health services for women, both public-biomedical and customary. In the following, I briefly retrace the story of Regina (a pseudonym), a rural woman who, as sister, wife and mother, has struggled to receive adequate health care before, during, and after pregnancies because of limited institutional-organizational support frameworks *and* her weakened status as a woman in Malaita today. Regina's story is not exceptional, but in various ways, it exemplifies women's continuing struggles with maternal health and MDG 5 goals, despite the promising numbers presented by official reports. Her story tells of shortages and priorities that further marginalize women, especially if their child is certain not to survive. This reflects a wider local and international trend towards prioritizing a child's health over that of the mother or considering a mother's health primarily in reference to that of her child (Jolly).

REGINA'S STORY

Regina is once divorced and currently married to her second husband in a predominantly Anglican village in the Northern Lau Lagoon. She married her first husband in her early twenties and had four children with him. She is very reluctant to talk about that period of her life. Regina's first husband was violent, especially so towards her. She left when she could no longer bear it, although with this decision she lost her children who remained with their father, which is the case for divorce in most patrilineal societies. Bride price not only secures a wife but also makes the couple's children members of the husband's lineage. If a woman does not give birth to at least two children, her husband's family is entitled to a "full or partial refund" or a "replacement" (for example, her family might choose to give her husband another daughter as a second wife, which recently happened in Regina's village). Today, it is possible for women to fight for their children in family court, and many men and women report that those who do go to court commonly win. Yet resort to courts is typically only available to those living in and willing to remain in town. In cases where the desire for divorce is mutual and the couple has had more than two children, children might also be split, with the father often, but not always, keeping the boys and the mother, the girls. Regina's only option was to leave her four children behind.

Regina is in a much happier marriage now. However, because her husband is younger than her and was known in his youth as a "warrior" (as far as such status is still possible today), witchcraft accusations persist—why would such a man choose a previously married, disgraced, and noticeably older woman unless she had bewitched him? Her husband's reputation protects her from prosecution as a witch but not from social exclusion. She belongs to none of the women's groups, and her family lives outside the immediate village boundaries.

Regina does come to the village daily. She takes care of not only her own household but also often that of her parents-in-law. She is also the woman most likely among her family to go to the markets voluntarily. She is among the few willing to paddle a canoe the approximately four-hour return trip and often takes it upon herself to sell fish caught by her extended family. This is risky, since markets, and especially fish sales, are busy, quick, and often very difficult to manage. Prospective customers rush to get the best fish and in the resulting confusion, some always disappear without paying. If this happens, she deducts the loss from her own fish sales while returning full amounts to those who asked her to sell theirs. She is proud of her status as a hard-working woman, and she never complains. Her willingness to labour and the cheerfulness with which she completes her work make her a valued member of her extended family; she is indispensable on an everyday basis. She does not rest and cannot and will not allow herself to be away for extended or "unproductive" periods of time.

Now in her late thirties, Regina has three children from her second marriage. Her last two pregnancies ended in miscarriages, one in the fifth month and one in the third. Her first pregnancy in her second marriage was a late miscarriage as well. Regina barely survived two of the miscarriages because her hemorrhaging would not stop. She fought for her life, in a cooking hut, so as not to make a mess or alert others of her pain. Only when she was barely conscious did someone call the parish priest. Regina is deeply grateful for the priest's intervention; he rescued her through prayer and helped her identify, at least in one of the two cases, the reason for her miscarriage—she had violated a customary food taboo, which was specific to her village of origin but not to her husband's family. The priest performed an exorcism, chasing away the last remnants of the *kastom* spirit, and, thus, removed the food taboo. The bleeding, in both cases, stopped after approximately two days. She survived.

Regina lives a two and one half hour dugout canoe ride from the nearest hospital at Malu'u. If an outboard motor (OBM) is available, the trip takes thirty minutes. If no other trip is scheduled, a return trip by outboard motor costs at least SBD 200 (around USD 26) in petrol, plus rental fees of between SBD 50 and 200, depending on which boat, motor and captain are available. A fare on an otherwise arranged trip is only around SBD 20. To put this into context, Regina's nuclear family only has access to cash income through microeconomic market activities that she cannot participate in regularly (perhaps only once every two weeks) and that others are often unwilling to participate in for her.[5] She is still breastfeeding her youngest child and does not feel comfortable being away too often for extended periods of time. Furthermore, going to the market only provides limited access to "cash." Of the SBD 30 to 80 that she earns on a good day, she spends a significant percentage immediately on other goods that are available at the market and are rare or more expensive in the village, such as cabbage (greens), betel nut and/or local tobacco, and some fruits, especially bananas for the children. Despite the monetization of many market activities, it remains primarily a trading zone; "saltwater goods" (fish, crabs, etc.) are exchanged for cash, and cash is exchanged for "bush goods" and vice versa. A cash return is often sought only for particular purposes at particular times, for example when school fees are due (between SBD 50 and 100 per child annually at the local primary school) or when a trip is being planned to distant Honiara.

A trip to Honiara takes six hours by truck and then an additional six hours by boat, costing around SBD 230 each way. For hospital visits, Honiara is likely more affordable in the long term. Malu'u is only a small township and most residents are from the same language group (To'abaita). Unless they are married to a man (and, to a lesser extent, woman) from To'abaita or government employees, few members of other language groups would choose or even be able to live there. Many do, however, live in Honiara or to a lesser extent in the provincial capital 'Aoke (Auki), where relatives can offer support during hospital visits. Kin provide food during hospital stays and shelter if patients are required to regularly seek medical care but are not admitted. Stays in Honiara are often lengthy. Although efforts are occasionally made to return to the village within four to five days, stays of two weeks to several months are much more common. Trips to Honiara quickly turn into "holidays"—a break from garden work and more convenient access to (private) toilets and showers, water, and electricity, among other things. Those who stay behind are generally suspicious of any claim that one will return swiftly from town.

Regina did not seek immediate or, in most cases, any medical care in Malu'u, 'Aoke, or Honiara for her miscarriages. She and her extended family did not deem it necessary. Who would take care of her children? Who would replace her labour in the gardens and household? Pregnancies (and miscarriages) are simply all too common to allow them to interrupt everyday life. Miscarriages especially are too expensive and, in their "normalcy," too unimportant to warrant either extended absence or the uncertainty of heading to Malu'u. Also, blood for transfusions is always in low supply at hospitals, and staff are reputed to avoid using it until, often enough, it is too late, especially for parturition and even more so during miscarriages when the life of the child cannot be saved. Regina is very much aware of this. In 2014, a young woman from her village died after being admitted to Honiara's National Referral Hospital for a miscarriage. Hospital staff procrastinated with giving her the necessary blood transfusions until her life could no longer be saved, despite continuing requests by family members to do so.

A retired midwife lives in Regina's village, and several men and women are knowledgeable in *kastom* medicine. However, Regina and many of the women with whom I talked preferred giving birth (and receiving pre- or postnatal care) in hospitals rather than in the village. Hospitals are looked at critically in view of ongoing shortages of staff, blood, and medication but so is *kastom* medicine. Many seem to trust local knowledge as much or more than biochemical medicine, and both systems are commonly treated not as contradictory but as equally valid and potentially complementary. That said, there are concerns about the effectiveness of *kastom* medicine after conversion to Christianity and the subsequent destruction of ties to ancestral lines and spirits. Without the correct prayers and rituals, knowledge of which has been lost or weakened through Christian conversion, *kastom* medicine as an attempt to "mediate between moral and physiological domains of experience" is considered to be less powerful than it used to be (Buchanan 10). This is not to say that hybrid *kastom*-Christian priests and lay healers have not created new intersections between *kastom* medicine and Christian spirituality, but skepticism remains. When the spatial separation of men and women was torn down and menstrual and birthing taboos were broken with the spread of Christianity, traditional knowledge and practices surrounding birthing were interrupted and on a metaphysical level, they became void. Within this context, hospitals and biochemical medicine have become the preferred resource for pregnant women.

In this vein, Regina sought medical treatment in Honiara when she was pregnant with her youngest child. The pregnancy had been a difficult one but she did not miscarry. Her family allowed, even encouraged and financially supported her to go to a hospital to ensure the survival of her child. Once Regina arrived at the National Referral Hospital, she had an ultrasound (to the envy of many other rural women) and despite the devastating news it brought, she is still proud and excited about having had this experience. She was pregnant with twins, but one had died in utero. The rest of her pregnancy and the birth were very difficult. She was confined to bed rest for significant periods and for short periods admitted to the hospital as well (in between she lived with relatives in town). Regina was told that the second twin might not survive if it was not born first, which luckily he was. A Caesarean section was never offered to her. Medical staff did, however, recommend that she have a hysterectomy after recovery from the birth. She was told that any future pregnancies would likely severely endanger her life and that having another live birth was doubtful.

Regina consulted with her husband and his family, and they agreed to the procedure. She had given birth to three healthy children, including two boys and, therefore, she had fulfilled the fundamental requirement of her "marriage contract." While waiting for her appointment, she remained in Honiara. It was simply too expensive and inconvenient to move between town and village for the surgery alone. However, when the date finally arrived, she was informed that the surgery had to be postponed further, a common practice when medical staff, medicine, and equipment are often in short supply. The new date was set for several weeks later. Regina did not feel comfortable waiting this long, since she had already been away from her family and responsibilities for a severely stretched period. She cancelled her appointment, returned to the village, and has not yet found an opportunity to reschedule the surgery. She has had two miscarriages since, and continues to worry that the next pregnancy may be her last.

About three days after her last miscarriage Regina had the opportunity to travel to Malu'u and return for free on the same day. The cost at the hospital itself would be minimal: SBD 2 to see a doctor and any prescribed medication is free, insofar as it is available. Also, one of her children was feeling ill with a cough and an elevated temperature, so her family agreed that she could take the child and visit the family planning centre at Malu'u hospital at the same time. The goal was to get a check-up after the miscarriage, perhaps obtain some medication, and potentially restart the conversation about a hysterectomy. Identifying a different means of contraception was not on the table.

Contraception (except for hysterectomies) appears to be rarely if ever talked about (at least not in semi-public spaces). Conversations immediately go quiet if the topic is brought up. The few short explanations I was able to get focused pragmatically on the difficulty of obtaining contraceptive methods and, more broadly, on the importance of motherhood and of women's obligation to bear their husband's children. With control over women's bodies already weakened in the disappearance of menstrual and related taboos, men appear unwilling to loosen the grip any further, while women are uncertain about the actual functioning of contraceptive methods. This is evocative of Smith's argumentation (this volume) concerning women's inability to make their own reproductive choices without having to ask their husbands or parents for permission and of Dureau's observations about attitudes towards family planning in Simbo (Western Province, Solomon Islands). Even though there is widespread agreement that high birth rates threaten the sustainability of subsistence gardening and fishing, which is also the case among Lau, attitudes towards contraception are in some places contradictory and, therefore, ineffective. Women prefer more "natural" contraceptive methods, state-run hospitals and health services advocate women-centred pharmaceutical products, and men are opposed to contraception that lies beyond their direct control (Dureau).

Regina arrived at Malu'u hospital on a Monday morning. Some women were already lining up at the family planning centre. She decided to see the general practitioner for her child first, to ask for some advice about her case and then to move on to the family health centre. About an hour later, she had learned that the family planning centre opened only once a week, on Fridays, and that no staff member with maternal health experience was currently available at the hospital. She talked to a few of the women standing around and was told that even on Fridays, the centre was not always open. They knew about its supposed schedule but were waiting at the centre nonetheless, just in case someone arrived during the course of the day (for a similar situation, see Yakong and McPherson this volume). Regina was unable to wait this long. She was dependent on when the other passengers on her OBM wanted to return, which was sooner rather than later, because the boat had been reserved for a different trip in the afternoon. She got medication for her child and after a second short consultation with the general practitioner, a standard all-purpose antibiotic for herself.

Regina would not return for another attempt. She recovered well from the miscarriage, which she attributes to spiritual support from the parish priest as well as the biochemical (antibiotic) treatment. She discussed with her family the possibility of heading to 'Aoke or Honiara for a hysterectomy, but they were uncomfortable about her leaving for a longer period of time. At this point her role was, first and foremost, that of a wife and mother with three young children, and she could not fulfill that role while away. Perhaps next year she would try again.

Regina agreed with this decision, but not to agree was not really an option either. Although she could have left, it would have likely meant a significant rift with her husband and his family. A woman's mobility depends significantly on decisions made by her husband, father-in-law, uncles-in-law and brothers-in-law. Even for movements within the village and surrounding garden areas, women are expected to notify a male relative, and particular emphasis is placed on this notification requirement if a woman is engaged or married. Young unmarried women are only allowed to go to gardens by themselves, and even in this context, it is preferred that they go with a female relative. For visits to markets, hospitals or to relatives, a woman must obtain explicit permission from immediate male family members.

This is especially the case if a woman wants to spend time in an urban space. Doubts about the morality of town, especially its sexual morality, are widespread. At least once a year, but if possible twice, Regina's Anglican village sends so-called rescue missions to Honiara. For one week, participants travel throughout town and visit village communities there. They discuss Christian morality and celebrate church services together. The goal is to remind urban residents of the importance of traditional *kastom*, Christian and hybrid values that focus on the sanctity of the family and motherhood and on the evils of alcohol and sexual promiscuity. With barely any medical services available in rural areas, fears of sexual misconduct among women in town constitute an important hurdle to women accessing female care providers. This is in addition to the restrictions already imposed on women's movements in order to retain their labour, especially the labour of a wife and mother.

By and large, Regina's husband and his family have been (comparatively) open to her exploring opportunities for medical care when necessary. A hysterectomy and the required travel are still a possibility once she is no longer breastfeeding her youngest child, and her daughter is old enough to help out in Regina's (thus her own) extended family's households. Importantly, should Regina get the surgery, her status would change from a fertile married woman to that of an "honorary man." She would be considered less sexually desirable and once her children are old enough to be without her for extended periods, she gains the right (agency) to move more freely without having to ask male relatives for permission for every movement. This status change makes this trip to town less "dangerous" because it is not as laden with fears of sexual immorality; at least, this is the case once the surgery is performed.

Regina is a valued member of her (husband's) family; she is often asked for advice, including by male family members, and many admire and also envy her mental and physical strength. Despite this, her choices, especially with regard to fertility (contraception), pregnancies, and motherhood are significantly limited by her physical and metaphysical position as woman. The risks associated with going to (urban) hospitals—shortages of staff, blood, and medicine—are intensified by restrictions placed on her mobility. With the spread of Christianity and emergent hybrid customs, ways in which the female body is controlled have changed but have not disappeared. On the contrary, with a weakened metaphysical status, women's dependence on men has grown and with that dependence, the challenges associated with pregnancies and births have also grown.

CONCLUSION: SHORTAGES AND PRIORITIES

In view of the experiences Regina and other women encounter with accessing adequate maternal health care, the numerical success of progress towards MDG 5 in Solomon Islands seems surprising, at least at first sight. Following the terms of MDG 5, Regina sought and received adequate prenatal care for her last "successful" pregnancy, despite the in utero death of one of the twins. She went to a hospital after her last miscarriage. Even though no maternal health staff members were available, she is satisfied with the service that she was offered insofar as she attributes her survival, at least in part, to the antibiotics she was prescribed. Regina also received advice about a type of contraception (hysterectomy), which she and her family consider a valid option and continue to pursue. Regina is alive; she has given birth to seven healthy children and has an overall positive attitude towards biochemical medicine. The situation does not *seem* too bad after all, especially considering Solomon Islands' classification as "least developed country" and its significant, ongoing challenges for improving public infrastructures and social services.

However, Regina's experiences also highlight substantial gaps in a perspective that focuses solely on MDG 5, which misses the wider context in which she must negotiate her survival and that of her children with her role expectations as woman, wife, and mother. Regina is aware of the shortcomings of Solomon Islands' public health system. She knows that she is subjected to often harmful decisions made by hospital staff in direct response to her needs (e.g., replacement blood in case of a miscarriage) or to the general situation (e.g., staff not showing up to work, unavailability of specialized medication), but she is not confident enough in any other option to reject the public health system outright. She is open to leveraging all options, which include *kastom* medicine and Christian prayer and their various hybrids as well as biomedical solutions. All options are in short supply, or, more accurately, they are unreliable at best: there are doubts about customary systems that are no longer based on strict adherence to ancestral ways; uncertainties about the extent, depending on the situation, to which Christian spirituality can replace, support, or combat *kastom* ways; and fears of inadequate service at public health centres, including a concern about their overriding focus on the physiological rather than the moral domain.

Regina does not have the luxury of rejecting any of these options. She is not allowed to move freely without rupturing the relationship with her husband's family, which would cast doubt on her sexual morality and on her commitment to her family and children as mother. Thus, she often cannot seek biochemical medical treatment when she deems it necessary. Financial resources are regularly limited and prioritized accordingly. With a high frequency of pregnancies, miscarriages and births, women's health appears to become affordable only in the latest stages of pregnancies when the child is endangered but survival is likely and, rarely, when the child has already been lost. In between and during pregnancies, Malaitan women are first and foremost wives and mothers, and, as such, they are responsible for the labour that this entails. "Holidays" in Honiara are only a last resort.

This is unlikely to change without improvements to the physical and metaphysical status of women (and therein MDG 3 and beyond) as well as a recognition that rural women's increasing role as domestic labourers significantly reduces their ability to seek even sub-par health care in non-emergency situations (see also Yakong and McPherson, this volume). More importantly, women's continued disenfranchisement on an everyday basis, in addition to increasing frustration with inadequate medical services at public health centres, may undermine the sustainability of the progress made towards MDG 5. Awareness of unsatisfactory medical treatment at public clinics is growing and so are the hurdles to rural women being allowed to expose themselves to the various potential moral dangers of an urban, "lazy," and promiscuous life. As long as women do not control their own bodies and mobility, or at least are unable to negotiate decisions with their husbands and extended families about their own and their children's health on a more equal basis, this danger will expand and women's (maternal and reproductive) health is likely to be sidelined further.

I thank Naomi McPherson and two anonymous reviewers for the advice and comments received to earlier versions of this chapter. I am especially grateful to the late Pierre Maranda and to David Akin, whose insights and guidance were more than generous and to the many Lau and Solomon Islander individuals who remain unnamed here to protect confidentiality. The twelve months of field research (2014-2015) that inform this paper were funded through a Vanier Canada Graduate Scholarship (SSHRC) and internal grants from Concordia University.

ENDNOTES

[1] Malaita province has seen the lowest level of economic development in Solomon Islands, with only little change over the past thirty years and a quickly growing and internally highly mobile population that constitutes the primary working force in many urban or peri-industrial centres across the country, as has been the case since the early twentieth century.

[2] Across Malaita, the extent to which becoming Christian has been associated with complete rejection of pre-Christian beliefs differs significantly. For example, the Deep Sea Canoe Movement (also in North Malaita) actively seeks to blend pre-Christian theologies and practices with Christian teachings, especially the Old Testament, as both are viewed as complementary rather than contradictory (Timmer).

[3] "A person's action on the piece of land (such as continual residence or farming), a person's relation to the *agalo* [ancestor spirit] of the land (such as following traditional taboos, contribution of pigs to the founding *agalo* in sacrificial feasts), and social relations with his/her community (e.g., harmony and cooperation)" (Guo 231).

[4] It is still common for women to move to their husband's village of

birth; however, marriages between couples from the same village, which used to be frowned on, are increasingly widespread.

[5]Market activities are customarily gendered, and they are still primarily a woman's domain. Among the Lau, men catch the fish (or other seafood) for the women to sell or exchange for vegetables at "bush markets" (Maranda, "Mythe, métaphore, métamorphose et marches").

WORKS CITED

Akin, David. "Concealment, Confession, and Innovation in Kwaio Women's Taboos." *American Ethnologist* 30.3 (2003): 381-400. Print.

Akin, David. "Ancestral Vigilance and the Corrective Conscience: *Kastom* as Culture in a Melanesian Society." *Anthropological Theory* 4.3 (2004): 299-324. Print.

Akin, David. "*Kastom* as Hegemony? A Response to Babadzan." *Anthropological Theory* 5.1 (2005): 75-83. Print.

Akin, David. *Colonialism, Maasina Rule, and the Origins of Malaitan* Kastom. Honolulu: University of Hawai'i Press, 2013. Print.

Buchanan, Holly R. "A Living Pharmacy: The Practice of *Kastom* Medicine in Honiara." MA Thesis. Concordia University, Montreal, 1998. Print.

Burt, Ben. "*Kastom,* Christianity and the First Ancestor of the Kwara'ae of Malaita." *Mankind* 13.4 (1982): 374-399. Print.

Dureau, Christine M. "Mutual Goals? Family Planning on Simbo, Western Solomon Islands." *Borders of Being: Citizenship, Fertility, and Sexuality in Asia and the Pacific.* Eds. Margaret Jolly and Kalpana Ram. Ann Arbor: University of Michigan Press, 2001. 232-261. Print.

Guo, Pei-yi. "Law as Discourse: Land Disputes and the Changing Imagination of Relations among theLangalanga, Solomon Islands." *Pacific Studies* 34.2/3 (2011): 223-249. Print.

Jolly, Margaret. "Introduction: Birthing Beyond the Confinements of Tradition and Modernity?"*Birthing in the Pacific: Beyond Tradition and Modernity.* Eds. Vicki Lukere and Margaret Jolly. Honolulu: University of Hawai'i Press, 2002. 1-30. Print.

Keesing, Roger M. *Kwaio Religion: The Living and the Dead in a*

Solomon Island Society. New York:Columbia University Press, 1982. Print.

Köngäs Maranda, Elli. "Le femmes Lau—Malaita, îles Salomon—dans lèspace socialisé." *Journal dela Société des Océanistes* 27.26 (1970): 155-162. Print.

Maranda, Pierre. "Mapping Historical Transformation through the Canonical Formula: The Pagan vs.Christian Ontological Status of Women in Malaita, Solomon Islands." *The Double Twist: From Ethnography to Morphodynamics.* Ed. Pierre Maranda. Toronto: University of Toronto Press, 2001.97-121. Print.

Maranda, Pierre. "Mythe, métaphore, metamorphose et marches: l'igname chez les Lau de Malaita, îles Salomon." *Journal de la Société des Océanistes* 114-115 (2002): 91-114. Print.

Mowbray, Jemima. "'Ol meri bilong wok' [Hard-working women]: Women, Work and Domesticity inPapua New Guinea." *Divine Domesticities: Christian Paradoxes in Asia and the Pacific.* Eds. Hyaeweol Choi and Margaret Jolly. Canberra: Australian National University E Press, 2014. Web. 2 June 2015.

Ross, Harold M. *Baegu: Social and Ecological Organization in Malaita, Solomon Islands.* Urbana: University of Illinois Press, 1973. Print.

Strategic Asia. "Millennium Development Goals Progress for Solomon Islands 2010." UNDP, 2010. Web. 2 June 2015.

Timmer, Jaap. "Straightening the Path from the Ends of the Earth: The Deep Sea Canoe Movement in Solomon Islands." *Flows of Faith: Religious Reach and Community in Asia and the Pacific.* Eds. Lenore Manderson, Wendy Smith and Matt Tomlinson. London: Springer, 2012. 201-214. Print.

Wardlow, Holly. *Wayward Women: Sexuality and Agency in a New Guinea Society.* Berkeley: University of California Press, 2006. Print.

World Health Organization (WHO). "Solomon Islands: Maternal and Perinatal Health Profile. Department of Maternal, Newborn, Child and Adolescent Health (MCA/WHO)." WHO, 2014. Web. 2 June 2015.

5.
Maternal Health (In)Equity in Mursi (Mun), Southern Ethiopia

Behind the Hype of "Harmful Cultural Practices"

SHAUNA LATOSKY

> Merging the traditional and the western medical system needs to be approached carefully, but the two can co-exist and complement each other in order to improve maternal health in Mursiland. (Baumann 4)

ETHIOPIA HAS ONE OF THE HIGHEST mortality rates associated with pregnancy and parturition (giving birth) in the world. In 2011, maternal deaths were at 676 deaths per 100,000 births (CSA, *Ethiopian Demographic Health Survey*).[1] An estimated 85 percent of all maternal deaths in Ethiopia are due to obstructed labour, obstetric haemorrhage, infection, abortion complications, pre-eclampsia or eclampsia, along with HIV/AIDS and malaria (FMOH). Despite global, national, and local maternal health initiatives, which are aimed at meeting Millennium Development Goal 5 on maternal health, death during childbirth is still unacceptably high in Ethiopia. This is especially the case in pastoralist and agro-pastoralist areas like the South Omo Zone, Southern Ethiopia. For the Mursi (Mun)[2], an agro-pastoralist people living in the Sala-Mago district of South Omo, maternal-newborn mortality is one of the most significant problems affecting Mursi women today (Baumann). With a population of roughly 10,000 people, and with only a few health facilities in their area, the percentage of infant deaths out of 303 births is roughly 35 percent (Kuhley, *Mursi Health Program* 6). Due to poor public transportation, poor communications, and fears associated with high hospital fees and culturally incompatible care, Mursi women in need of emergency or operative intervention still have no reliable access to emergency obstetric care (EmOC).[3] As the public health literature on maternal health already suggests, a large proportion of maternal deaths could be prevented "through timely interventions that have proven to be effective and affordable" (Austin et al. 1-2; Jackson and Yaliso et al.).

Very little analysis, however, has been carried out to follow up why maternal health programs fail to adequately address maternal-newborn health on the ground, especially in agro-pastoralist areas of Southern Ethiopia. In this chapter, I begin by critically engaging with the rhetoric of "harmful cultural practices" in South Omo and argue that beneath the "harmful cultural practices" hype are the neglected maternal health needs of Mursi women (LaTosky, "Lip-Plates, 'Harm' Debates"). More specifically, my aim is to provide insights into the deep dysfunction that continues to plague access to health care, despite "accelerated solutions" (FMOF) in Mursi—and other agro-pastoralist communities—and large donor investments in South Omo over the last decade. I conclude that no amount of international funding for maternal health care services in South Omo will bring change unless future efforts focus on gaining a more complete understanding of the contexts of agro-pastoralist women's lives (e.g., their parturition practices, and the health priorities that women themselves identify) and unless the onus is put on donors and development partners to follow-up *if* and *how* maternal health services are being implemented.

THE MILLENNIUM DEVELOPMENT GOAL ACCELERATION FRAMEWORK (MAF): AN ACTION PLAN FOR REDUCING MATERNAL MORTALITY AND MORBIDITY IN PASTORALIST AREAS

The Federal Ministry of Health (FMOH) confirmed that insufficient progress had been made over the last decade in achieving the fifth Millennium Development Goal (MGD 5) to reduce maternal mortality (FMOH 15). In response, the MGD Acceleration Framework (MAF), endorsed by the United Nations Development Group, was developed and implemented by the FMOH as an action plan that would "concentrate resources and interventions in communities where maternal deaths are high" (12). These priority intervention areas include the four emerging region states (Afar Regional State, Benishangul-Gumuz Regional State, Gambela Regional State, Somali Regional State) and "pastoral community zones" in Oromia Regional State, and Southern Nations, Nationalities, and Regional State (SNNPR). As described by the FMOH,

> This Action Plan, developed specifically for pastoralist communities, complements the national roadmap on maternal health and seeks to operationalize implementation of interventions tailored to specific contexts of pastoralist communities in Ethiopia. (18)

The FMOH has recognized "the lack of an appropriate health service package for pastoralist communities and the need to develop a viable strategy for delivery" (35-36).[4] According to the "MAF Plan of Action" for pastoralist community zones in SNNPR 2012/2013 to 2015/2016 (84-88; see Appendix A for full text), the following "Priority Interventions" have been included as having the highest priority in pastoralist communities[5]:

> Enhance skilled birth attendance (SBA)
> Improve emergency obstetric care (EmONC)
> Improve antenatal care (ANC)
> Enhance family planning services (FPS)
> Promote maternal health education, awareness, and advocacy
> Strengthen infrastructure and partnership.

Although the Action Plan seems promising, no guidelines or suggestions yet exist as to how, when, and with whom these "priority interventions" and "accelerated solutions" are being or will "be tailored to the specific contexts of pastoralist communities" (FMOH 18). Effective strategies for tailoring the MGD Accelerated Framework to the diverse cultural contexts of pastoralists and agro-pastoralists (from Afar and Borana to Bodi and Mursi) will include understanding traditional beliefs and practices around giving birth, engaging with women about their experiences of both traditional and modern maternal health care, and learning how

EmOC services could be made to be more culturally compatible. Inge Baumann's research (*Indigenous Childbirth*), conducted under the auspices of Serving in Mission (SIM) and the Ethiopian Federal Ministry of Health (FMOH), is an excellent example of how health research can contribute to tailoring action plans to meet the needs of agro-pastoralist communities.[6] Within the Mursi context, for example, a key strategy to reducing maternal mortality in Mursi, as Baumann suggests, is to understand the practices of traditional birth attendants (TBAs) and to provide training for them:

> Generally when thinking about the content of the training for Mursi TBAs, their belief system and the way of looking at the wholeness of human beings, health and disease needs to be taken in account. The trainers have to be aware that approaching the training with a western medical worldview might not be understood and applicable for the Mursi context. It is advised that, before designing the programme further, research should be carried out on the belief system. (Baumann 63)

Although Baumann's research makes clear the necessity of culturally appropriate strategies for improving maternal health in Mursi (see, also, LaTosky, *Predicaments of Mursi Women*), there is a growing trend in South Omo to prioritize campaigns against traditional "harmful cultural practices," often at the expense of priority interventions, such as those outlined in the MGD Accelerated Framework (MAF). Most programs and research on maternal health in South Omo include "harmful cultural practices" as part of their agenda but rarely do they contextualize them or differentiate between levels of risk or include statistical data to indicate their potential harm. Moreover, the direct correlation between certain "harmful cultural practices" (HCPs) and maternal health in pastoralist communities is often unclear. For example, it is generally assumed that early marriage, abduction, tonsillectomy, lip-plates, milk teeth extraction, uvulectomy, prelacteal feeding,[7] postpartum seclusion, and so on, "may have a direct or indirect effect on maternal and newborn health" (Berhan and Berhan 125), yet the correlation seldom is made clear, let alone verified with empirical evidence.[8] Whereas the eradication of "harmful cultural practices" is not listed anywhere in the MAF as a "priority intervention" to reduce maternal mortality in pastoralist communities, "harmful cultural practices" campaigns are plentiful in Mursi and South Omo in general and obscure the many practical and cost-effective solutions that could accelerate improvements in maternal health (LaTosky, "Lip-Plates, 'Harm' Debates").

THE HYPE OF "HARMFUL CULTURAL PRACTICES" AT THE EXPENSE OF EMERGENCY OBSTETRICAL CARE

AMREF [African Medical Research Foundation] has become synonymous with "sewing women's lips," not with "saving women's lives." (Olisarali and Milisha Olibui, Personal interview)

The government of Ethiopia manages 42 percent of health sector spending, whereas the majority of health sector resources are financed and already earmarked by donors (WHO, "Comprehensive Analytical Profile: Ethiopia"). Between 2011 and 2012, ETB 7.63 billion was spent on the health sector in Ethiopia, a number that is estimated to increase to ETB 13.89 billion (roughly USD 68 million) in 2014–2015 (FMOH 15). Since 2007, for example, the African Medical and Research Foundation (AMREF) alone has spent millions of donor dollars (especially from Canada, USA, and UK) on maternal health programs in the South Omo Zone[9] of Southern Nations Nationalities and Regional State (SNNPR).[10] For example, the estimated annual budget for South Omo in 2008 was USD 1.68 million (AMREF). The aim of AMREF's interventions in South Omo has been to implement community outreach services, improve the skills of health extension workers (HEWs),[11] raise women's awareness of child health services, and improve transportation services to get women in need of emergency obstetrical care to deliver in hospitals. However, the experiences of Mursi women and local health workers show that AMREF's maternal and newborn health programs have not yielded improvements in maternal health outcomes in the Sala-Mago district.[12] During my fieldwork in 2014, Mursi women (and men) reported that the only influence felt by AMREF was its campaigns to eradicate "harmful cultural practices" like the wearing of lip-plates by Mursi women and adolescent girls. As I explain elsewhere:

> AMREF's work on reconstructive surgery of Mursi women's lips appears to be beneficial to some women, but, their "project in focus" ("Project in Focus") misuses medical information in two ways: First and foremost, it underrates the real medical needs of the Mursi. AMREF's rhetoric about the harmfulness of lip-plates overshadows the real life-threatening concerns of Mursi women today. Secondly, the exaggerated focus on lip-plates, which quickly loses credibility in the light of the experiences and existing knowledge about lip-plates shared by Mursi women, does not support the claim that grave health consequences await girls and women.
>
> (...)
>
> During recent conversations with Mursi women in Maregge about how they [the Mursi] prioritize health risks for women, lip-plates were never mentioned, whereas maternal and infant health were considered top priorities. Among the most harmful and potentially life-threatening diseases affecting Mursi women and children today, they included: malaria, pneumonia, typhoid, diarrhoea, meningitis and tuberculosis. Milisha Olibui, the only trained Mursi health practitioner, added HIV/AIDS to this list and explained that, "if NGOs like AMREF were to prioritize harm in Mursi, to improve projects in pastoralist areas, in Mursi this would require an ambulance, mobile clinics and locally trained Mursi health workers to reach the most remote areas in Mursi." As he continued "So far, AMREF has done a good job of improving the clinic in Hana (Bodi), and although it continues to help in Meganto, supplies and staff are never there. The only reliable clinic in Mursi today is still [the mission clinic] in Mako, otherwise we must get patients to the Jinka hospital, which is almost impossible in emergency situations" (LaTosky, "Lip-Plates, 'Harm' Debates 183-184).

The government of Canada's Muskoka Initiative (a commitment to improving maternal, newborn and child health issues [MNCH]) and the Canadian International Development Agency (CIDA) have donated several million dollars (from 2012 to 2014) to focus on MNCH in South Omo, "with activities encompassing things such as training for Health Extension Workers, the mobilization of community members for Community Conversations outreach and the provision of key material supports, for example, three ambulances are being deployed to the program area" (Carmichael, E-mail to the author). However, despite a decade-long request from the Mursi for free ambulance service in their area at the time of writing, transportation had only been offered to Mursi women who accepted a small payment from AMREF to have their stretched lower lips stitched (LaTosky, *Predicaments of Mursi Women*; "Lip-Plates, 'Harm' Debates"). One Mursi woman who had recently delivered her third set of twins explained that she might have agreed to go with the other women who had their lips sewn if it meant also taking her son with her to be treated at the hospital. She further explained that if only she had access to a hospital during her second delivery of twins, they both would have survived (see Figure 1 below). The biggest inequity for Mursi women is that despite significant funding from AMREF Canada, for the purchase of three ambulances for South Omo, the delivery and distribution of basic transportation services remains unevenly distributed. For instance, to date, no ambulance service is available for the Mursi in the Sala-Mago district, yet ambulances are being made available to new government employees and migrant labourers flowing into Mursiland to work in the newly state-run sugarcane factories and plantations along the Omo River in Sala-Mago. In short, nothing has changed for Mursi women who most need the service in order to access EmOC care, which is only available in Jinka.

JINKA ZONAL HOSPITAL

The Jinka Zonal Hospital is the closest hospital (roughly forty-five kilometres away) that can provide Mursi women with emergency obstetric care (EmOC). The hospital in Jinka has many of the same problems that plague other health care facilities in rural areas of

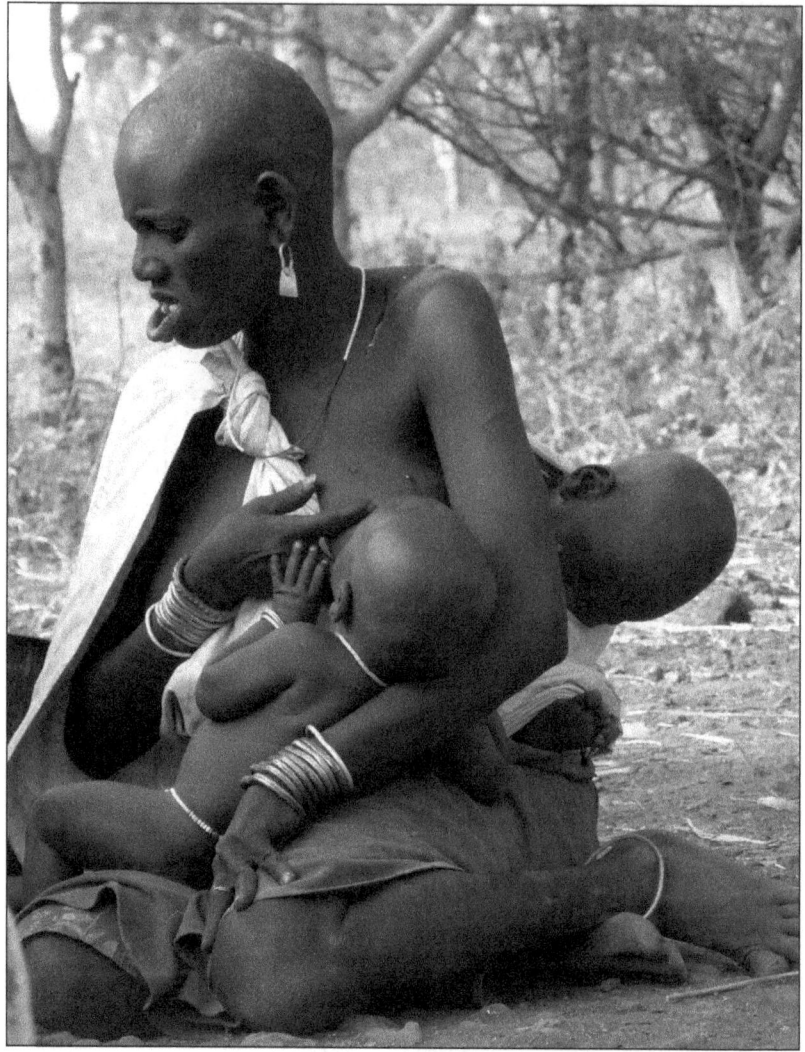

Fig. 1: Mursi woman after delivering her third set of twins in 2014.
Photo ©S. LaTosky, 2015.

Ethiopia: a shortage of qualified staff, a shortage of obstetric care equipment due to budget deficits, and poor management. As a result, the hospital has relied on the Norwegian Lutheran Mission to overcome the labour shortage by inviting surgeons, obstetricians, and midwives to run the obstetric and surgical ward and to help train local staff members in EmOC. Some stay for periods of months, and some surgeons have stayed on for years or have returned for subsequent terms. The Norwegian Lutheran Mission has done an excellent service over the years, but emergency obstetric care still suffers from overcrowding, lack of funding, and material and staff shortages, despite efforts to place volunteer medical staff (e.g., neonatal nurses). The next hospital is in Arba Minch, which is three hundred kilometres north of Jinka.[13]

COMMUNICATION PROBLEMS AND CULTURALLY INCOMPATIBLE CARE

Most Mursi women who arrive in Jinka are high-risk patients who had not attended any antenatal services and arrive at the hospital in labour in extremis (Milisha Olibui, Personal interview). In 2009, I experienced first-hand what it is like for a Mursi woman by the name of Hoitigolinyi to arrive at the Jinka hospital in labour.[14]

> We were only one kilometre from the hospital when she looked up and told me that the baby was on its way. I yelled at Gallo to stop the car and saw the head crowning. Cupping it carefully, a baby girl slipped into my hands.... I ran to get a nurse to cut the umbilical cord.
>
> When the doctor arrived, I explained to him that it was taboo in Mursi for men to see women's private parts. He assured me that he would try to make it comfortable for her. I asked for a sheet for her legs but instead, the nurse brought a small cotton cloth with which I tried to keep her covered. The swinging doors into the hallway of the maternity ward opened and closed, exposing us to the curious eyes of those walking by. I explained to her that she would need a few stitches. She was scared and resisted opening her legs. She began to tremble and the nurses became impatient as she continued to resist. One became rough and rammed her legs wide open. I squeezed her hand and could feel her pain and the utter helplessness, as the two other nurses held her down on the table. It was all over within seconds but traumatic nonetheless. She wanted nothing more to do with this place. When the nurse insisted that she should have the obligatory HIV/AIDS

test, Olisarali (her husband) refused. Nobody wanted to be there a minute longer in the crowded room with women from Hamar, Ari and Maale. (LaTosky, *Predicaments of Mursi Women* 228)

Shortly after Hoitigolonyi delivered a healthy baby girl, I visited one of the surgeons from the Norwegian Lutheran Mission to exchange insights regarding the culturally incompatible care that Mursi women experience (e.g, lying down to deliver, opening one's legs, exposing one's body to male birth attendants, etc.) and to address communication challenges that extended beyond language to cultural and economic factors—from burying the placenta in Mursi and food preferences to paying for hospital fees and transportation to get home (Baumann). The surgeon explained that the hospital was working closely with the mission clinic in Mako, which had already made recommendations to have local Mursi translators and TBAs accompany women to the hospital and to help teach health care workers a few skills necessary to facilitate culturally appropriate care. Furthermore, it provided a car service whenever possible for women requiring emergency obstetrical care (sometimes for a small fee, which could be paid at a later date). These were in line with recommendations that public health researcher Baumann made in her research on designing culturally appropriate training for Mursi traditional birth attendants. As Baumann suggests, "it should be the responsibility of the SI Mission health programme to advocate for the provision of expansion of maternal health services for the Mursi" (66). Although the volunteer program was eventually phased out, when the Norwegian doctors who had taken it up returned to Norway,[15] the SIM clinic has continued to make significant strides towards improving maternal and newborn health in Mursi, despite the numerous challenges it has faced over the years (LaTosky, "Predicaments of Mursi Women" 226).

HEALTH POSTS IN MURSI

Serving in Mission opened the first remote health post in Mako (also called Makki), Northern Mursiland in 1999. Since its establishment, one health post has been built in Meganto, Mursiland in 2008[16] and in 2013, a new health post was built for migrant labourers in Romo, Mursiland. Although the Romo health post was built primarily to serve the growing number of sugar plantation workers, it also provides basic health services to Mursi patients. As I observed in 2014, overall, the clinic was marked by the poor quality of care provided by inadequately trained staff, by poor financial management (e.g., no receipts were issued to patients) and by culturally inappropriate treatment (e.g., drugs administered without the patient's clear understanding of how to use them).[17] As with the health post in Meganto, the Romo health post has increasingly been met with suspicion by the Mursi. In 2014, I wrote the following in my journal after visiting the new health post:

> In Romo, a lowland area in Mursiland, there is one corrugated shack along the main road to Omo that has become the only clinic to serve the hundreds of migrant sugarcane plantation workers that have taken up residence there since 2012. The clinic also serves Mursi and some Bodi and Suri who live in Bodi. During my second visit to the clinic, I heard the cries of a young girl in the back room where most patients stand to get their penicillin shots, which are given out like candies here for a flat rate of ETB 100. The young girl had miscarried and almost died of an infection that she developed shortly after. She was on IV antibiotics and her family was there to give her the traditional *shalu* (gruel) for post-partum women. When her father was told the amount he would have to pay, he had the same look on his face as a father in America, whose health insurance would not cover a 5000-dollar chemotherapy dose to try and save his daughter's life. He turned to me and asked if I could give him ETB 400 of the 600 needed to cover her treatment. The heavy reality in the room was plastered all over the walls. Posters bearing signs with hearts and slogans in English and Amharic on how to prevent HIV/AIDS were already peeling away at the corners. A young man from northern Ethiopia sat cupping the bleeding gash close to his eye as the result of a stone that fell from one of the

trucks delivering rocks to one of the sugar cane factories near the Omo. A young girl from Arba Minch, who wore skinny jeans (that my female friends from Mursi found too revealing) came from the local bar where she worked as a hostess, complaining of a headache. Both of the migrant workers were given priority over the Mursi and Bodi patients who clearly share the burden of fast-track development in South Omo. (Field journal, Romo, 20 July 2014)

In remote areas like Romo, there is very little oversight and control by the FMOH, let alone international donors in charge of funding basic health services. Mursi women's experiences and my own observations suggest that new health posts, such as the one in Romo, are not the answer to addressing deficits in maternal health care so long as emergency obstetric care is not available

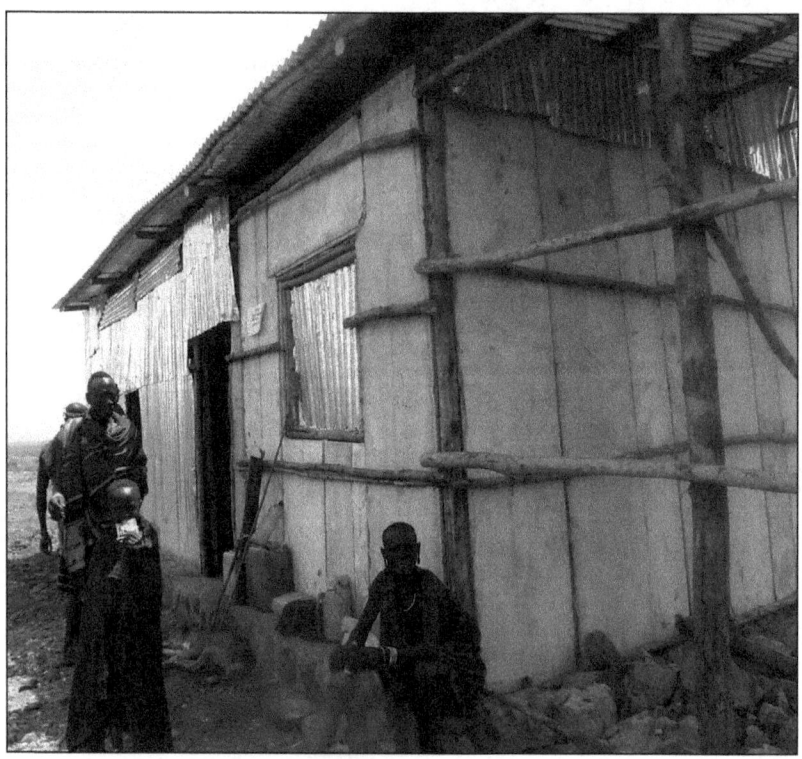

Fig. 2: New health post in Romo, Mursiland.
Photo ©S. LaTosky, 2014.

and so long as the quality of care, clinical skills, and management remain poor (see Figure 2).

The SIM clinic in Mako has proven to be the most reliable over the years and remains the only clinic where basic antenatal care (ANC) is available.[18] The budget for the clinic is low (approximately USD 12,500 per year)[19] but highly effective. The SIM clinic has earned a reputation for being committed to maternal and newborn health issues, which is in line with the Ethiopian government's MGD 5 agenda and its more recent "MGD Accelerated Framework." However, very little has been done to formally acknowledge or reward their efforts, which include training Mursi to become health workers, educating, and training women (and men) about the importance of antenatal and postnatal checks, informal training for TBAs, assisting Mursi women to seek emergency obstetric care, making them aware of the "waiting maternity home" at the Jinka hospital, motivating TBAs (and translators) to accompany mothers with life-threatening complications to the hospital, implementing mobile vaccinations programs, HIV awareness, and voluntary counselling and testing (Kuhley, *HIV/AIDS Survey in Mursi*). Although this is a single example of one site in Mursi, the intervention not only has been cost-effective but has also had a positive impact on raising awareness in the area of maternal morbidity and mortality. During a two-year period, for example, 240 pregnant women who visited the clinic received at least one antenatal check-up, while 76 women received at least one postnatal check-up and a total of 7 women received assistance to deliver (Kuhley, *Makki Health Program 2008/2009)*. At the clinic in Mako, where I volunteered for several days in 2006, there was a general attitude of respect towards women and an understanding that for Mursi women, parturition is perceived as a normal practice that a woman should perform at home. Often recommendations were given to women and TBAs as to how parturition can be made safer at home. This requires first and foremost an in-depth understanding of traditional Mursi birthing practices, which I discuss briefly in the next section.

The different examples of health care facilities in Mursi indicate that "increasing the access to and utilization of facility-based maternal care alone does not necessarily translate into maternal outcomes" (Austin et al. 2). SIM's commitment and involvement in maternal and newborn health is, however, so far unprecedented in Mursi. Instead of concentrating on "harmful cultural practices," charging Mursi women high fees, or providing care that is culturally incompatible and quite often disrespectful, maternal and newborn health care has been at the heart of the SIM's work. Moreover, SIM operates with a budget that is a mere drop in the bucket compared to the millions of dollars of donor money that has reached South Omo, via AMREF and other government and non-government organizations, who, so far, have had little impact on meeting the urgent needs of agro-pastoralist women in the Sala-Mago district.

TAILORING THE MGD ACCELERATED FRAMEWORK TO THE MURSI CONTEXT

Most Mursi women in life-threatening situations often still have ambiguous feelings towards a hospital birth, as Hoitigolonyi's experience shows. Mursi women prefer home birth to hospital birth and call on traditional birth attendants (TBAs) called *nyeria* (sing. *nyere*) when it is their first labour, or when labour is prolonged, or if there are signs of danger, such as a retained placenta or bleeding (Baumann). The position assumed during delivery at home is mostly kneeling and holding onto a tree, whereas in hospitals women have to lie on their backs and stretch their legs open, which they do not like to do, since it exposes their private bodies to birth attendants who are often male. As one *nyere* in Mako explains:

> All women have to give birth in the bush, before the child comes out we all go together with her to the bush ... because there the children and men cannot see us, and we need a tree, we have to find a strong tree and then the mother can grab the wood and give birth. (Baumann 45)

Most Mursi women do not receive postnatal check-ups in clinics or hospitals[20] and prefer the supportive care and traditional food that they get at home after they have given birth. A Mursi woman remains in her house by the fire for up to one month and is served gruel (*shalu*), which is high in vitamin A. During this time, other women grind for her and fetch her firewood, water, and even certain plants that when placed near the fire, act as a natural insect repellent. Yet some government organizations and NGOs refer to this period of postpartum seclusion (found in many agro-pastoralist groups) as "harmful" to women's health (Women's Affairs). The Mursi, on the other hand, see this as an essential time of rest that helps to maintain and promote the health and well-being of the mother and newborn child (LaTosky, *Predicaments* 230-231). During this time, a husband cannot have sexual relations with his wife and, typically, they will wait for at least two years before having another child. That is, Mursi women's traditional healing practices attend many of the potential postpartum complications—such as anaemia through the provision of vitamin A supplementation, family planning through postpartum sex taboos, and provision of insecticide to prevent malaria. Any program that plans to take seriously Mursi women's maternal health must also take traditional practices into account (see Figure 3 below), rather than assuming that traditional practices are harmful and will negatively affect health outcomes.

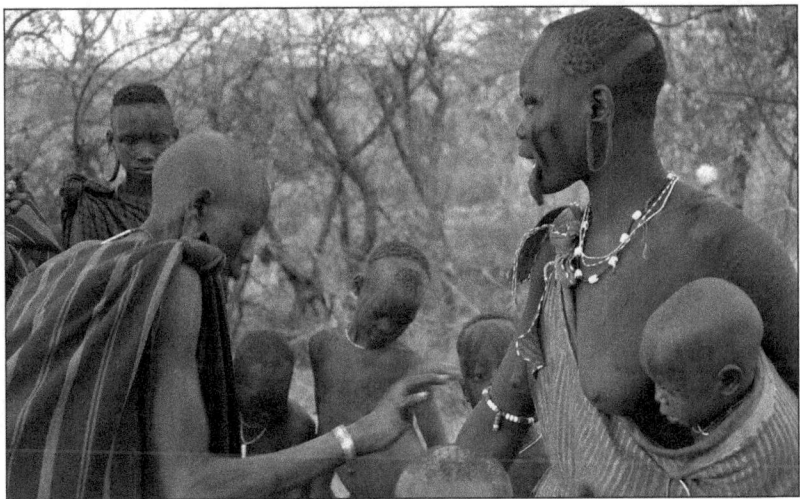

Fig. 3: Mursi healer applying special clays to ward off illness.
Photo ©S. LaTosky, 2014.

For example, Baumann's research is the only research to date that identifies traditional practices in Mursi that are beneficial to women and should be encouraged (e.g. support from TBAs, vertical birth position, herbal treatment for retained placenta, etc.). It is also the first study to make practical and concrete suggestions as to how indigenous practices might be improved—for example, antenatal care screening as part of TBA training, understanding the benefits of breastfeeding, not only to the child but also as a way to stimulate uterine contractions after delivery, or to reduce the chance of a newborn being fed cow's milk, since it is taboo to breastfeed so long as there is a retained placenta. Other suggestions include encouraging women to have tetanus toxoid injections in pregnancy, providing vaccinations after pregnancy, and ensuring that TBAs have razor blades (Baumann 58-61; LaTosky, *Predicaments* 226-227).

Baumann's study contextualizes both the favourable and less favourable aspects of the traditional system rather than placing the blame on "harmful cultural practices" officially listed and targeted by certain government and non-government organizations working in South Omo (59). For Sala-Mago district, the following "harmful cultural practices" have been listed: lip-piercing, postpartum seclusion, and cutting the belly of the mother, which is presumably referring to "fetonomy," since Caesarean practices are unknown among agro-pastoralists, such as the Bodi and Mursi[21] (Women's Affairs; LaTosky, *Predicaments of Mursi Women*). In contrast, according to the Mursi and researchers working on Mursi health, the most "harmful" issues facing women, which are also said to be the cause of most of the maternal deaths in Mursi, is a retained placenta (Baumann 47-48) and no reliable access to EmOC (LaTosky, "Lip-Plates, 'Harm' Debates").

In short, tailoring the Millennium Accelerated Framework to Mursi women's needs requires a commitment to understanding traditional childbirth practices and women's experiences at modern health care facilities. Although this paper does not claim to provide all the answers for what a tailored approach should look like, as a starting point, such an approach should add to MAF's "priority interventions," training for traditional birth attendants, who are also skilled birth attendants in their own right, as Baumann's research has already suggested. The Millennium Acceleration Framework could also tailor its "prioritized acceleration solutions" to the

Mursi context, for example, by supporting mobile health teams that would include locally trained Mursi health workers, by rewarding and learning from role models like the SI Mission for their good practices and promotion of maternal health in Mursi and, finally, by granting the Mursi their decade-long wish for free ambulance service for women in urgent need of emergency obstetric care.

CONCLUDING REMARKS

Improving Mursi women's maternal health and reducing the high maternal and infant mortality have been pencilled in to agendas but have not been a priority of the Federal Ministry of Health. The framework for accelerating the Millennium Development Goals has been a way of recognising that pastoralist communities continue to be neglected (FMOH). However, more ethnographic research is needed to clarify the factors that currently prevent international funding and strategic action plans from bringing sustainable change to the quality of maternal care for women in agro-pastoralist areas in Southern Ethiopia. As I have tried to show, programs must be adapted and embedded within the local context, as the SIM has effectively done over the last decade by focusing on the health priorities of Mursi women rather than the priorities or agendas of outsiders. Mursi women are not nearly as interested in having their lower lips sewn as they are in having equal opportunities to make choices about accessing emergency obstetric care.

ENDNOTES

[1] According to the 2011 national Ethiopian Demographic and Health Survey (EDHS), the 2011 Maternal Mortality Rate (MMR) has not changed from the 2005 MMR of 673/100,000 births. This controversial figure contrasts greatly with the World Bank data, which show a MMR of 350/100,000 births in 2011 (WHO, UNICEF, and UNFPA). The MDG goal for 2015 is 267/100,000 births (CSA and ICF International).

[2] "Mun" (sing. Muni) is a self-designation, whereas "Mursi" is the

name commonly used by outsiders and in the literature.

³An estimated 99 percent of Mursi women deliver at home with the help of traditional birth attendants (TBAs) (Milisha Olibui, Personal interview). Adequate records have been maintained at the Jinka Zonal Hospital and would provide a good source of information for accurate comparison later on. However, at the time of writing, no hospital data were available that show the number of Mursi women who use maternal health services, especially emergency obstetric care. This estimate is based on records made available from the clinic at the SIM mission in Mako, Mursiland.

⁴For the complete "MAF Plan of Action – Pastoralist Community Zones in SNNPR 2012/2013-2015/2016," see Annex 5 (FMOH 84).

⁵According to the FMOH, "pastoralists ... occupy 60 percent of the territory and constitute about 12 percent of the total population, making the country one of the most pastorally populous in Africa" (35).

⁶Since Baumann's research, no detailed assessment or analysis of maternal and newborn health in Mursi has been conducted, let alone one that includes women's experiences of maternal health programs (compare LaTosky, *Predicaments of Mursi Women*).

⁷Prelacteal feeding (feeding any other substance before first breastfeeding) is common in many parts of Ethiopia and is carried out for a number of different reasons.

⁸According to Berhan and Berhan, it is difficult to say whether or not, for example, the common practice of prelacteal feeding found throughout Ethiopia can be attributed to increased neonatal mortality rates rather than multiple factors (127). For maternal health and harmful cultural practices in Ari and Maale, see also Ergao et al., 116-7.

⁹South Omo Zone includes Sala-Mago, Hamer, Benna-Tsemay and Kuraz districts.

¹⁰AMREF's donor and co-funding donors in South Omo Zone include CIDA/AMREF Canada (CAD three million from 2012 to2014); ET–Ethiopian Delegation/ Band Aid, JOAC, GOAC, OPAL, AMREF NL (EURO 1,105,010 from 2008 to 2011); DFID (GBP 499, 954 from 2009 to 2012); Allan & Nesta Ferguson Charitable Trust Medicor Foundation (GBP 500,000 from 2007 to 2011) (AMREF "Original Project Proposal to DFID").

[11] In the Sala-Mago *woreda* alone, 20 percent of public basic service (PBS) money is said to be for health extension workers (WHO, *The Partnership* 22).

[12] Although Sala-Mago district is included in AMREF Canada's maternal health funding program for South Omo, most AMREF projects on community-based maternal health in South Omo focus on communities in South Ari and Maale districts (Ergano et al.), in which government representation is high; see Pastoralist Health Care Systems Strengthening Projects in South Ari and Mali (AMREF). It is important to note that to date, the Mursi still have no government representatives (e.g. member of parliament).

[13] Another clinic is in Hana, approximately ninety kilometres from Mursi; however, emergency obstetric care is not available.

[14] Most women arrive in Jinka without anyone who can speak Mursi or who can translate for them, although young Mursi girls and boys at the boarding schools are sometimes called on to assist.

[15] At that time (2009), only two Mursi who could speak fluent English, and only a handful more could speak Amharic. This made the translation project difficult to sustain, especially since there was no budget to pay translators (or TBAs).

[16] The health post in Meganto is considered by the majority of Mursi to provide inadequate and unreliable care, which is common in remote pastoral areas like South Omo (Ergao et al. 112).

[17] One suggestion that I made to the health assistants, for example, was to visit the SIM clinic to understand how they administer drugs to a largely non-literate population (e.g. using sun-moon symbols to explain dosages).

[18] During interviews with Mursi women in need of antenatal care in Maregge in July 2014, women still preferred to walk to the clinic in Mako (a one-day walk) than to visit the health post in Meganto (a one hour walk), which often had a shortage of supplies and where women said there was a low trust in the abilities of the health extension workers.

[19] According to one SIM quarterly report, a total budget of ETB 566,990 (roughly USD 25,000) was raised for a two-year project period 2008 to 2010 (Kuhley, *Makki Health Program 2008/2009*). The missionaries themselves raised a significant proportion of this budget.

[20]Ergao et al. claim that most community-based health care services in rural Ethiopia provide ANC service, basic medicines, and so forth free of charge; however, this has not been the experience of Mursi women in South Omo (14).

[21]In the event of fetal death in utero, fetonomy is sometimes carried out by a male expert. Although fetonomy is only indirectly labelled as a "harmful cultural practice," ironically, it is the last possible resort to try and save a woman's life when no other possibility exists (Baumann 47; LaTosky, *Predicaments of Mursi* 227). No statistics exist on the number of women whose lives have been saved by this procedure.

Appendix A: "MAF Plan of Action – Pastoralist Community Zones in SNNPR 2012/2013-2015/2016" (FMOH 84-88)

Priority Intervention	Prioritized Acceleration Solutions
Enhance Skilled Birth Attendance (SBA)	1. Encourage HEWs [Health Extension Workers] to send pregnant women to health centres/hospitals for delivery, and immediately refer them when danger signs become apparent
	2. Support the establishment of cost-effective and culturally sensitive maternity waiting homes/centres close to HCs [Health Centres]/hospitals
	3. Support the establishment and operation of an effective mentoring system for new graduate HWs [health workers]
Improve Emergency Obstetric Care (EmONC)	1. Make the health facilities (HCs and hospitals) fully ready and accelerate the placement of BEmONC [Basic Emergency Obstetric and Newborn Care] and CEmONC [Comprehensive Emergency Obstetric and Newborn Care] services in hospitals
	2. Avail appropriate means of transport/ambulance service
	3. Introduce the use of mobile call service for seeking help and info
	4. Advocate, promote and implement EmONC [Emergency Obstetric and Newborn Care] and free maternal health services at all levels of HFs [Health Facilities]

Improve Antenatal Care (ANC)	1. Recruit more mature female HEWs to deliver ANC [Ante Natal Care] and other maternal health services
	2. Prioritize provision of ANC in the HEP [Health Extension Program]; provide essential supplies and make health care provision user/mother-friendly
	3. Support establishment and operation of mobile health teams (avail camel, solar power, refrigerator, tent, etc.)
	4. Establish a reward and sanction mechanism for performance of health personnel
	5. Strengthen user feedback systems for performance
Enhance Family Planning Services (FPS)	1. Conduct intensive advocacy targeting religious leaders, elders and political leaders so that they openly promote and support the use of FP [Family Planning] methods
	2. Provide specific skill training for nurses in contraceptive methods, especially LAPMs [Long-Acting and Permanent Methods
	3. Avail comprehensive FP services in health facilities and strengthen the supply chain
Promote Matenal Health Education, Awareness, and Advocacy	1. Develop IEC strategy specific to localities to enhance timely health-care-seeking behaviour
	2. Create community awareness about the benefit of skilled attendants at delivery
	3. Enhance the awareness of men, women, and community about the risk, need, and availability of EmONC and FP services
	4. Promote advocacy for the use of FP among community religious and political leaders and youth
	5. Reward role models for their good practices and promotion of maternal health
	6. Raise awareness about maternal health through regional mass media, including the educational mass media, CC, "folk" media and facility-based health education
	7. Ensure home visits by HEWs during pregnancy and postnatal period and mentoring by peer mother groups and model mothers
	8. Mobilize community, traditional, and religious leaders to increase demand for ANC, SBA [Skilled Birth Attendant], PNC [Prenatal Care], FU [Follow up] and EmONC
	9. Work closely with religious leaders for integration of maternal health into religious teachings
	10. Promote and strengthen sharing of experience among regional actors and service providers

WORKS CITED

African Medical and Research Foundation (AMREF). "Annual Programme Performance Synopsis." Hawassa, Ethiopia. 2008. Print.

African Medical and Research Foundation. "Project in Focus: Reconstructive Surgery for the Most Remote Communities." *AMREF News*. 2011. Print.

African Medical and Research Foundation. "Original Project Proposal to DFID." *DFID GPAF Impact Proposal Form (for Round 2)*. *Amref Health Africa*, 10 Jan. 2012. Web. 4 March 2015.

Austin, Anne, Ana Langer, Rehana A. Salam, Zohra S. Lassi, Jai K. Das, Zulfiqar A. Bhutta. "Approaches to Improve the Quality of Maternal and Newborn Health Care: An Overview of the Evidence. *Reproductive Health* 11.2 (2014): n.pag. Web. L 1 March 2015.

Baumann, Inge. *Indigenous Childbirth: Towards a Strategy for the Design of Culturally Appropriate Training for Mursi Traditional Birth Attendants in Ethiopia*. MCommH, University of Liverpool, 2011. Print.

Berhan, Yifru and Asres Berhan. "Reasons for Persistently High Maternal and Perinatal Mortalities in Ethiopia: Part II—Socioeconomic and Cultural Factors. *Ethiopian Journal of Health Science* 24 (2014): 119-136. Web. 13 Aug. 2015.

Carmichael, Todd, AMREF Canada Director. Message to the author. 27 Feb. 2014. E-mail.

Central Statistical Agency Ethiopia (CSA) and ICF International. *Ethiopia Demographic and Health Survey 2011*. USAID, 2013. Web. 15 March 2014.

Federal Ministry of Health (FMOH). *MDG Acceleration Framework (Ethiopia). Accelerated Action Plan for Reducing Maternal Mortality. Federal Ministry of Health and UN in Ethiopia. United Nations Development* Programme, UNDP, 2014. Web. 15 March 2014.

Ergao, Kebebe, Medhanit Getachew, Dawit Seyum, Kassahun Negash. "Determinants of Community Based Maternal Health Care Service Utilization in South Omo Pastoral Areas of Ethiopia." *Journal of Medicine and Medical Services* 3.2 (2012):112-121. Print.

Kuhley, Thomas. *Mursi Health Program: Data, Survey, and Information*. Mursi Health Station, Makki: SIM Ethiopia. 2002. Print.

Kuhley, Thomas. *Mursi Health Program: Physical Accomplishment Report 2008/2009*. Mursi Health Station, Makki: SIM Ethiopia, 2009. Print.

Kuhley, Thomas. *HIV/AIDS Survey in Mursi*. Mursi Health Station, Makki: SIM Ethiopia, 2009. Print.

Jackson R. *The Three Delays as a Framework for Examining Safe Motherhood in Kafa Zone, SNNPR, Ethiopia*. Ph.D. dissertation, Deakin University, Australia, Addis Ababa University, Ethiopia, November 2007. Print.

LaTosky, Shauna. *Predicaments of Mursi Women in Ethiopia's Changing World*. Cologne: Koeppe Verlag. 2013. Print.

LaTosky, Shauna. "Lip-Plates, 'Harm' Debates, and the Cultural Rights of Mursi (Mun) Women." *Interrogating Harmful Cultural Practices. Gender, Culture and Coercion*. Eds. Chia Longman and Tamsin Bradley. Surrey: Ashgate, 2015.169-191. Print.

Serving in Mission. "Makki Health Program." SIM. 2015. Web. 20 Feb. 2015.

Olisarali and Milisha Olibui. Personal interview. February-July 2014.

WHO, UNICEF, UNFPA. "World Bank Trends in Maternal Mortality 1990–2010: WHO, UNICEF, UNFPA and the World Bank Estimates." Geneva: WHO. 2012. Print.

Women's Affairs Office. "Traditional Harmful Practices". Trans. Sophia Thubauville. South Omo Zone. Women's Affairs Office, 2009. Print.

World Health Organization (WHO). "Comprehensive Analytical Profile: Ethiopia." WHO, 2014. Web. March 2014.

World Health Organization (WHO). *The Partnership for Maternal, Newborn and Child Health*. Geneva, Switzerland: World Health Organization. 2011. Print.

Yaya, Yaliso, Kristiane Tislevoll Eide, Ole Frithjof Norheim, Bernt Lindtjørn. Maternal and Neonatal Mortality in South-West Ethiopia: Estimates and Socio-Economic Inequality. *PLOS ONE* 9.4 (2014): 1-12. Print.

6.
Maternal Health Services Miss the Mark

An Ethnographic Case Study in Rural Ghana

VIDA NYAGRE YAKONG AND NAOMI M. MCPHERSON

THE CONCEPT OF "PRIMARY HEALTH CARE" (PHC) was introduced at the 1978 Alma Ata Conference as a means for achieving health for all in resource-poor nations by the year 2000 (Hall and Taylor; Fendall). The main purpose of the PHC concept was to make essential health care available, accessible, affordable, and culturally acceptable to individuals and families, regardless of individual social position. Theoretically, strong emphasis was placed on full community participation and respect for indigenous knowledge. Provision of services was proposed to be based on sound scientific and practical methodologies acceptable to all stakeholders of health. Not surprisingly, the year 2000 passed without the much expected goals achieved, just as the MDG goals are not being met in 2015. Access to health care for all failed to take place because the majority of people residing in "challenging contexts" (Crichton), particularly those in rural settings, still have limited access to basic health care. After three decades of primary health care, maternal and infant mortality rates are on the increase in most resource-poor nations (UNICEF; WHO; WHO, UNFPA, and The World Bank).

HEALTH CARE REFORMS AND SERVICE DELIVERY

The introduction of PHC resulted in health care restructuring, new initiatives, programs, and policy developments and implementations in sub-Saharan Africa and across the globe that aimed to increase access to basic health care for the majority of citizens

(Awoonor-Williamsa et al.). Based on the realization that PHC was not realizing the goals of maternal health, especially in community-based health planning and service (CHPS), new initiatives aimed at reorienting health care with more community level involvement were introduced. Some of the key initiatives were designed to improve basic and maternal health care access and were specifically aimed at bringing general and reproductive health care closer to rural residents.

In Ghana, for example, the CHPS concept is viewed as one of the best ways to make health care more accessible to rural peoples. However, despite the strategic and concerted efforts within various health care systems and the implementation of these new initiatives, health care disparity remains a significant challenge across Africa and other challenging contexts nations, which share the highest percentage of the global disease burden, with specific reference to reproductive health care (UNICEF; Davis et al.). Although all governments and nations have committed to playing a significant role in achieving these goals for reproductive health care, recent studies from 181 countries across the globe show that reproductive health care and maternal and infant morbidity and mortality ratios still remain a major challenge to most health care systems in resource-constrained nations; most significantly affected are sub-Saharan Africa and some parts of Asia and Latin America, despite the declaration of the United Nations' Millennium Development Goal 5 (MDG) to address such specific maternal health related issues (Davis et al.; Hogan et al.; Maine and Rosenfield).

WOMEN'S PERSPECTIVES ON FACTORS AFFECTING ACCESS TO SERVICES

Access to general and reproductive health care in resource-poor nations remains a challenge, despite the existence of health care facilities, a perceived reorientation of health service delivery, and the concerted efforts of local health care systems to increase access in many countries (Wogaing, this volume; Gage; Simkhada et. al.; Yakong et al.). Several studies have attributed the lack of or limited access to maternal and reproductive health care to a number of issues ranging from physical or geographical location, and socio-economic and socio-cultural factors to maternal age and marital status, religion and belief systems, and health care system factors (McPherson, "Modern Obstertics"; "Women, Childbirth and Change;" Yakong et al.). Although efforts have been made to improve some of these factors over the past decades, many studies, such as those included in this volume, suggest that not much has been achieved and that change has been slow. Based on Yakong's life experience in Ghana, her ethnographic field research in the Talensi-Nabdam region of northern Ghana, and her experience as a nurse, we discuss some of the issues faced by rural Ghanaian women accessing general health and maternal health care services.

THE ETHNOGRAPHIC SETTING

In rural Ghana, geographical access remains a major challenge affecting health care access. In 1990, well over 70 percent of Ghanaians lived over eight kilometres from the closest health care facility, a distance considered too far by health care standards (Gabrysch and Campbell; Nyonator et al.). Apart from the long travel distance, which prevents the majority of women from accessing health care, other complicating factors include the non-availability or the high cost of transportation, the poor quality road network linking towns to rural settings—compounded by seasonal flooding limiting access to the already-existing poor roads—and the dispersed rural settlements common in rural Ghana in particular (Ghana Ministry, *Vision 2020*; Nyonator et al.; Yakong et al.). Women who live in the study area as well as midwives working in rural communities stated that distance, poor roads, and unreliable transportation negatively affect their access to service delivery at different stages in their reproductive lives, including prenatal care, labour and delivery, and postnatal care.[1]

There are a number of health care facilities in the Talensi-Nabdam study setting, both private and public, which provide maternal and reproductive health services. The nearest health care facility for residents in this geographic setting is estimated to be ten to fifteen kilometres away (Yakong). Nearly all residents travel on foot to access care because transport is not easily accessible and women have to be able to walk the distance. It is more challenging for people living in this area to access emergency care, such as during labour and delivery, because it is nearly impossible for women in labour, especially difficult labour, to walk this distance.

In sub-Saharan Africa, more women access services from a health care professional during the prenatal period than during labour and delivery (Darmstadt et al.; Mills and Bertrand). During interviews, most pregnant women indicated that they accessed prenatal services when they could walk the distance but stopped prenatal visits when their pregnancy got more advanced because they found it difficult to make the return trip on foot. For example, Tiipogbire, a twenty-four-year-old mother of two lived about ten kilometres away from the nearest health care facility:

The two times that I was pregnant I tried my best and went to the prenatal clinic for care. Each time I went, they [nurses] asked me to come back for a check-up regularly, which I did try my best [to do]. But when I was getting closer to giving birth, I found it tiring to walk that long distance. So I stopped attending.

In terms of a home versus a clinic birth, Tiipogbire said:

When I was attending the prenatal clinic, the nurses warned me not to give birth at home. I thought they were not really thinking about when and what time labour would start and how I am going to be able to make it there. Even though I would have liked to go to them for delivery, there is absolutely no way I could get there. How do I get there, especially if labour begins in the night? I just laughed in my head when they insisted that I should not give birth at home, without considering the distance. I guess they do not even think about what we have to go through to get there. No cars come here, so what are they talking about?

Tiipogbire had both her babies at home with the help of a traditional birth attendant (TBA).

Teni, a twenty-nine-year-old woman who was carrying her second pregnancy at the time of interview related that:

You know, it is easy to walk while pregnant even though sometimes I feel tired to do that but I have been going for prenatal care ever since I realized I was pregnant. But I do not have plans to give birth at the clinic. Let's not even talk about that. The nurses keep on saying that no one should give birth at home. Would you have walked that distance yourself while in labour? I do not know when labour will start and whether at that time, we can have access to a vehicle over here to take me.

Although it appeared that women were committed to accessing care for their personal benefit, they are not always able to do so, as is expected by their health care providers. The challenges associated with travel distance and access to transport during labour or in any emergency situation cannot be underestimated; women's decisions are dependent on these factors, which are beyond their control.

AVAILABILITY AND ACCESS TO TRANSPORTATION

Lack of available and accessible transportation in most parts of northern Ghana is common and, regardless of the nature of the emergency or the medical situation, is a major barrier preventing access to emergency obstetric health care in rural Ghana (Oiyemhonlan et al.). Common types of available transport are bicycles, motorbikes, and donkey carts. The Talensi-Nabdam district public health sector provides services for a population of approximately 100,000, yet at the time of Yakong's research, the district's public health system possessed one ambulance for emergency use by the entire population. On several occasions, the ambulance was mechanically faulty and had no fuel or a readily available driver. If the ambulance had been available to move, the cost of fuel, paid for by clients, would have been more than they could afford. The cost is much higher when transport involved private commercial vehicles, such as taxi cabs, due to the poor condition of the road network. Study participants revealed that in the unlikely event that a taxi was accessible, most drivers—in all cases, males—were unwilling to take women in labour because they might soil their cars with blood. Drivers who did take women in labour charged much higher fares to cover cleaning their cars in the event of a stain.

Such factors discourage families from attempting to access any form of transportation to carry labouring women to clinics unless the labour is complicated and cannot be managed at home by a TBA. Tampoka—a twenty-nine-year-old woman, who due to difficult labour had her first childbirth at the clinic three years ago—shared her experience of getting to the clinic.

> *My labour started in the night until dawn. My family decided to send me to the clinic but we could not get any car. My brother-in-law rode a bicycle to the nearest market to look for a taxi, but there was none because it was not a market day, so he continued to another town much further. The driver was reluctant to come when he realized that it was a labour case. My brother-in-law pleaded with him that his refusal could result in the death of the woman and baby. He agreed and came but was really mad at me, yelling at me to make sure I did not soil his car with blood. It was a nightmare. He also charged us so much that my husband had to borrow money from neighbours, and we struggled to pay back over several months.*

Tempoka, a twenty-three-year-old primipara, wanted to go to the clinic because she was told at the prenatal clinic that she would likely encounter problems if she attempted to give birth at home. However, her wishes did not come true. Even though her family supported her attending the clinic despite the distance, they could not find a car. Tempoka related that "unfortunately my labour started in the night, and we had no way to get a car to take me to the clinic. But you know, by God's grace, I gave birth safely with the help of TBA."

Although donkey carts can serve to carry women to the clinic in the absence of a car, these carts were never mentioned in women's stories as another means of transport. When asked why they did not use a readily available and less expensive donkey cart to go the clinic, Tempoka agreed with Teni who related that, "when a donkey cart carries a patient to the clinic, it is rare that the patient would survive." Six focus group discussants responded to the same question regarding the use of donkey cart, and they all laughed, rolled their eyes, and whispered to one another. One woman, echoing the consensus of the group, said, "here it is believed that when you use a donkey cart to the clinic, it is almost like a dead case already. Because of how people think about it, no one wants to use a donkey cart to carry a sick person." This belief has discredited the use of donkey cart for transporting patients in the absence of a motor vehicle. Overall, women tend to access maternal health services for prenatal care more often than they do for labour and delivery because they can walk and do not need expensive transportation.

WOMEN'S WORKLOADS

In addition to distance issues, workload was cited as another factor limiting women's access to maternal health. All six focus group members indicated that they found it difficult to take time during the farming season to attend prenatal care, despite their intentions to do so. Bane, an eighteen-year-old woman, stated, "The farming season is normally full of work and asking for permission from husbands to attend clinics when one is not sick is interpreted as being lazy. I try to go sometimes but not all the time." Dokpoka, a nineteen-year-old woman, added:

> *Unless I am sick, I just forget about going to clinic at this time of year [farming season]. You walk all this distance to the clinic, and you are still expected to come back and go to the farm. No! I just pray that I am not sick. You know how men feel that one just wants to find an excuse and go to the clinic and leave work?*

Kolpoka, a twenty-seven-year-old woman, told Yakong that:

> *I do understand that going to the clinic has benefits for pregnant women, but I do not have control over work schedules at home. It is my husband who determines what*

> *should be done and at what time. When you, as a woman, do not abide by what they [husbands] ask you to do, it can become a problem. Just because one is pregnant does not mean that you do not work. They [husbands] tell you that pregnancy is not a disease to be going to the clinic every time while neglecting your part of the work at home. They say that you are simply lazy.*

Dougpoka, an eighteen-year-old woman, was carrying her third pregnancy at the time of our interview and had already lost two pregnancies because of ill health added:

> *Well, I tell you, I have been to the clinic only once and now that it is farming season, I am not sure if I can continue to go again, even though the nurses want me to come regularly. I know the next time I go back I am going to have a problem with the nurses because they do not understand these things. You dare not tell them that it was because of work that you could not come. They will yell at you and say that you are not serious about your own health. So you know what, when I go back again and they ask why I did not come, I will simply keep quiet. They will say all kinds of things but I know what I am going through. They will never understand it anyways, so why talk?*

Women's heavy workload and household responsibilities can be a barrier to accessing health care, a factor not often discussed or considered. Dougpoka's description reveals that health care providers do not understand rural women's living reality and how their situation might be a barrier to accessing health care. Rather, nurses blame the women for self-neglect, which, in turn, can further discourage women from accessing care.

MATERNAL AND CHILD POSTNATAL CARE

Typically, when women give birth at the clinic, they are required to report back after two weeks for assessment by a professional midwife to ensure that mother and baby are doing well. In the case of a home birth, TBAs, although banned from practice, are expected to immediately accompany women whom they assisted to the clinic to report so that nurses can assess the woman and the baby, who normally receive their first immunizations also. Most women access such care because they feel they can now walk the distance and because they want immunizations for their baby. However, in recent times, the health care system established that women who give birth at home and then access postnatal care are charged a fee, which is intended as punishment for women who home birth. The pressure on women to give birth attended by "skilled birth attendants" (MDG 5) arises from the belief that the increasing rates of maternal mortality are a result of home deliveries, mostly performed by TBAs (Kruske and Barclay). Although the intended purpose may be laudable from the perspective of the health care providers, the financial burden becomes an obstacle to women's postnatal care and the child's immunization. It also ignores issues that prevent women from accessing care. Poagbil, a twenty-three-year-old woman who delivered her baby at home a few weeks before our interview, lamented:

> *I am not sure if I want to go to the clinic because I do not want to be charged a fee for giving birth at home. I do not see what I have done wrong to be punished. I wanted to go because of the immunization for my baby, but what is happening makes me feel like not going. Plus, I do not have the money to go and pay [the fee].*

In a related issue, Nagbire, a thirty-three-year-old mother of five children, stated:

> *Although I have had all my children at home with the help of a TBA, I normally take them to the clinic as soon as possible to get assessed and immunized. After all, it is not difficult to walk the distance after birth; but now that nurses are charging fees, I do not think that it is fair. They charge you for giving birth at home. So my plan is not to go this time after birth, unless the child is sick.*

SOCIO-CULTURAL AND PERSONAL HEALTH BELIEFS

Studies in Ghana, and in other resource-poor nations, such as those described in this volume, show that socio-cultural factors and personal beliefs have a huge influence on health care decisions (Jansen; Mills and Bertrand; Shaikh and Hatcher; Yakong). For example, many Ghanaians believe that when women have sex while breastfeeding, the breast milk becomes polluted by the sperm and affects the baby's health. Thus, women may not seek birth control methods when they are breastfeeding because postpartum abstinence is encouraged rather than sex with birth control methods. Also, during labour, women are expected to stay out of contact with bad spirits and persons believed to have been involved in "sinful behaviour," such as adultery, because the mothers or their newborn babies may become ill or even die if exposed to such "bad" people (Yakong). In the event that a woman is on her way to give birth or is at the clinic postpartum, there is the possibility that she and her newborn may not be able to avoid coming in contact with such people. Noah, a forty-nine-year-old mother-in-law, was hesitant about her daughter-in-law giving birth at the clinic for this reason:

> *You know, there are all kinds of people living with dirt [adultery] these days and when these kinds of people see a woman in labour or a newborn baby, it can be harmful. I do not know who is going to be there at the clinic, so I do not want to expose my daughter-in-law and baby to such people. She can go for prenatal, but I am not sure if I want her to go there and give birth.*

Food-related taboos are also identified as a reason for not wanting to give birth at clinics. Immediately following her home birth, a woman is given hot water mixed with millet flour and shea butter to drink. This water is required to help expel blood clots and dirt postpartum and to initiate breast milk. Women who give birth at the clinic are given cold water to drink, which they believe can cause ill health and limit the immediate production of breast milk. Nabil, a fifty-year-old mother-in-law, for example, decided that because of the dispensing of cold water, it was not safe to allow her daughter-in-law to give birth at the clinic.

The inappropriate handling of placentas and the refusal to allow women to carry them home for cultural rites and appropriate burial also influence women's decisions whether to give birth at the clinic (Moyer et al.; Yakong). Cultural beliefs hold that improper handling and non-burial of the placenta can cause the baby ill health. Customarily, when a woman gives birth at home, the placenta is placed in a small new pot with a lid that the mother carries close to her lower abdomen into a designated place outside of the main house—normally a place used as compost for the family—for burial. This placenta must not come into contact with dirt or ants. Should that happen, the baby is likely to fall ill. Families are able to identify in later years and generations to come, how many children were born into the family, including all those who died, by a physical count of the placenta pots in this designated area. Care is taken not to break any of these pots. Women found it difficult to express their feelings about placentas being handled disrespectfully at the clinic because health care providers associate such things with local superstition. For example, Lamisi, a twenty-five-year-old woman, said:

> *When I asked the nurse to protect the placenta for me because I would like to carry it home, she yelled at me and said, "What do you mean I should protect it? Is it food? You people come here with all these weird beliefs." So I just kept quiet. I was not sure how she handled it afterwards, even though I was able to get it to take home with me.*

Studies in rural Ghana have confirmed nurses' refusal to release placentas to families and its possible consequence on maternal health care in northern Ghana (Moyer et al.). Nurses are unwilling to provide any reasons for their refusal, only suggesting that those who demand their placentas are superstitious and backwards in their thinking. Being unsure what nurses do with the placentas creates fear and generates reluctance to birth at the clinic.

Some women held a strong belief that taking pills, such as vitamins, calcium or iron, normally given to them during prenatal checks, will help them build "strong blood" to carry their pregnancy to term and help the baby grow well (McPherson "Modern Obstetrics"). Naabmah, a nineteen-year-old woman who just had her first baby at the time of our interview, said she went to the clinic regularly for care, despite the distance; she wanted to get the pills for strong blood. Her friends who had prior experience with pregnancies had shared the information regarding pills and strong blood. However, Naabmah said:

> *I already knew that I was not going to give birth at the clinic, but I went there for prenatal care so that I could get the pills that they said ... will help you get strong blood to carry the baby. Why would I struggle to get there to give birth when there is a TBA in our neighbourhood to help me? Most of these babies you [the researcher] have seen here were not born at the clinic. I just wanted the pills.*

Assipoka, a twenty-eight-year-old woman, was expecting her baby in the next few days and wanted to be among the first to be interviewed. She thought that she might not get the chance once the baby came. Assipoka decided to have her baby at home and explained why:

> *I have three other children and this will be my fourth one. It is my neighbour who is a TBA and always assists me. Even though in all my pregnancies I went for prenatal care so that I can get the pills for strong blood, I do not go there for delivery. This TBA has done this work even before I married into this area. There has never been a problem with her doing it. I know that the nurses hate to hear this but I did not see it necessary to travel all the way there to do the same thing that can be done right here in my house.*

True to her words, she gave birth a few days after our interview, assisted by her TBA neighbour. As culture demands, Yakong visited Assipoka in her home, where mother and baby were doing fine. Despite policy changes that bans her practice, Boodsomah, a seventy-four-year-old TBA who firmly protests the ban, continues to provide services to women in her family despite the directive.

In some clinics, women were unhappy that midwives and community health nurses required them to purchase new clothing for themselves and their unborn babies, a practice that conflicts with cultural beliefs around preparation for labour and delivery. Buying new things for unborn babies is widely believed to lead to miscarriage. When clinic staff insisted that pregnant women should purchase new clothing for unborn babies and themselves, Tempoka said that she

> *was shocked when she [nurse] said that I should buy new things for an unborn baby. We believe that you cannot bring baby things for a baby yet to be born. You could lose your pregnancy if you did that. I do not know where she [nurse] is coming from. What I know in terms of preparing for confinement is that you gather firewood, shea butter, and foodstuff and ingredients so that after birthing your family can use these things to take care of you, but not clothing.*

Based on their own training, midwives and community health nurses believe that they are educating women on preparation for confinement, which includes buying new items to prepare for babies as well as gathering rugs used by women to collect blood. They are also required to bring cakes of soap and Dettol for the nurses as a form of payment, although in principle midwives are not supposed to take payment. Informed by Western ideologies around childbirth classroom learning, theoretical knowledge, and textbooks have influenced midwives' practice and their expectations of women. Midwives are disconnected from local cultures and inappropriately apply these cosmopolitan ideals in local non-cosmopolitan contexts.

In addition to cultural inappropriateness, these demands place a financial burden on women who, unlike nurses, have no means of income to purchase the items nurses request. As Tampoka said:

> *I find it difficult to get money for all these things. I cannot even count all these things to my husband and ask for money to buy them, and I do not want to borrow money*

to do all these things because, immediately following birth, I cannot do other things that I have always done, such as selling firewood to earn more income to repay those debts. I may consider stopping the clinic visits.

Some women changed clinics and walked longer distances because of these demands, hoping other clinics would offer much more respectful services and, possibly, fewer demands and embarrassing practices, such as the display of rugs for others to view. Assipoka told us that she moved to her current clinic, much farther from her home, to receive prenatal services. When asked why she changed, she replied:

I came here because I could not deal with that nurse anymore. She kept on asking me to bring all these items to the clinic, which I could not afford to do. I tried to explain to her, but she would not listen. She insisted that every pregnant woman must bring those things. She yells a lot and does not care what your situation is. I just wanted to try this place, too, and see what they [nurses] do.

According to Midwife Adisa, "we ask [pregnant women] to get these things ready before they give birth, so they have something decent to wear thereafter." This means that, from the midwives' perspective, there is nothing wrong with asking women to do this because the women benefit from having new clothing to wear.

HEALTH CARE PROVIDER-PATIENT RELATIONSHIP

Poor health care provider-patient relationships are consistently identified by women as a factor influencing their decisions to access maternal health care services. This factor is a long-standing issue affecting service use in resource-poor nations (D'Ambruoso et al.; Ghana Ministry of Health, *Programme of Work*; Jewkes et al.; Moyer et al.; Oiyemhonlan et al.; Shaikh and Hatcher; Yakong et al.). In Ghana, the poor health care provider-patient relationship dynamic affects all levels of care but is most appalling in rural settings where access to health care and options for providers is limited. Poor attitudes toward patients are also attributed to power differentials and discrimination by health care providers, who assume a higher social positioning compared to rural residents (Moyer et al.; Yakong et al.). Moyer et al. found that in northern Ghana, women who had less money, were uneducated, and lived in rural settings were treated disrespectfully when they visited health care facilities compared to their counterparts in a different socio-economic position. Nurses and other health care providers place themselves above community members and tend not to respect those beneath their status. These attitudes translate into physical, verbal, and emotional abuse. Women in our study cited a number of examples of being abused by health care providers: from being judged, ignored, called names, yelled at, and disrespected to receiving physical beatings during labour. This abuse affected the women's desire to visit health care facilities. For example, Bogremah, a seventeen-year-old married woman who was pregnant for the first time when interviewed, related that

> *When I went for prenatal care, the nurse asked me why I was pregnant at this age. She said, "you young girls of this modern time will not sleep in the night." I felt so embarrassed and did not want to go back there again. When she asked me questions because I was already feeling bad, I could not answer them to her satisfaction, so she was yelling at me.*

During labour, Bogremah's experience was no different from her prenatal experience:

> *When I was in labour, I said I was not going back to that clinic again, so my mother-in-law took me to a different clinic, but it was no different. She [nurse], too, ignored me when we got there. She was angry that I did not remove my underwear before coming in. She shouted at me and said, '"do you think you are going to give birth in your underwear? If you were shy, you should not have had sex in the first place." She said she was busy, and if I did not co-operate she was going to leave me alone or I could go*

> back home. I do not know if I would like to go to any clinic for any care in the future. I felt so bad.

Yenpoka, a thirty-nine-year-old woman, recalled her experience when she went to seek prenatal care at another clinic during pregnancy.

> I met a nurse at the office who was busy doing something. I greeted, but she did not respond, so I was afraid to ask more questions. I decided to sit outside and wait. All I saw was that she came out and closed the office door and was leaving for home. I approached her, and she yelled at me and asked why I was sitting outside there if I needed her? I simply apologized because she would not even allow me to explain. I felt like a little girl before her, even though she was just a young woman.

Azumah, a thirty-four-year-old mother of three, tearfully recounted her experience of being slapped in her face during labour at the clinic.

> I started to push when she asked me not to, but I knew the baby was coming because this is not my first time of giving birth. When I told her that the baby was coming, she sat somewhere and shouted, "do not push it is not time." But I had to and she just rushed in and slapped me in my face. I shed tears that day, not because of the labour pain but because of how she treated me. You know I am not just a little girl for another woman to do this to me.

When it came to how their relationships with providers influenced their decisions to access care, a poor nurse-patient relationship was a common theme in most women's narratives and a strong factor in women's maternal care decisions. Most women preferred to seek support from TBAs who they felt treated them more respectfully, which corroborates previous findings on women's preferences for TBAs over nurses (Yakong et al.). Women commented they would go to clinics if forced to or if they were in trouble with difficult labour.

INCONSISTENT SERVICE AVAILABILITY

In principle, the Ghana Health Service mandates rural clinics to provide twenty-four-hour service; however, in practice, the situation is different. During fieldwork, Yakong randomly visited a number of clinics to have conversations with nurses to learn about their work. One Sunday morning, she drove to a clinic that posted twenty-four-hour service to find it closed to the public. The main gate was locked with a huge padlock, and the nurses' residence was also locked. No work would be done on that day. Yakong sat with women at the church during their service and saw several patients coming to the clinic, carried on bicycles or on foot supported by relations. Some of the patients seemed desperate and knocked at the big clinic gate, despite the padlock hanging there. When asked, women at the church confirmed that the clinic was supposed to be open for twenty-four-hour service. However, they also noted that the absence of nurses at the clinic was routine. One woman remarked:

> *Well, this is what happens over here most of the time, especially at the weekend and in the night. Nurses are supposed to stay here in the village but they do not. You see that house over there [pointing] that is their house. Most of the time, when you run there in the night, you find nobody, and you will have to look for another clinic somewhere. That is, if you have the means of transport to do so, especially if a woman is in labour, you know that cannot wait.*

Another woman said,

> *This is not new, but we cannot talk about it to anybody. I mean, we cannot report because we are afraid that if we do, it may even be worse, so we just pray that whenever we go with a patient and they are there, we count ourselves lucky.*

Some of the women said the nurses go to the market to do business to earn more income. One woman added that, "you know today is a market day over here, so they may be at the market. They go to do business for more money."

The irregularity of service provision was a common theme affecting most clinics in the study area, which, in turn, resulted in lack of confidence in the health care system. Tampogremah, a woman in her late thirties, was leaving a clinic when we arrived to conduct interviews, but she shared her experience of birthing and labour a year ago:

We cannot rely on these people [nurses] for our health needs. I came here last year while in labour to be attended by the midwife. When I arrived I was told the midwife had gone to Bolgatanga [a city] and would not be back until the next day. Because my house is not too far from here, I was able to get back home but delivered on my own.

An older woman narrated her experience when, accompanying her daughter-in-law, they had to visit three different clinics before a nurse attended her labour.

We first visited clinic A where we were told that the nurse did not come to work that day. Then we continued to clinic B where we were asked to go to clinic C because the clinic B nurse had gone for a meeting in the town. At clinic C we found a nurse who finally referred us to Bolgatanga [a regional hospital in the city] because we were too late and she was closing. I tell you, if we had known this, we would have just stayed home. It was because they [nurses] said we should not let her give birth at home that we had to go through all this.

This inconsistent service availability contradicts Ghana health service policy and commitment to providing maternal health services targeted at reducing the high maternal mortality rates in rural settings. The concept of community-based health planning and service (CHPS) was initiated to ensure regular availability of service in rural settings in order to bridge the health care access gap between urban and rural settings (Awoonor-Williamsa et al.).

The irregular service availability results in community members' lack of confidence in the health care system and reinforces the low use of services intended to benefit the people.

MISSION VERSUS PUBLIC HEALTH CARE SERVICES

Countrywide, there have been huge differences between mission health services and public health services over a number of issues ranging from resource allocation—material, logistical, budgetary, and human—to quality service provision and patient-centred care (Ghana Ministry of Health *Vision 2020*). Anecdotal and public opinion show that compared to public health service, patients receive quality care and reliable service from mission health services (Barlow; Gibbs and William, this volume). Although this argument has often been disregarded and considered anecdotal for political reasons, all the women in this study preferred travelling long distances to attend a particular mission clinic rather than a public clinic that was closer to them. Mission staff members were available, regardless of the time of day or night, medicine was stocked. An onsite ambulance was ready for emergency patient referrals, and a relatively collegial staff-client relationship existed. Christiana, a mission clinic midwife, confirmed that, compared to the other public clinics, their clinic got more mothers seeking maternal health services. However, even though their services were perceived as having quality, she worried about the concomitant increase in workload experienced by their limited staff, which might affect their ongoing ability to provide quality service. Christiana mentioned that "we depend on the public sector for staffing, and there is lack of equity with regard to human resource allocation by the public health sector to us." During our interview, she also revealed that for some obscure reason, all public sector nursing staff members were being withdrawn from the mission sector, leaving the workload too high for her to manage alone. Another midwife who practised in a different mission clinic also confirmed that women who attend her clinic do so for similar reasons as mentioned above. Although pleased their clinic services met the needs of patients, she worried about the long-standing and unhealthy relationship between mission and public health service clinics and the negative implications for maternal health.

> *Doctors and nurses from the public clinics where we [mission staff] are supposed to refer patients for further management, refuse to take our patients simply because those patients chose to come to our clinic. Because of this, patients who come here will also be refused there on referral. Some patients who end up going there are treated badly by the staff, the reason being that they came to our clinic first.*

Thus, the endemic conflict between these two health sectors has severe negative implications for ordinary Ghanaians in general and pregnant women in particular, who suffer the consequences of the conflict. This needs to be addressed from a higher authority level, such as the Ghana Ministry of Health and Ghana Health Service as well as the local government, if maternal health and rural health are to see some level of improvement and contribute toward the achievement of the MDGs (Ghana Health Service; Oiyemhonlan et al.). In northern Ghana, women feel obliged to bear as many children as they can to satisfy their social role because of the social value placed on children (Oiyemhonlan et al.; Yakong; Pollock, this volume). However, the majority of women confirmed that they opted for birth control methods, even though their husbands and other kinfolk did not support birth control use. They accessed birth control methods because of the lack of resources available to care for their children properly and the hardship of raising them almost completely on their own. They cited limited access to and inadequate food supplies, the high cost of medical bills, and education as reasons to access birth control, despite family members' opposition.

However, lack of information about possible and actual side effects of various methods also discouraged many women from using birth control. A number of women mentioned severe and irregular bleeding as reasons for declining birth control methods. Midwives confirmed that those women who used birth control preferred "injectables" (depo provera) so that their husbands would not discover that they had used birth control. At this point, it was not clear if side effects were particularly related to their use of depo provera or if their experience would have been different with other methods. For example, Assipoka stopped using birth control after three months because of severe irregular bleeding, as she told us, "I had no idea that this would have happen to me when I take them and the nurse did not tell me about what to expect." Although midwives refuted this claim, inadequate patient education regarding birth control methods and their proven side effects as well as other medical conditions during pregnancy are a barrier to women making decisions about their maternal health care and choosing to access services, which contributes to underutilization of services (Oiyemhonlan et al.; Yakong). Information deficit leads to uninformed decision making, which affects not only birth control but also other maternal and child health services.

Why some nurses in these settings routinely deny information to help patients properly understand and utilize services remains an issue with negative implications for rural women. Through personal experience and observation, Yakong discovered that some nurses (although they would not admit this) have various knowledge deficits and are unable to provide information to their clients. For example, during her field research, Yakong attended a child welfare clinic so her two-month-old baby could receive immunizations. First, the community health nurse charted the baby's weight incorrectly; then, the nurse who immunized the baby did not share any information with the mother (Yakong in this instance) regarding potential side effects and what to do should they occur, a routine practice that should occur with every immunization. Although as a community health nurse, Yakong knew what to expect and what to do, she wanted to challenge nurses' knowledge and practice. Thus, when she enquired about what to expect, Yakong was shocked to be told that "nothing will happen after the immunization." While at the clinic, Yakong observed that scales used for weighing pregnant women during prenatal checks were not balanced and, as a result, wrong weights were assigned to them, a practice that puts these women at risk. Although Yakong brought these malpractices to the attention of the clinic manager, it is not yet known whether there was any change in practice. Lack of information sharing and malpractice among nurses in rural Ghana are pervasive issues cutting across all areas of service implementation. The consequences of these occurrences for patients are immeasurable.

Women's decisions about using and accessing birth control in rural Ghana are also influenced by religious beliefs and even by health care providers acting as a gatekeepers of morality (Lema; Stanback and Twum-Baah). As Tempoka said,

> *I went there [clinic] to take birth control injection, but the nurse would not give it to me. Instead, she started to talk to me about something called "natural birth control," which I did not understand. But anyways, she said here in their clinic, what they do is tell people to do natural birth control. So I could not get it.*

Although Government of Ghana population policy states that birth control methods should be accessible to all citizens at all times, religious beliefs and personal morality prevent free access to such services, regardless of women's reproductive health needs. In a number of countries across sub-Saharan Africa, when providers use their personal religious and moral values to deny services to women, the consequences for their reproductive health can be severe (Lema). Such practices contribute to the high maternal morbidity and mortality ratios in sub-Saharan Africa and remain a key challenge to achieving MDG goals on maternal health.

GENERAL HEALTH POLICY ISSUES: RESTRICTIONS ON TRADITIONAL BIRTHING

Traditional birth attendants (TBAs) are usually respected and trusted older women who have given birth and have acquired midwifery skills through observation and apprenticeship with other practitioners (Abodunrin et al.; Davis-Floyd; Kruske and Barclay). They apply their knowledge and skills to assist their family and their community members who need their services. Often, they will provide their services free of charge but, if offered, will also accept gifts from families whom they have helped. These gifts may range from food, such as chickens, to help with farm work.

Although these highly experienced women provide important services to their community members, TBAs are labeled non-skilled and unprofessional because they do not meet the requirements of midwifery according to the standards of cosmopolitan obstetrics (Davis-Floyd). Not so long ago, as Kruske and Barclay note, the services of TBAs were viewed by the World Health Organization (WHO) and other international health related agencies to have a positive impact on the reduction of maternal and infant mortality in resource-poor nations. In the 1970s, these agencies supported the design and development of training programs for TBAs so that they could practice in their communities within the context of biomedical science. Training usually took about two weeks, and when they went back to their various communities, TBAs were expected to know everything about performing safe deliveries. Unfortunately, by 1997, policy makers within WHO (Kruske and Barclay) blamed TBAs for increasing maternal mortality, and all training programs and funding was withdrawn, resulting in the creation of the moniker "skilled attendants," part of the later MDG 5, which excluded TBAs. Research evaluating the practices of TBAs in Ghana concluded that training TBAs had no impact on maternal health and, thus, further investments were not worthwhile (Smith et al.).

Notwithstanding the above criticisms and conclusions on the practices of TBAs, on a yearly basis, globally, approximately sixty million women give birth at home and another fifty-two million births occur without a skilled birth attendant (Darmstadt et al.). In resource-poor nations, studies show that most rural women give birth at home with support from TBAs (Abodunrin et al; Amoako et al.; Shaikh and Hatcher). In the upper east region of northern Ghana, where this study was conducted, recent studies show only 35 percent of deliveries are attended by professional health care providers (Moyer et al.). Because of policy, however, TBAs are no longer permitted to practise in rural communities (Yakong), leaving the great majority of rural women with no assistance at all.

During interviews, both women and TBAs worried that the restrictions placed on the practice and the withdrawing of TBA services would have serious negative impacts on maternal health.

Tangmah, a twenty-seven-year-old woman, who delivered her baby at home supported by a TBA said:

Without her [TBA], my baby and I would have been dead by now. I would not have been able to get to the hospital as they [nurses] expected me to do in the middle of the night when labour started. They [nurses] would not help women at home to give birth, even if you call them. But the TBA was right there when we called her and in no time the baby was delivered.

Another participant strongly argued that she did not understand why TBAs should not be allowed to work when they are the only providers women can easily access when they need them. She indicated that she would never go to the clinic unless the TBAs in the community refused to attend her labour. Apart from the fact that women in her community have easy access to TBA services, she also felt that TBAs offer quality care and knowledge. For example, Lariba, a twenty-five-year-old woman, said:

I never heard that any woman died in the hands of the TBA in this community ever since we [women] have been working with them. But I hear that women die through childbirth at the hospital too, so what are they talking about?

Apart from women's confidence in working with them, TBAs themselves felt that forbidding them from providing services that contributed to their families and communities was an abuse of their rights and obligations. Seventy-four-year-old Boodsomah, a practising TBA with decades of experience, stated in an interview that

I have assisted several women both within my own family and the outside community to give birth without any problem. I enjoy doing it. I have never failed in assisting a woman to deliver. But now the doctors [from the cosmopolitan health care system] say it is not safe to assist women at home to give birth. They say it is safer for a pregnant woman to go to the hospital than to be helped at home. I

> *continue to assist my daughters-in-law [the entire clan] to give birth at home. What I would not do is to assist other women outside the family. None of my children have been to the hospital to give birth. I feel bad that I cannot help other women outside the family to give birth and feel that my rights have been taken away. I feel irresponsible that I cannot help people in my community who need my help.*

When Yakong asked how she learned her skills, she explained, as she would to a younger kinswoman:

> *My daughter, this is women's work. I just learned at home as an older woman. It is expected that every old lady knows how to do this thing. You do not need any training to begin with. It is natural. Some time ago, the health care system gave us [TBAs] some training on how to help women give birth safely. We went to Bolgatanga for about two weeks to learn how to do deliveries.*

Although she did not mention the benefits of this training, it appeared that it did provide some useful information, especially on aspects of hygiene, which improved their TBA practice. Before being forced to stop assisting women at home, TBAs were required to accompany the woman and baby to the clinic and render a report. As Boodsomah stated:

> *After a woman gives birth, I get someone to write the date, and I accompany the woman and her baby to the clinic to report to the nurses and for documentation. What is wrong with this? Then about two years ago, they called all TBAs and gave us some things (soap and disinfectant) to use for our hands and the baby's cord to prevent infection. After a year again, they told us not to help women in labour. Now we are expected to accompany women in labour to the clinic or call them [nurses] to come for the woman. The clinics are very far from this village. So my question or concern: is the woman in pain or suffering or not? And how long is it going to take them to come*

for the woman? I have heard them, but I will continue to help my own family. As I talk now, I just delivered one of my daughters-in-law last night, and I feel really tired and sleepy. She finally gave birth in the middle of the night.

These respondents' remarks as well as studies in Ghana and in other resource-poor nations suggest the majority of women in rural settings prefer the assistance of a TBA to that of a professional midwife (Yakong et al.; Spangler). When asked what she thinks of this contrast, Boodsomah stated that

Most women who have been to the clinic complain that midwives beat them up during labour. I think that is inappropriate. How do you beat up a woman who is carrying another human being inside? Women continue to tell me that they prefer my support. They say that midwives treat them disrespectfully.

When asked what will happen to the future generations with regard to birthing skills and practices, Boodsomah responded:

Well, it is good for women to go to the hospital. They say it is safer. But I am worried that older women's knowledge is fading out. Older women are now reluctant or afraid to even practise doing it. The majority of older women are losing their skills to support women in labour because of the fear they put in us. My fear is how it would look in the future. Also, it may take a long time for nurses to come for a woman in labour because our village is far from the clinics. I think they are putting women and babies at risk.

MIDWIVES' PERSPECTIVES ON REPRODUCTIVE HEALTH CARE

The general perception of the four midwives interviewed was that women's access to maternal health care had improved since they took over. Three of the midwives had been working in their new public health stations for the past two to three years; the mission midwife had been at her clinic almost seven years. They believed they were doing everything possible to break barriers that prevented women from accessing care, such as reaching out to them and improving their interpersonal relationships with women. However, they collectively identified barriers to effective service delivery, including: limited transportation, the poor road network, inadequate staff, few supplies and little equipment to work with, a lack of funding to effectively run the clinics, few innovations to improve practice, a dearth of patronage by community members, a paucity of incentives, and the isolated nature of the places in which they work. They noted an increase in women attending prenatal and postnatal services, but labour and delivery service usage was not increasing. They expressed concern that women did not report to access care immediately following pregnancy. However, on early prenatal reporting, another midwife pointed out that in the culture of the community members, it was against their beliefs to report early pregnancy to an outsider. It is believed that the pregnancy might spontaneously abort if divulged prematurely.

Regarding transportation, with the exception of the mission clinic's single ambulance, the four facilities relied on motorbikes as their means of transportation (Yakong). Motorbikes were used for outreach clinics, staff meetings outside the clinics, and other activities related to work. But if a woman had been in labour at home and her family had sent for help, the midwife could do little because motorbikes could not have carried a woman in labour. At the time of our interviews, midwives did not attend labour at home either. For example, Samantha, one of the midwives stated:

> *I was called to attend a woman who gave birth at home in one of the villages and she had retained placenta. I was able to get an ambulance from a different clinic, but it took a little while to get it. On our way, we got stuck. We had to continue the rest of the journey by foot, but it was also too far. We managed to get there anyway, but it was a bit late; though she did not die, she suffered a lot. These are some of the problems we have here that sometimes makes it difficult to do our best. Imagine in an emergency*

> situation like this where, as a midwife, I could help but how can I if I cannot get there at the right time? I have encouraged women to use donkey carts because these are able to travel the rough roads where cars cannot go, but there is a wide belief that when donkey carts carry patients, those patients will not survive.

Adisah, another midwife, stated that,

> We [midwives] give women our [cell] phone numbers to call us if they are in labour, but even if they call, we do not have the means to go. We only have a motorbike which cannot pick a woman in labour. So, yah, it is difficult to really do what we are here for.

The majority of the women interviewed did not appear to have access to cell phones, and there is no commercial phone system available to community members. Based on Yakong's observations and insider knowledge, it is unrealistic for midwives to provide residents with cell phone numbers to call them when their family member is in labour because very few people—and those few are mostly men—have access to cell phones.

With regard to irregular service, two midwives agreed that they were supposed to provide twenty-four-hour services to residents but because of family commitments and heavy workloads with limited staff, they often get tired and have to alternate with other staff. Samantha, who was the only midwife among the other staff, commented:

> My family live in Bolgatanga and I work here [at the village]. I go on weekends to see my little boy and come back on Mondays. But I leave my [cell] phone on so, if there is an emergency, the other staff will call me to come back.

Another midwife confirmed that Samantha goes to Bolgatanga for the weekend, resulting in no one on weekend day duty to attend to labour or any other medical condition. Christiana, who works at a mission clinic, provides twenty-four-hour service.

> *I live here every day and attend to all the labour cases that come here. Even though I get tired because I am the only one here, I still do my work. I may be cranky because I am tired but I make sure that no woman struggles to get here to find I am not here to help.*

Whereas women stated they went to the clinics but no nurses were available and so they no longer bother to attend, some of the nurses said that they feel demotivated when they "sit here every day and no patient comes for their services." This is a particular issue for midwives working in the public sector. Sub-Saharan Africa is experiencing an acute shortage of health workers, particularly midwives and other categories of nurses (Gerein et al.). This shortage reflects Ghana's experience and may be associated with the fact that the majority of older midwives are retiring from service and younger staff members do not willingly accept postings to rural areas. Similarly, the maternal health care service delivery in rural Ghana rests mainly in the hands of midwives and nurses, and most facilities are understaffed and those few staff members are overworked (Oiyemhonlan et al.). The few staff members also appear unmotivated because of their heavy workloads as well as a lack of incentives to work in rural areas. These may be two key reasons for midwives' poor attitudes towards women. Midwives also impose illegal demands and fees on mothers to compensate themselves for being in deprived areas rather than in urban areas, where nurses may have more opportunities for advancement in their careers. Another important issue affecting midwives who live and work in rural settings is a lack of quality education for their children because schools in rural settings do not offer the quality education these midwives wish for their children. This means that midwives with school age children will have to leave their families in towns while they work in villages so that they can have access to quality education. This could account for why staff members are often absent at their clinics, as they have to travel between work place and town where their families live to offer them needed support. It may also be a difficult experience for young unmarried staff to work at these rural settings because it is difficult to find men that they might potentially marry.

Two midwives admitted that poor attitudes towards mothers and the abuse of some women by health care providers can turn women away from accessing care. However, they rationalized the tendency of midwives to abuse women. For example, Christiana confirmed that

> *Sometimes I hit them because they do not listen to commands when you ask them not to push because the baby is not ready. I focus on getting the baby out alive and when a woman is doing something that goes contrary to that, I do not accept it. As a midwife I get hurt when I deliver a dead baby. I am attached to what we do.*

Adisah shared that:

> *Yes, I shout at them. If you come and misbehave, especially as I am alone, particularly in the evening or night when I am tired, I shout. Also, if the labouring woman is not co-operating, I yell. I am afraid the baby would die or the woman will get a tear. I shout to correct them so that I can have a safe delivery. At times, when the woman is misbehaving, and you try to tap her a little so that she can relax, then they say you are beating them.*

However, Samantha disagreed with the idea of shouting at and beating women in labour. She felt such practices inappropriate and unprofessional. "I have given birth myself, and I know what it is when a woman is in labour." Despite her disagreement, she confirmed that at some places women are beaten. She shared a story about referring a woman to another hospital for further treatment.

> *I referred a woman to another place after delivery. She was bleeding seriously and would not allow me to examine her for clots, if any, so that I can bring them out to stop the bleeding. And I am not used to forcing or beating women. I know that going into the vagina to scoop out clots is very painful, but you have to. Besides that, you can get some bruises around the vagina and those bruises*

can cause pain too. So I called an ambulance and referred her to the hospital. When she came back to child welfare clinic, she told me that she was beaten like a donkey at the Bolgatanga regional hospital. She said they used forceps (I am sure it was a delivery forceps) to hit her. On the day she came to the clinic, I was delivering another woman who had similar problems, and I wanted to inspect for clots and she was not allowing. That woman rushed in and told the other woman to better allow me to do it because if she goes to the Bolgatanga regional hospital, they will beat her like a donkey.

Although midwives were somewhat frustrated by the multitude of challenges that they faced in their work, as a group, they generally appeared committed to providing services to benefit women in their areas of practice.

CONCLUSION

As in other resource-poor nations, in rural Ghana, factors influencing women's maternal health care decisions and service access are complex. These factors present several negative consequences for women in their reproductive years. This study, as in previous studies (Oiyemhonlan et al.; Yakong et al.), reveals several layers of barriers that intersect to impede women's access to health care as well as impede a health care provider's ability to deliver effective and efficient maternal health services to rural women. These findings challenge health care policy makers' understanding of local contexts and how these contexts might influence health care policies that they put in place. There is also a need for the Ghana health care sector as well as in local governments to modify and improve conditions that are unfavourable for access and service delivery in rural areas. For example, the poor road networks need improving, access to public transport system should be improved, and provision of resources and logistics would go a long way to increase access and enhance service delivery in rural Ghana.

Also, the socio-cultural context of women's lives discussed in this chapter reveals that viewing rural women's lives outside of their lived reality presents serious misconceptions that can complicate how health policy formulation and implementation are carried out to meet women's health needs. The nature of women's daily and seasonal work and the cultural construction of gender roles make it challenging for women to realize their own health goals. They must conform to societal norms, beliefs, and values of patriarchal cultures that mandate women's lives are defined and directed by male others, especially their husbands. Policy makers and implementers, such as maternal health care providers, need to be cognizant of women's lived reality and take these social realities into consideration to find ways to support Ghanaian women's access to health care in rural settings. As this chapter and others in this volume show, unless cultural and contextual issues are addressed, MDGs aimed at improving maternal and child health in challenging national contexts will miss the mark. With the demise of traditional reproductive and birthing knowledge replaced by a culturally unsafe cosmopolitan system of reproductive care, the possibility exists that women will continue to abandon the health care system in rural settings, which will exacerbate a situation of poor maternal and child health, increase maternal and child mortalities, and, ultimately, negatively affect the achievement of MDGs and future Sustainability Development Goals.

ENDNOTES

[1]In Ghana, midwives who offer maternal and child health services in rural settings are either registered general nurses with an additional midwifery certification or registered midwives without a general nursing certificate. Other nurses with related backgrounds who offer the same services include community health nurses or community health officers. Although somewhat different with regard to background and levels of education, these categories of health care providers are generally referred to as "nurses" by the general public. Traditional birth attendants are not referred to as midwives; they are simply addressed as traditional birth attendants. Although Yakong interviewed only midwives with regard to health care providers, we will use the title "nurses" or "midwives."

WORKS CITED

Abodunrin, Olugbemiga L., James O. Bamidele, Adenike I. Olugbenga-Bello, and Dauda B. Parakoy. "Preferred Choice of Health Facilities for Healthcare among Adult Residents in Ilorin Metropolis, Kwara State, Nigeria." *International Journal Health Research* 3.2 (2010): 79-86. Web. 10 June 2012.

Amoako, Fiifi Johnson, Sabu S. Padmadas, and James J. Brown. "On the Spatial Inequalities of Institutional Versus Home Births in Ghana: A Multilevel Analysis." *Journal of Community Health* 34 (2009): 64-72. Web. 2 Oct. 2011.

Awoonor-Williamsa, John Koku, Elias Kavinah Sory, Frank K. Nyonator, James F. Phillips, Chen Wang, and Margaret L. Schmitt. "Lessons Learned from Scaling Up a Community-Based Health-Program in the Upper East Region of Northern Ghana." *Global Health Science Practice* 1.1 (2013): 117-133. Web. 3 Nov. 2013.

Crichton, S. and B. Onguko. "Appropriate Technologies for Challenging Contexts." *On the Move: Mobile Learning for Development*. Eds. S. Marshall and W. Kinuthia. Charlotte, North Carolina: Information Age Publishing, 2013. 25–42. Print.

D'Ambruoso L., M. Abbey, and J. Hussein. "Please Understand When I Cry out in Pain: Women's Accounts of Maternity Services during Labour and Delivery in Ghana." *BMC Public Health* 5 (2007): 140. Web. 10 July 2008.

Darmstadt, Gary L. et al. "60 Million Non-Facility Births: Who Can Deliver in Community Settings to Reduce Intrapartum-Related Deaths?" *International Journal of Gynecology and Obstetrics* 107 (2009): S89–S112. Web. 11 Aug. 2010.

Davis-Floyd, Robbie. Global Issues in Midwifery: Mutual Accommodation or Biomedical Hegemony? *Midwifery Today* 1.17 (2000): 68-69. Print.

Davis, Thomas P Jr., Carolyn Wetzela, Emma Hernandez Avilanb, Cecilia De Mendoza Lopes, Rachel P. Chase, Peter J. Winch, and Henry B. Perry. "Reducing Child Global Undernutrition at Scale in Sofala Province, Mozambique, Using Care Group Volunteers to Communicate Health Messages to Mothers." *Global Health Science and Practice* 1.1 (2013): 36-51. Web. 9 May 2013.

Fendall, F. R. E. "Declaration of Alma-Ata." *The Lancet* 312.8103:

(1978): 1308. Web. 7 Apr. 2010.

Gage, Anastasia J. "Barriers to the Utilization of Maternal Health Care in Rural Mali" *Social Science and Medicine* 65.8 (2007): 1666–1682. Web. Feb. 2008.

Gabrysch, Sabine, and Oona M. R. Campbell. "Still Too Far to Walk: Literature Review of the Determinants of Delivery Service Use." *BMC Pregnancy and Childbirth* 9.1 (2009): 34. Web. 15 Aug. 2013.

Gerein, Nancy, Andrew Green, and Stephen Pearson. "The Implications of Shortages of Health Professionals for Maternal Health in Sub-Saharan Africa." *Reproductive Health Matters* 14.27 (2006): 40–50. Web. Jan. 2007.

Ghana Health Service. *Annual Report. Ghana Health Services.* Ghana Health Services, 2010. Web. 15 June 2013.

Ghana Ministry of Health. *Medium Term Health Strategy Toward Vision 2020.* Accra: Government of Ghana, 1999. Print.

Ghana Ministry of Health. *The Ghana Health Sector Programme of Work.* Accra: Government of Ghana, 2006. Print.

Hall, John J., and Richard Taylor. "Health for All Beyond 2000: The Demise of the Alma Ata Declaration and Primary Health Care in Developing Countries." *Medical Journal of Australia* 178.1 (2003):17-20. Print.

Hogan, D. P., B. Berhanu, and A. Hailemariam. "Household Organization, Women's Autonomy, and Contraceptive Behavior in Southern Ethiopia." *Studies in Family Planning* 30.4 (2010): 302–314. Web. 7 July 2011.

Jansen, I. "Decision Making in Childbirth: The Influence of Traditional Structures in a Ghanaian Village." *International Nursing Review* 53 (2006): 41-46. Web. 2 May 2007.

Jewkes R., N. Abrahams and Z. Mvowhy. "Why Do Nurses Abuse Patients? Reflections from South African Obstetric Services." *Social Science and Medicine* 47.11 (1998): 1781-1795. Print.

Kruske, Sue, and Barclay Lesley. "Effect of Shifting Policies on Traditional Birth AttendantTraining." *Journal of Midwifery and Women's Health* 49.4 (2004): 306–311. Web. 5 Nov. 2006.

Lema, V.M. "Conscientious Objection and Reproductive Health Service Delivery in Sub-Saharan Africa." *African Journal of Reproductive Health* 16.1 (2012): 15-21. Web. 12 Mar. 2011.

Maine, Deborah, and Allan Rosenfield. "The Safe Motherhood Initiative: Why Has It Stalled?" *American Journal of Public Health* 89.4 (1999): 480-482. Web. 8 Sept. 2010.

McPherson, Naomi. "Modern Obstetrics in a Rural Setting: Women and Reproduction in Northwest New Britain." *Urban Anthropology and Studies of Cultural Systems and World Economic Development*. Special Issue: Women and Development in the Pacific. 23.1 (1994): 39-72. Web.11 June 2009.

McPherson, Naomi. "Women, Childbirth and Change in West New Britain, Papua New Guinea." *Reproduction, Childbearing and Motherhood*. Ed. Pranee Liamputtong. New York: Nova Science Publishers, 2007. 127-141. Print.

Mills, Samuel, and Jane T. Bertrand. "Use of Health Professionals for Obstetric Care in Northern Ghana." *Studies in Family Planning* 36.1 (2005): 45–56. Web. 4 May 2006.

Moyer, Cheryl A., Raymond Akawire Aborigo, Gideon Logonia, Gideon Affah, Sarah Rominski, Philip B. Adongo, John Williams, Abraham Hodgson, and Cyril Engmann. "Clean Delivery Practices in Rural Northern Ghana: A Qualitative Study of Community and Provider Knowledge, Attitudes, and Beliefs." BMC *Pregnancy and Childbirth* 12 (2013): 12-50. Web. 10 August 2013.

Nyonator, Frank, Koku John, Awoonor-Williamsa, James Phillips, Tanya C. Jones, and Robert A. Miller. "The Ghana Community-Based Health Planning and Services Initiative for Scaling Up Service Delivery Innovation. *Health Policy and Planning* 20.1 (2005): 25-34.Print.

Oiyemhonlan, Brenda, Emilia Udofia, and Damien Punguyire. "Identifying Obstetrical Emergencies at Kintampo Municipal Hospital: A Perspective from Pregnant Women and Nursing Midwives." *African Journal of Reproductive Health* 17.2 (2013): 129-140. Web.11 May 2013.

Shaikh, B. T., and J. Hatcher. "Health Seeking Behavior and Health Service Utilization in Pakistan: Challenging the Policy Makers." *Journal of Public Health* 27.1 (2005): 49-54. Web. 8 June 2007.

Simkhada, Bibha, Edwin R. van Teijlingen, Maureen Porter, and Padam Simkhada. "Factors Affecting the Utilization of Antenatal Care in Developing Countries: Systematic Review of the

Literature." *Journal of Advanced Nursing* 61.3 (2007): 244-260. Web. 28 Oct. 2008.

Smith, Jason B., Nii A. Coleman, Judith A. Fortney, Joseph De-Graft Johnson, Dan W. Blumhagen, and Thomas W. Grey. "The Impact of Traditional Birth Attendant Training on Delivery Complications in Ghana." *Health Policy Planning* 15.3 (2000): 326-331. Web. 15 July.

Spangler, Sydney A. "'To Open Oneself is a Poor Woman's Trouble': Embodied Inequality andChildbirth in South–Central Tanzania." *Medical Anthropology Quarterly* 25.4 (2011): 479–498. Web. 12 Mar. 2012.

Stanback, J. and K.A. Twum-Baah. "Why Do Family Planning Providers Restrict Access toServices? An Examination in Ghana." *Curationis* 27.1 (2001): 37-41. Web. 20 Apr. 2010.

United Nations (UN). *United Nations Millennium Declaration. 2000.* UN, n.d. Web. 5 February 2013.

United Nations. *Millennium Development Goals Report 2012.* UN, 2012. Web. 15 Apr. 2013.

World Health Organization (WHO). *En-gendering the Millennium Development Goals (MDGs) on Health.* WHO, 2003. Web. 13 June 2012.

World Health Organization (WHO), UNICEF, UNFPA and the World Bank. *Trends in Maternal Mortality: 1990 to 2010.* WHO, 2012. Web. 10 Sept. 2013.

Yakong, Vida Nyagre. "Rural Ghanaian Women's Experiences of Seeking Reproductive Health Care." MSN Thesis. University of British Columbia, 2008. Print.

Yakong, Vida Nyagre, Kathy L. Rush, Joan Bassett-Smith, Joan L. Bottorff, and Carole Robinson. "Women's Experiences of Seeking Reproductive Health Care in Rural Ghana: Challenges for Maternal Health Service Utilization." *Journal of Advanced Nursing* 66.11 (2010): 2431–2441. Web. 15 July 2011.

7.
Giving Birth in Douala, Cameroon

A Real Challenge

JEANNETTE WOGAING

THE MOTHERHOOD EXPERIENCE IS SOCIALIZED everywhere, and maternal mortality is a historical fact present in all human societies. In Cameroon, a girl or woman who is pregnant dies every two hours, according to a joint report of the United Nations Funds for Population (UNFPA) and the Ministry of Public Health, Cameroon. The 2011 Cameroonian Government Demographic and Health Survey revealed a maternal mortality rate (MMR) of 782 deaths/100,000 live births. The ever increasing mortality of girls and women in the course of giving birth is a public health problem that led us to question the why and how of these deaths.

Very few historical and anthropological studies have investigated the deep causes of all these avoidable deaths (De Brouwere et al.). Following the international meeting concerning the Millennium Development Goals (MDG), and MDG 5 in particular—regarding the amelioration of maternal mortality in Cameroon, and in view of the recent national statistics on maternal mortality in Cameroon—I sought to understand why Cameroon is among the countries that did not achieve MDG 5 by September 2015.

MATERIAL AND METHODS

Sociocultural practices alone cannot explain the multiple dimensions and the silence that surround maternal death in Douala town. Thus, in order to understand the why and the how of maternal deaths in Douala, I chose to focus on five obstetrical services in different settings, with different structures, and at different levels of maternal care in the city of Douala. These are the Laquintinie Hospital, Ndogbati Protestant Hospital, Cité des Palmiers District Hospital, Saint Thérèse Health Centre, and the Bomono Integrated Health Centre. My study took place from March 2008 to December 2010. The ethnographic data collection was done via interviews, life stories narratives, and case studies with 100 parturients and mothers, plus twenty medical and paramedical personnel. The interviews were conducted with the help of an interview guide or script. The data analysis was combinatory, as I opted for a comprehensive and interpretative method that relies on a quantitative approach. This enabled our research team to analyse expectant mothers' narratives and health care personnel narratives based on their respective experiences.

SOCIOCULTURAL PRACTICES LINKED TO PREGNANCY AND CHILDBIRTH

In all societies, there are beliefs and strategies regarding the protection of obstetrical life. Sociocultural practices might include a set of forbidden foods and behaviours that favour the conservation of the pregnancy and lead to a favourable outcome during childbirth. These cultural practices came into existence long before the development of modern obstetrics. They are not very different from present-day biomedical considerations that consist of antenatal consultations, which aim to monitor the normal progress of the pregnancy and to ensure a happy parturition for both mother and newborn. Despite the biomedical obstetrical revolution, many cultures have maintained traditional ideas and practices, which vary from one culture to another, about pregnancy, gestation, and delivery. In many cultures, a girl or woman is "never alone [but] ... develops her individual experience in the midst of a community. The stages [of delivery] are anticipated and codified: childbirth takes the form of an initiative travel, at the same time social and cultural" (Knibiehler 36). Among the interviewed populations (Bamiléké, Basaa, and Duala), it is striking to realize that they all insist on the necessity of some secrecy surrounding pregnancy. Secrecy is also maintained by virtually all the Bantu populations, with the aim of hiding the pregnancy of the future mother. The pregnant woman must not talk about her pregnancy to strangers, who could make the pregnancy disappear by causing a miscarriage. To talk about a pregnancy means exposing it, thereby risking losing it. In Cameroon as well, this fetal seed-life is very fragile; thus, "we must avoid to make it flow," says Mama Jane, a postmenopausal multiparous woman from Laquintinie Hospital. The verb "to flow" symbolizes the bodily fluids that flow from the womb during a miscarriage.

In Cameroon, generally, the pregnant girl or woman is faced with all sorts restrictions, be they of gesture, posture, behaviour, or food types. The multiplicity of ethnic groups in the country makes a synthesis difficult, as "the exhaustibility of a list of restrictions and prescriptions linked to pregnancy ... is rendered impossible by the variability of cultural areas. Every ethnic group, every clan, or even every family proposes its detailed scheme" (Ewombé-Moundo 58). Traditionally, the risks linked to birthing, such as poor fetal presentations, are materialized by the names some children are given; indeed, it is said that they "come" with their name. Boy babies who birth with footling presentation during delivery are named "Tachum" or "Tchumtchoua," and footling presentation girl babies are named "Matchum." The prefix or suffix "-Tchim" means "to fall" in the Ghoma'la language. In traditional society, these presentations indicate to the *makumou*, "the one who traditionally welcomes life," that she must be more careful with the labouring woman and the child to be born.

A mother who dies during childbirth is neither forgotten nor tabooed. Her offspring will bear a specific name "Wacweu," which means "something thrown away." That is, the mother who died during the delivery process, thus, discarded or abandoned her seed. Among the Bamileke, the Basaa, or the Duala, the names of certain individuals bring to mind their birth circumstances. Furthermore, the names attributed show that the outcome of the delivery was not favourable for the mother; the names also highlight the existence of maternal deaths and the difficulties faced by certain women in procreation (Mayi-Matip 73). Nowadays, apart from some sociocultural practices, few children bear names that relate to their birth or delivery outcome. Besides sociocultural practices, there are other factors linked to modernity that must be taken into account when analyzing maternal mortality rate in Douala.

HOSPITAL DIMENSION OF CHILDBIRTH

In urban and even rural settings, pregnant girls and women aspire to give birth to their children in a hospital environment, where they are received primarily by women health care workers. The health care structure itself is organized as a three-level pyramid. At the base is a health cabinet or a community health centre. At the local or community level, health centres are made up of integrated health centres and health cabinets. The health care providers here are essentially nurses and midwives who take care of basic health needs, promote and provide immunization for children aged zero to five, and give anti-tetanus vaccines for the parturient women and girls. In these centres, women of reproductive age and normal vaginal deliveries can benefit from basic obstetrical care. The Bomono Integrated Health Centre and the Catholic Health Centre correspond to these classification criteria.

District hospitals and divisional health structures make up the intermediate level. Every district and division (peripheral or intermediate level) has a district hospital or a divisional medical centre of varying capacity. These constitute the first reference point for the health centres and cabinets and have at least one medical doctor and a pediatrician. Pregnant girls and women are able to meet a medical doctor here, in addition to receiving basic obstetrical care. The Cité des Palmiers district hospital fits in this category.

At the third or regional level are public and private hospitals, which are the reference centres for the district and divisional hospitals. Laquintinie Hospital and the Protestant Hospital belong to this category. These hospitals have a capacity of more than two hundred beds and facilities for specialized care from physicians who are at the top of the health pyramid. Women and girls experiencing pathological or high-risk pregnancies can receive specialized obstetrical care at these hospitals. A girl or woman can give birth here by Caesarean section, with help from a medical doctor, and her pregnancy could equally be followed up by a specialist, such as a gynaecologist obstetrician. In this public sector, women do not need to pay extra fees to receive specialized care.

In these different health structures, the available equipment is still rudimentary, and the pharmacies are not well supplied, a reality that renders emergency intervention inefficient. Even though the community might be involved indirectly, pregnancy for women is, first of all, an individual experience, the business of the woman carrying the fetus. Ideally, a pregnancy is hidden throughout the first trimester. Only personal motivations prompt girls or women who think they are pregnant to seek confirmation of the pregnancy from medical or paramedical personnel. Furthermore, the pregnancy develops in a context where there is no social security. Listening to her body remains the principle element whereby a woman is able to determine that she is pregnant. For some, in the absence of sympathetic signs or due to lack of time or a previous experience, one of the most reliable ways of confirming pregnancy is to do an echography [ultrasound]. In Cameroon, less than one in every ten pregnant women has an echography (Ntjam 54). Melanie, a primiparous woman at the Protestant Hospital, related that "at the beginning of my pregnancy, I did not have time. I am a *gendarme* [police officer]. I therefore started by doing an echography to have a confirmation of my state. I then went to the hospital later."

In this study, women's obstetrical behaviour was determined by several variables, including age, the number of children, civil status, and profession. These elements are equally indicators that lead to varied obstetrical behaviours. Often, fetal gestational age at the first antenatal consultation marks the first contact with a health structure for virtually all the girls and women. Augustine, a primiparous woman at the Protestant Hospital, noted that she accessed antenatal care "at two weeks" gestation. Whereas Dipocko, a primiparous at the Integrated Health Centre, said that she "went to the hospital at three months [gestational age]." The two main reasons that pregnant women give for their late antenatal consultations were their lack of means or their lack of decision-making power. It is possible that those who come after the first trimester of their pregnancy are ignorant of the fact that the uterus is not always the site of the pregnancy, as the ovum or embryo can implant itself outside the uterine cavity, thereby developing into an ectopic pregnancy. Extra-uterine pregnancies represent the "first cause of maternal mortality in the first trimester of pregnancy" (Leke et al. 693).

THE DELIVERY ROOM:
A FEMININE AND FEMINIZED SETTING?

Globally, traditional cultures present a history of childbirth as an entirely feminine universe of experience and practice. Child birthing practices are perhaps the oldest labour a woman accomplishes for herself or in assisting another woman (Bartoli). Historically, Cameroonian men were not allowed to be present when women are in labour and during delivery. In the light of historical narration of the women interviewed, only older women and those well experienced in birthing took part in deliveries.

Today, every woman goes to the hospital based on her understanding of the risk linked to pregnancy or her expectations of hospital care. Women expressed their primary fears to be long and difficult deliveries, placental retention, and bad positions or "*mal* presentations."

At the traditional level, the birth attendants, or those who "received life," had in common the fact that they all belonged to the cultural group within which they practised. This offered psychological security or cultural safety to the parturient, since attendants knew the ways and customs of their soil. Birth attendants' knowledge was acquired by personal experience and, at times, through an apprenticeship with an experienced maternal relative (Wogaing, *Maternité et décès maternels*).

In the past, men were excluded from the place of delivery for reasons of their incompetence and to maintain feminine decency. Today, in delivery rooms in Cameroon, women remain the most numerically represented portion of the personnel, thus constituting the pivot of obstetrical practice in hospital settings. Paradoxically, however, future mothers, no matter their status, complain about the women health care personnel. Claire, a primiparous woman at the Catholic Health Centre, remarked that "when you get to the hospital, you are poorly welcomed. The nurses shout a lot. They are impulsive and impatient. I would rather deal with men." The women prefer being in the good hands of masculine delivery personnel because they are more understanding and patient (Wogaing, *Rethinking Childbirth*). Thus, Annick, a primipara at Laquintinie Hospital, noted that "if I were to choose who should conduct my delivery, I would never choose a woman." Cathy Flore, a multipara at the Catholic Health Centre, stated she "hates women during delivery." These mothers-to-be, like Ngo, another primipara at the Catholic Health Centre, say that the men are "more affectionate and less aggressive than the women." Whether they are unmarried, married, or a co-wife, these future mothers remain convinced that the attitude of nurses contributes ineluctably to determining the outcome of parturition (see Figure 1), much more than their own personal omissions—not attending antenatal consultations after the first trimester of pregnancy or delivering without any laboratory tests—might determine their outcome

The "Happy" Ones

The "happy ones" are women who respected all their cultural food taboos and behavioural patterns. Socially, they survived all the hazards linked to parturition by benefiting from the goodness of nature. They have no scars. These are women who have "normal" pregnancies and spontaneous deliveries.

At Laquintinie Hospital, Marcela, a pauciparous woman—one who has already experienced birth three times—related, "I have always given birth normally. This is my third delivery without any cut or tear." The "happy ones" come from all social classes, independent of their anthropological characteristics. They can give birth anywhere and with the help of any courageous person. For this to happen, according to Mama Njock, a post-menopausal, grand multiparous woman, all the assisting person needs is to "keep her head and to have a clean sharp object to cut the umbilical cord, wait for the expulsion of the placenta, and then let her rest." Their "cherub" is in good health. Concerning the "happy ones," Diarra remarked that these are parturients who had the grace to have "a so-called simple delivery by the nurses and needed no manoeuvres from the [nurse] and no transfer. All the management ... was done at the delivery unit under the sole responsibility of the [nurse]." Socially, the factors favouring this "happy" situation are sometimes random events, such as the woman's behaviour during her pregnancy and childbirth, or the fact that parturition happened to be in good hands. Nevertheless, there exist also "bruised happy ones."

The "Bruised Happy Ones"

Those women described as the "bruised happy ones" are physically healthy after delivery, but their neonates are sick or "badly done;" that is, they are neonates with imperfections, handicaps, or infirmities right from birth or are infants who die in the course of birthing or immediately postpartum. Cultural explanations for these outcomes are that these mothers did not observe their ways and customs for the conservation of their pregnancy and the neonate's survival. Medical causes of these neonatal deaths are multiple: fetal distress, congenital malformation, poor fetal presentation, inappropriate management of delivery, a nosocomial (hospital acquired) infection or sudden death of the child. The women are psychologically affected because of the infant's health condition or by the death of their baby, but they are happy to have escaped death themselves.

Ngo Mbog, a primipara pregnant with twins, delivered within physiological norms but, unfortunately, lost her babies. "While being pregnant, I was impatient to hold them in my hands.... They were hardly born that they have already gone back. What can I do? What have I done?" Ngo Mbog's situation had several causes. Despite a prematurely dilated cervix, she travelled on foot to the clinic and then gave birth prematurely in a setting that lacked incubators. I also noted at the clinic the absence of a delivery plan in place for a primipara pregnant with twins.

The "Near Misses"

The "near misses" are those women who deliver "abnormally" but, as their name may suggest, they narrowly missed death at the end of the birth process and postpartum. They are divided into two main categories and two subclasses: those who give birth vaginally and those who give birth abdominally by Caesarean section, often called the "operated" or surgical patients.

The vaginal "near misses" are parturients who deliver abnormally and whose delivery can start at one health structure and end up in another obstetrical unit. An "abnormal delivery" is one whereby the parturient, in addition to delivery complications, is subjected to obstetrical mutilations that, according to De Forts (67-68), include episiotomies, obstetrical tears, infections, and obstetrical fistulae

(Skard 112-3). The abnormal delivery is described as difficult or toilsome and may require the use of forceps and other instruments. Complications often result from the social pressure incurred by the future mother (often due to her socioeconomic status), whereas the mutilations are often associated with the woman's physiology, such as her pelvic structure and by her obstetrical past history. Other complications can result from factors such as fetal weight, the pathological position of the fetus, and impatience on the part of the nurses.

Jade, a primipara at Laquintinie Hospital, underwent an episiotomy, as do those who sustain obstetrical tears. She remarked that "the nurse told me that I was at risk of sustaining a tear, so she preferred cutting me." Thus, Alida, a primipara at Protestant Hospital, related that she "had a big tear during the expulsion phase. I thought I will die. My child drank amniotic liquid." These mothers are found in all social classes, independent of their anthropological characteristics. In contrast to the "happy ones," for whom delivering is "natural," for those who experience "near misses," childbirth is a battle (De Sardan et al.) and the outcome is not always to the advantage of mother or child. The delivered women may survive, but without their baby (the "bruised ones"), or they may survive it with their baby. The child, however, may or may not be in good health but born sick or handicapped. In fact, the pregnancy can just "as well lead to unpredicted *in utero* deaths or deaths at birth, unless fate hounds more insidiously on them that they may not give birth to 'counterfeit' children" (Soussan 119).

The "Operated"

The "operated" are those women, found in all socio-economic classes, who when vaginal delivery is impossible, give birth by Caesarean section or C-section, a surgical operation that consists of extracting the fetus via an incision of the abdominal wall and the uterus. C-sections are often necessary in cases of fetomaternal malformations, such as a mother with small pelvis and a big fetus or the foetus is in a transverse position. The child may be in good health, sick, or handicapped. More and more, the prognosis of Caesarean delivery is determined during the antenatal consultations as a function of imaging technology (obstetrical echography).

C-Section Perceptions and the Neonate's Fate

Therese, herself a "near miss," says that for some "happy ones" and "near misses," "delivery by C-section means poor delivery." Furthermore, "this delivery mode presents greater risks," as Antoinette, a pauciparious and "a happy one" at Protestant Hospital, further emphasized:

> *When you give birth by C-section, it is dangerous. It is really very risky. Imagine you get to a hospital; they have to operate on you; there is no light. You are aware of our repetitive electrical failures. There is no stand-by generator. What do you do? You are really exposed. Or, if a woman comes in labour and then the nurse discovers that she cannot give birth normally, you must deliver by C-section and the medical doctor is not available or some members of his team are not present, what do you do? There are even some cases whereby the doctor wants his money first! If you do not have money, you can die like a joke. Women who give birth by C-section are really in danger.*

Narratives vary among those who had to face a C-section, based on the circumstances of the obstetrical surgery. It all depends on their preparation for delivery, as some are sensitized well ahead of time to the possibility of a Caesarean section, whereas others are only informed of the delivery mode when they are already in labour. Catherine, a pauciparous, C-section surgical patient at Protestant hospital, was operated on for the third consecutive time. The first experience was traumatizing and, in her own words, she was very afraid and still retains a bad memory of the event:

> *It is the third time that I give birth by C-section. My gynaecologist told me that I have a narrow pelvis but I do not bear big babies: 3.5kg, 2.5kg, and 2.9kg. My first C-section was at Laquintinie Hospital. I was really afraid. Even to shave your pubic hair the nurse asks for CFA 5000 [USD 11]. The doctors ... or at least the members of the team did not inform me of anything. I found the nurses really cold. When I was placed in the reanimation room, it was*

terrible. You will call for the nurse and nobody will come. It took some little motivation to get their attention. I assure you that the attitude of the personnel can precipitate your death.

For those who are informed they would undergo a Caesarean section, at the time of the transfer to or even in the delivery room, the situation is pathetic. They are broken; some even cry out loud when the prognosis is announced. When the nurse who prepares the surgical patient is "cold" or "lukewarm," the situation is even worse. Since she is not ready financially, the patient does not benefit from a psychological management of her situation. Some women are often preoccupied by the opinion that their in-laws will have of them at the end of this process. Those who do not have the financial means lose all their self-esteem because they are not up to the task of a "normal delivery." Their in-laws will only see them as "vulgar" spenders who take advantage of childbirth to ruin the husband. I took part in the preparation of a paucipara woman awaiting a Caesarean section, and this excerpt from my notes, taken at the time, reflects her dismay:

She cried so much, the nurse did not know what to tell her in order to appease her. Her worry was what her husband and her in-law family will say as regards her delivery. She will not stop crying out: "Last time I gave birth without problems [referring to her vaginal delivery]. What happened this time? What will my husband say?" The nurse brought the person who accompanied the mother to the hospital into the delivery room to try to reason with her as well. As for the nurse, she did not want the patient's blood pressure to rise because she explained, a high blood pressure will not favour a C-section. Such news, instead of calming the patient, was rather troublesome for her as she had not been prepared for a Caesarean section.

A minority of the "happy ones" and "near misses" said that the essential thing is to give birth, regardless of the delivery route chosen by the child to enter into the world. The important issue here is that the pregnant woman must be informed and that the health care personnel provide psychological assistance. A C-sectioned patient at the Protestant Hospital and at the Laquintinie Hospital remarked that whether it was programmed long ago or not, "one must be prepared for any outcome and be sensitized no matter the time. In fact, it is the fear of not waking up after the surgery that scares the women. The medical doctor must inform the women as to the why and how of the C-section." But, as noted above, in the case of the "near misses" who deliver vaginally, the outcome is not always to the advantage of the mother-child pair because "C-sectioned" patients emerge either alone or with their neonate, who might be "badly done."

What often seems absurd is that despite the risks taken by the woman to bring forth a child, when she leaves without a baby, she is the person who feels guilty. The long-awaited child gave up along the way, unable to survive passage through the vaginal walls during delivery. It is as though "the needs and efforts of the mother did not coincide with those of the foetus" (Flanagan 83). Either the baby dies in utero or a few minutes after delivery, leaving the mother at a loss. She does not have the time to recover from labour pains and all other related sufferings, yet already she mourns for her baby. Moreover, she does not have the right to express her pain, her suffering. Most often she hears herself repeating: "One does not mourn for a neonate! He did not want to stay; it was a bad child! You will have another one." The social pressure and the obligations linked to her feminine role impel her to conceive again in the following months, as soon as her menses resume. The womb is not recovered but already she must be seeking a new pregnancy. Compared to the "bruised happy ones," some "near misses," despite the trauma their bodies went through, step out with live and healthy babies, just like the "cherubs" born to the "happy ones." But the most unjust situation is that of the future mother who loses her life in a bid to give life or who dies for refusing to be a mother.

The *"Damned"*

The "damned" are those who die in the course of their pregnancy or during childbirth. There are two distinct categories of the "damned." The first category consists of those who decided to carry their pregnancy to term and become mothers but who die during birthing. Their newborn baby may be in good health, sick, or might also end up dying. The second category consists of those who refuse motherhood and voluntarily interrupt their pregnancy by abortion (Cazenave 157). As with the previous categories, the "damned" are found in all social classes.

Women who had an abortion go against "the foundations of ... society, that is, the famous myth of motherhood as being the sole and unique identity of women" (Desmarais 52). For the "damned," childbearing is war; delivery implies the possibility of dying.

The second category of "damned," women who decide to interrupt their pregnancy, is in contrast with warriors, those who fight to defend their territories or ideas. On the one hand, they do not want to be "women," in the cultural sense of the word, mothers. But they have made the choice not to become mothers in an environment where abortion is not legalized, where having babies is an obligation, but also where abortion is stigmatized and can be perilous to one's health and life. Even though women are exposed to the dangers linked to delivery or abortion, the risk seems to be least in the case of an accepted pregnancy since, at the end of the day, women who deliver have respected their social contract, whereas those who refused have remained "themselves," by rejecting the cultural definition of womanhood. Unfortunately, those who die in the course of abortion do not have time to triumph and, to an extent, are the martyrs of motherhood and of the female sex. My analysis shows that culturally, the appearance of the "bruised happy ones," the "near misses," and the "C-sectioned" marks, among other things, a partial failure of the culture, whereas the "damned category" materializes as a total failure of culture. In reality, the existence of these categories also depends on the woman's social status and malfunctioning of the health system (see figure 1).

As for the parturient women who die during delivery or abortion, their death permits them to find some peace from those nurses who used to shout at them. They give to the delivery room that quietness the nurses had been requiring of them. Some partners, who were hoping for boys and not girls, remain speechless.[1] The father, who deplored his daughter's state as a cohabitating single

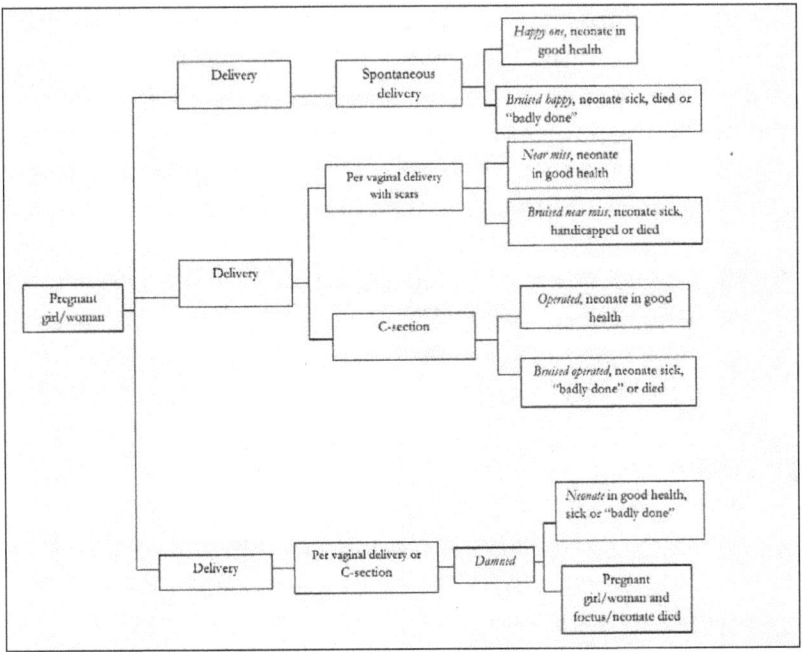

Fig. 1: The Various Issues of Delivery in Douala, Cameroon

mother, did not have the time to say goodbye to his daughter, who was actually making him a grandfather.

Chloe was living with the father of her child and she died after giving birth due to an eclampsia crisis. Ingrid and Marie Astride, while seeking to become mothers, also found death in the delivery room of Laquintinie Hospital. This hospital, because of its status as a category three "reference hospital," served as the only health structure possessing data that could be used for a retrospective analysis, with emphasis on the anthropological characteristics of the admitted patients. Marie Astrid, a primapara, gave birth to a live baby boy at the Deido District Hospital, a little after midnight on September 4, 2008. At 11:45 a.m., she was evacuated from the Deido District Hospital to Laquintinie Hospital for immediate postpartum eclampsia and her febrile state. I found her lying on a delivery table. She had an intravenous line. Since she could no longer communicate, I had no idea of how long she had been there, staring into emptiness.

Marie Astrid died there of postpartum eclampsia; she did not have the same luck as the "happy ones" or the "near misses." She "gave birth normally!" said her father, who was inconsolable. "Who will take care of this boy she did not have time to know." So many questions remained unanswered. At reception, I learned that her relatives were seeking a means to have her transferred to the recovery room for intensive care. The nurse considered that the parents had delayed in taking the young mother to the hospital.

> *That's how they [parents] are. When they are transferred, they delay before coming. When they arrive, they don't have money for emergency management; afterwards, they will accuse us of neglecting the patients. It is very easy to make us bear the cap. If this woman had done all her laboratory tests in the course of pregnancy, maybe we could have avoided all what is happening now. We do not have the necessary equipment to reanimate her. She must be taken to the reanimation service. We have told her parents! We do not know what they are waiting for to take her there."*

When I went to meet Marie Astrid's mother who came with her and was waiting at the reception, she told me,

> *I don't understand what is happening. At Deido [District Hospital], we were asked to take her to Laquintinie. That is what we have done; we have bought what they asked us to; a little while later, they told us to take her to the reanimation service. [She cries]. I don't know anymore, she gave birth normally! The nurses do not tell us anything; do we know anything in medicine? Are they not to do what is necessary?*

The delivery room did not have oxygen at that time. The parents estimated that it was the duty of the health personnel to take Maria Astrid to the recovery room. "Do we work here? We are just strangers! ... We brought her into the ward, they saw what was wrong; it is in their place to take her where they say she has to go!"

For Marie Astrid's parents, taking her to recovery was a logical follow-up, part of the care that she needed. But it was not their duty to take her there. It was a responsibility the health care personnel should have assumed. Moreover, if the personnel of the Deido District Hospital could not manage her case, it was the duty of the doctors at the delivery room of Laquintinie Hospital to take care of her. The parental obligation was to take their daughter to a specialist, which they did. Accusations were coming in from every direction. According to the parents, although they had paid, their daughter had not received any care since their arrival at the delivery room. Marie Astrid had received first aid, but she presented with respiratory distress that could not be managed in the delivery room because it did not have the appropriate equipment for such care, necessitating an immediate transfer to the reanimation service. This is how, from hesitations to accusations and counter-accusations, Marie Astrid was not taken to recovery and could not, therefore, benefit from intensive care. Marie Astrid passed away at 2:30 p.m. in the delivery room of a reference hospital.[2]

Marie Astrid gave birth in a district hospital and then to a "referral" health structure for the health centres and health cabinets. A referral health structure[3] must provide basic obstetrical service and on-duty personnel capable of managing cases of complications, such as eclampsia, postpartum haemorrhage and respiratory distress. But due to many inadequacies, Marie Astrid was transferred—actually taken there by her parents—to Laquintinie Hospital for better management. At the Laquintinie delivery room, the nurses and institutional actors in charge of childbirth obviously have the same training as those working in the maternity ward where Marie Astrid gave birth (Deido District Hospital). However, once the doctor on duty has done his rounds, he only comes in when he is invited, which implies that when a patient is in an emergency situation, the nurse is the first contact with that patient. The nurse thus makes the initial diagnosis before deciding whether or not the specialist should be called. In this case, only professional conscience or an acknowledgement of one's limitations comes into play in the decision-making process. Furthermore, the delivery room had no communication system that could enable personnel in the room to contact outside resources without them having to leave the room themselves.

Clearly, even if the nurse did have personal cell phone, she would not have put her communication credits at the disposal of the consulting community. The responsibility in this case falls on the patient or the person accompanying her. This is the situation in which Marie Astrid's parents found themselves when, because of a lack of equipment, they had to get their daughter out of the delivery room to the recovery service. Thus, the failures and malfunctions common to this setting precluded saving Marie Astrid, who was considered *a priori* to be in good hands. Marie Astrid lay on the table for over two hours without any decision being taken about her situation. Everything happened as though the urinary catheter inserted in Marie Astrid represented a sort of palliative care. I suggest that if the delivery room had been supplied with adequate equipment and with competent personnel readily available for the management of obstetrical emergencies, Marie Astrid would still be alive. If the health personnel had considered her case as an obstetrical emergency, Marie Astrid could have been saved.

Ingrid's situation differs from Marie Astrid, but both narratives have in common the fate of the two parturients. At term in her pregnancy, Ingrid's common-law spouse brought her to the delivery room at 4:30 p.m., where she was received by the on duty nurse (a man this time). In the entry registers, I noticed she was hospitalized for severe anaemia. The delivery nurse auscultated her (listened to her internal organs) and asked the family to buy two pints of blood. As with every reference hospital, the Laquintinie Hospital has a blood bank but to obtain a pint of blood, it is not enough to pay the corresponding code at the cashier's desk. One must resort to a family donor who is there specifically to donate blood to save the life of that particular kinsperson.[4] Thus, for a pint of blood, every patient must bring two donors and disburse a sum of money, varying between CFA 10, 250 to 15, 000 (between USD 23 to USD 33), depending on whether or not they are hospitalized in the health system. When there is no one available on site, as a last resort, one must call on remunerated donors. While studying the representations of blood among the Bamileke, Basaa and Duala as well as the influence of these representations on blood donation, Ngo Billong (56) noticed that remunerated donors are never far away from the blood banks. Ingrid's family was ready to pay the necessary price to save her and her baby: "At the Laquintinie Hospital, you will find their phone contacts and they will ask you to pay a caution of CFA 5000 [USD 11] per donor depending on the stock of blood that had been tested and secured ... At times, the bids may go as high as CFA 15, 000 [USD 33] for a pint of blood." Sometime later, one of her parents brought back the requested pints of blood.

The delivery nurse transfused the first pint of blood, after which there was no real change, so he proceeded to place the second pint, also to no avail. Despite the transfusion, Ingrid was going pale, and the nurse noticed that there was no blood loss by any natural orifice to alert him. Ingrid seemed rather calm, with no noticeable panic or fear on her face; she seemed not to take notice of anything happening around her. She seemed absent and febrile. The nurse was constantly taking her blood pressure and reporting that it was normal. For this reason, she had not been placed on the delivery table but on a bed in the labour room. Three hours later, the nurse noticed that there was still no amelioration, so he called the medical doctor on duty who, after making his diagnosis, opted for a C-section to try and rescue the mother and the baby. Unfortunately, Ingrid died at around 9:45 p.m., before the surgery could be done in the theatre. Then her family began to talk; below is an extract of the words spoken by Ingrid's sister:

> **Sister:** *My [brother]-in-law had the bad habit of beating her up. This afternoon, he quarrelled with my sister. In fact, it was because of a dispute between her and another mistress of my [brother]-in-law. A fight broke out between the two of them. It is possible that he gave her a kick in the belly. Afterwards, she started feeling pains. I don't know if it is that kick that ended up being fatal?*
>
> **Nurse:** *So why did you not say anything when you brought her here?*
>
> **Sister:** *It is my in-law who brought her! I only got the story afterwards!*
>
> **Nurse:** *What a pity! We could have done an echography.*

She was really very pale. Despite the two pints of blood that we gave her, there was no amelioration because she was emptying herself on the inside! The result is there; in spite of all our efforts, we could not save the mother or the child. You will be the first to say that, at Laquintinie, we neglect patients. Meanwhile, you are the ones lacking any consideration for your relatives. Where are we now?

Allegedly, Ingrid had been a victim of domestic violence by her partner. All that was left to do was to take her corpse to the mortuary. For these girls and women, pregnancy and childbirth constitute a warrior's journey (Des Forts 25-32). These women's deaths, being at the same time unpredictable and also avoidable, remain a source of questioning. These deaths take place in an environment where the women only aspire to be women, and as mothers they desire to live this new phase of their lives.

CONCLUSION

At the end of this research on childbearing and its outcomes, what stands out is that the fate of parturients is favoured by factors that are at the same time sociocultural and biomedical or hospital linked. Food and behavioural restrictions during pregnancy are not obstacles to accessing modern obstetrical care and delivery. The "happy ones" have "normal" pregnancies, spontaneous term deliveries, and their babies are in good health. The "bruised happy ones" are physically healthy after delivery, but their neonates are sick or "badly done." That is, born with imperfections, handicaps, infirmities, some of whom end up dying as neonates. The vaginal "near misses" are parturients who deliver abnormally. In addition to delivery complications, they are subjected to obstetrical mutilations. They may survive without their babies (the "bruised ones") or survive with babies who may be in good health or who may be sick or handicapped; again, some may end up dying. The "operated" are those who give birth by Caesarean section. Their neonate might be in good health, sick or "badly done" and end up dying. "The damned" are those who have died during pregnancy or delivery, along with their baby. Sometimes, their neonate can survive in good health or survive as "badly done."

Mothers must give birth in a humanized and humane setting, where there will be more "happy ones;" a place where the midwife, who remains a practitioner with limited competence, will present complicated cases to the gynaeco-obstetrician within proper clinical time frames to ensure the rescue of the "near misses." Such an approach will reduce the number of the unfortunate "damned."

Urgent measures need to be taken, and the Cameroon health system must be reorganized and restructured to ease delivery in a hospital setting, where there are trained personnel who are highly qualified to receive life. Even now, with the pyramid structure of health care and hospitals, health care in Cameroon still "misses the mark" in providing good maternal and reproductive health care for all women.

ENDNOTES

[1] Even though I did not mention the preference of a baby boy, one of the interviewees at the district hospital maternity burst into tears when the nurse announced that she had just given birth to a baby girl. "Another one!" she said with tears. "My husband will kill me! She is the fourth," she declared crying. She first refused to take care of her newborn. The paramedical team members in the maternity ward had to mobilize themselves around her to convince her to take care of the baby and to explain to her human reproduction as well as the genetic factors that determined the sex of a child.

[2] A "reference maternity" is a service or obstetrical unit whose personnel and technical facilities offer quality care to pregnant women. The "reference" hospital, in addition to the medical personnel and technical facilities, offers specialized health care.

[3] In 2008, Laquintinie Hospital did 3,853 deliveries, an average of 321 deliveries per week, or eight to eleven deliveries per day. The lowest figure was 260 births in February 2008, compared to 428 births in May 2008. For the same period, at the Cité des

Palmiers District Hospital, the delivery room recorded 525 deliveries for an average of 43 births per month. The real proportion of deliveries was 30 to 61 deliveries per month, an average of one to two births per day.

[4]There equally exist benevolent donors who are individuals who freely give their blood in hospital centres.

WORKS CITED

Bartoli, Lise. *Venir au monde*. Paris: Payot et Rivages, 2007. Print.

Cazenave, Odile. *Femmes rebelles. Naissance d'un nouveau roman africain au féminin*. Paris: L'Harmattan, 1996. Print.

de Brouwere, Vincent, René Tonglet, and Wim Van Lerberghe. *La Maternité sans Risque dans les pays en développement: les leçons de l'histoire*. Antwerp, Belgium: Studies in Health Services Organisation & Policy, 1997. Print.

de Sardan, Olivier, Jean-Pierre, Adamou Moumouni, and Aboubacar Souley. "L'accouchement c'est la guerre—De quelques problèmes liés à l'accouchement en milieu rural nigérien." *Le bulletin de l'APAD 17, Anthropologie de la santé*. 2006. Web. 6 Mar. 2009.

des Forts, Jacqueline. *Violences et corps des femmes du Tiers-Monde*. Paris: L'Harmattan, 2001. Print.

Diarra, Aïssa. "La Production de la violence au fil des décisions dans quelques services publics de santé maternelle au Mali." *Le bulletin de l'APAD 25, La Violence endémique en Afrique*, 2007. Web. 23 Aug. 2010.

Desmarais, Louise. "L'avortement ou l'envers d'un mythe." *Espaces et temps de la maternité* Eds. Francine Saillant et Christine Corbeil. Montréal : Remue-ménage, 51-67. 2002. Print.

Ewombé-Moundo, Elisabeth. "La Callipédie ou l'art d'avoir de beaux enfants en Afrique Noire." *Grossesse et petite enfance en Afrique Noire et à Madagascar*. Ed. Suzanne Lallemand. Paris: L'Harmattan, 1991. 41-60. Print.

Flanagan, Géraldine Lux. *Les Neuf premiers mois de la vie*. Paris: Robert Laffont, 1963. Print.

Knibiehler, Yvonne. *Histoire des mères et de la maternité en occident*. Paris: Presses Universitaires de France, 2000. Print.

Leke, Robert J., N. Goiyaux, T. Matsuda, and P. F. Tonneau. "Ectopic Pregnancy in Africa: A Population-Based Study." *Obstet. Gynecol.* 103.4 (2004): 92-97. Print.

Mayi-Matip, Théodore. *L'Univers de la parole*. Yaoundé: CLE, 1983. Print.

Ngo Billong, Germaine. *Le Sang dans ses représentations chez les Duala, Basaa et Bamiléké et leur influence sur le don de sang: l'apport anthropologique*. Mémoire de Diplôme d'Etudes Approfondies en Anthropologie de la santé. Douala: Université de Douala, 2008. Print.

Ntyam, Marie-Chantale. *Handicap et intégration au Cameroun: représentations parentales du handicap et mise en apprentissage des enfants handicapés*. Thèse de Doctorat en Psychologie Clinique, Université de Picardie Jules Verne, Amiens. 2008. Print.

OMS [WHO]. *Statistiques sanitaires mondiales*. OMS, 2012. Web. 23 Aug. 2010.

Skard, Torild. *Afrique des Femmes, Afrique d'Espoir*. Paris: L'Harmattan. 2004. Print.

Soussan, Ben Patrick. *La Grossesse n'est pas une maladie*. Paris: SYROS, 2000. Print.

United Nations Funds for Population and Minister of Public Health, Cameroon. *Plaidoyer pour la réduction de la mortalité maternelle et néonatale au Cameroun*. FNUAP, 2009. Web.23 Aug. 2010.

Wogaing Jeannette. *Maternité et décès maternels à Douala (Cameroun): Approches socio-anthropologiques*. Thèse de doctorat en anthropologie, Université de Strasbourg/Université de Douala. 2012. Print.

Wogaing Jeannette. *Rethinking Childbirth: The Male Gender as Preferential Model during Delivery*. Douala, Cameroon: Revue ABA, University of Douala. In press.

8.
Throwing the Mother Out with the Bathwater

Vanuatu's Breastfeeding Initiative in Theory and Practice

CHELSEA WENTWORTH

THE PROMOTION OF BREASTFEEDING as a means to reduce child malnutrition has been a cornerstone of public health policy for nearly forty years (Labbok and Krasovec; van Esterik). The Baby-Friendly Hospital Initiative was created in the 1980s through the joint efforts of WHO and UNICEF, as they attempted to combat growing fears that mothers across the globe were breastfeeding in decreasing rates, contributing to poor child health, growth, and development outcomes (Black et al.; de Onis et al.; Pérez-Escamilla). The program was designed to help mothers begin breastfeeding immediately after birth, ideally within the first hour, to breastfeed exclusively for the first six months, and to continue breastfeeding with complementary foods through the first twenty-four months of the child's life (de Onis et al.). As the use of infant formula as a breast milk substitute in both the developed and the developing world was on the rise, the Baby-Friendly Hospital Initiative sought to address this problem directly through a uniform set of standards and practices implemented at hospitals worldwide.

Although often referred to as simply the Baby-Friendly Hospital Initiative (BFHI), recent recognition of the benefits of breastfeeding for maternal health and the need for lactation support for mothers have prompted a change in the name to the Mother and Baby-Friendly Hospital Initiative (MBFHI). In the past several years, some hospitals have received this MBFHI certification; however, the name change has not been widely adopted, and even on the WHO website, the program is still commonly referred to simply as the BFHI with no distinct information marking specific changes for the MBFHI. This inconsistency of the role of the mother in the name and in the implementation of the program is indicative of the treatment of mothers in Vila Central Hospital, the MBFHI-certified hospital in Vanuatu.

In this chapter, I examine the Mother and Baby-Friendly Hospital Initiative as it is interpreted and implemented in Vanuatu, a small Pacific Island nation. Drawing on extensive ethnographic fieldwork conducted in 2010, 2012-13, and 2015, I look at the ways that breastfeeding and bottle feeding are discussed among mothers and health care practitioners. I argue that with increased pressure at Vila Central Hospital to promote and support the goals of the MBFHI, nurses, doctors, nurse aides, midwives and other hospital staff, whom I group under the term health care practitioners in this chapter, create a place where bottle feeding is interpreted as failure and laziness on the part of the mother. These data reveal that negative discourse on the quality of care mothers provide to their infants affects future interactions between mothers and health care practitioners. Negative discourse sets the mothers on a course of distrust and poor interaction with health care practitioners. Subsequently, this influences mother's attitudes towards health services and the level of trust for the advice provided to them and their young children.

HEALTH DEMOGRAPHICS, CHILDHOOD MALNUTRITION, AND THE MDGS IN VANUATU

Situated to the west of Fiji and northeast of Australia, Vanuatu is an archipelago comprised of 83 islands, nearly all of which are inhabited. With great cultural diversity, the roughly 260,000 people living in Vanuatu—the ni-Vanuatu, as they have been calling themselves since they gained independence in 1980—speak over 110 distinct languages. From 1906 through 30 July 1980, both the French and British colonial governments jointly administered the islands as a colony, then called the New Hebrides (Rodman). Although still labeled as one of the Least Developed Countries (LDC) in the world, Vanuatu has seen rapid population growth, particularly in the urban centre of Port Vila, its capital (Vanuatu Young People's Project). As people move from the outer islands to Port Vila in search of employment and access to cash, the increasingly congested city is experiencing rising unemployment, land scarcity, crowded living conditions and, subsequently, has the highest rates of childhood undernutrition in the country (Knowles). Port Vila is also the site of the largest hospital in the country, Vila Central Hospital (VCH). First certified through the BFHI, VCH was unable to meet the requirements of re-evaluation and lost its accreditation. However, in December 2012, it celebrated the success of certification in the MBFHI. The Ministry of Health hopes eventually to certify two other hospitals in the country, on the islands of Tanna and Santo.

The research presented in this paper was part of a larger study examining the social, economic, and environmental factors that contribute to persistent problems of childhood malnutrition in urban and peri-urban Vanuatu. Drawing on data collected from interviews, participant observation, surveys administered at visits at well-baby clinics, dietary journals, and a visual-cognitive elicitation project, this research yielded an array of data on the factors that influence infant and young child feeding in an area with a high prevalence of food insecurity. Much of these data address questions beyond the scope of this paper. However, I have written about other aspects of this project elsewhere, including how children use community feasts as a coping mechanism for food insecurity (Wentworth, *Feasting and Food Security*; "Public Eating, Private Pain") and the influence of kin networks on child nutrition, as children are cared for by a number of extended family members (Wentworth, *The Influence of Kin Networks*).

Childhood malnutrition is a significant problem facing many developing countries around the world. Despite nutrition education programs, Vanuatu continues to experience high rates of undernutrition in children, birth to age five, expressed as underweight (low weight for age), stunting (low height for age) and wasting (low weight for height). Working with UNICEF, WHO, and AUSAID, the Vanuatu Ministry of Health has conducted several nation-wide surveys of maternal and child health (Knowles; Vanuatu). The most recent survey was completed in 2007, with summary results presented in Table 1. When compared to the previous survey in 1996, there was no statistically significant change in the rates of underweight, stunting, and wasting in children. The 2007 Vanuatu Nutrition Survey revealed that across Vanuatu, of children under five years of age, 11 percent are underweight, 26.3 percent are stunted, and 5.8 percent are wasted. However, children living in the city of Port Vila have rates of malnutrition higher than the national averages. This is particularly troublesome when examining the rates of stunting, which indicate chronic, long-term malnutrition is highest in Port Vila at 29.5 percent of children under five[1] (Knowles). Using Port Vila as the nexus of this research was critical to understanding the economic, environmental and, cultural factors contributing to the chronic problem of malnutrition where it is most severe.

Vanuatu's averages are slightly better than global averages for developing countries, but they are not yet achieving the targets of the Millennium Development Goals (MDGs) for malnutrition in children. Furthermore, these numbers have *not* demonstrated that the situation has improved as compared with earlier nutrition surveys dating back to 1996 (Shuaib and Rahman). To have no statistically significant change over a ten-year period indicates a serious problem in the context of the MDGs, which strive to halve the number of children suffering from hunger. Based on these surveys, Vanuatu has not made any measurable strides toward achieving this goal. However, since the last survey data was collected, efforts have been made to change this, particularly in the area of breastfeeding as a critical source of infant nutrition.

Both nutrition surveys collected data on the rates of initial breastfeeding, and Vanuatu has high rates of initial breastfeeding. Rates are particularly high in Port Vila, which is likely due to the larger numbers of women who give birth in the hospital and receive breastfeeding education and support at that time. The 2007 survey revealed that the national average of children who breastfed within one hour of birth was 72 percent, and 82 percent of infants are breastfed within their first twenty-four hours of life. The averages for Port Vila were slightly better than the national averages in which 85.9 percent of infants are breastfed within the first hour of birth, and 91.2 percent breastfeed within their first twenty-four hours (Knowles). The 1996 National Nutrition Survey shows that 10 percent of infants were exclusively breastfed for their first six months. However, the 2007 Multiple Indicator Cluster

Table 1: Birth to Age Five Child Malnourishment in Vanuatu (Knowles)

		Weight for age: % below -2 SD	Weight for age % below -3 SD	Height for age: % below -2 SD	Height for age: % below -3 SD	Weight for height: % below -2 SD	Weight for height: % below -3 SD	Weight for height: % above +2 SD
Region	Tafea	6.7	1.7	25.8	9	1.1	1.1	6.2
	Shefa	8.9	0.6	23.4	5.7	4.4	0	3.2
	Malampa	11.6	1.8	26.8	7.1	2.7	0.9	3.6
	Penama	14.4	0.8	27.1	5.1	7.6	2.5	4.2
	Sanma	13.4	3.6	28.6	9.8	10.7	1.8	1.8
	Torba	14.6	4.1	17.1	4.1	6.5	2.4	1.6
Cities	Port Vila	10	3.6	29.5	12.8	8.9	5.3	8.5
	Luganville	18.2	1.7	22.3	9.1	8.3	0.8	6.6
Area	Urban	11.4	3.2	28.2	12.1	8.8	4.5	8.2
	Rural	11	1.8	25.9	7.3	5.2	1.2	3.7
Vanuatu Country Total		11	2.1	26.3	8.2	5.8	1.8	4.5

Survey (MICS) indicates that 39.7 percent of infants are breastfed exclusively for the first six months. Survey administrators of the MICS state that because of the differences in the way the questions were framed in each of the surveys, it is difficult to compare these data. However, they do suggest that the differences between the two surveys do not show statistically significant changes, as percentages for both datasets fall within the 95 percent confidence interval (Knowles).

It is important to note that despite advances in nutrition education administered throughout the country, the situation had not improved, and it was unlikely that Vanuatu would achieve the Millennium Development Goals for childhood malnutrition and hunger. Millennium Development Goal Target 1c was to halve, between 1990 and 2015, the proportion of people who suffer from hunger; it focused on global data that showed undernourishment as a key indicator of hunger. Growth stunting is a particularly important indicator of hunger and undernourishment, as it indicates chronic hunger rather than short-term malnourishment that could be caused by an acute disease, such as diarrhea. Stunting indicates a much more severe problem of undernourishment that is measured in a child's stature. Stunting can indicate irreversible brain damage and developmental delays that can have a significant impact on an individual's economic success later in life, a country's future GDP, and sustainable development (Sheeran; Victoria et al.). A joint report from UNICEF, WHO, and The World Bank found that "since 1990, the global prevalence of stunting has decreased 36 percent, from an estimated 40 percent (95 percent confidence limits: 38 percent, 42 percent) in 1990 to 26 percent (24 percent, 28 percent) in 2011" (de Onis et al. 9). Although this is not quite achieving the MDG of halving the rate of hunger as measured by growth stunting, it does show significant progress toward that goal globally. Those countries deemed the Least Developed Countries (LDCs), including Vanuatu, have also been making progress toward this goal globally but at a slower pace. The de Onis et al. report reveals that

> the prevalence of stunting in LDCs decreased from 60% (52%, 67%) in 1990 to 38% (35%, 42%) in 2011. This

decline accounts for an estimated decrease from 53 million stunted children in 1990 to 48 million in 2011 (an 11% decrease). Again, while stunting prevalence is decreasing, the increase in under-five population in the LDCs results in a continuing increase in the number of stunted children in the LDCs. (12)

To contextualize this within the region of Oceania, the prevalence of stunting was 40 percent in 1990 but has only decreased to 35 percent in 2011, indicating that much less progress has been made here than globally (de Onis et al.). In the Pacific Island region, countries are far from reaching their MDG or child nutrition. Even in their own reports, UNICEF and the WHO focus on sub-Saharan Africa and Asia as areas of primary concern—and it is true that there are a greater number of the world's population of children living in those areas. However, it does raise the question as to what kind of interventions, levels of funding, and programmatic oversight are provided to Pacific Island countries to aid in their public health interventions concerning child malnutrition.

BREASTFEEDING: THE SILVER BULLET?

In the face of these significant obstacles related to child malnutrition and the grim realization that Vanuatu and many of the world's Least Developed Countries, particularly those in the Pacific region, will fail to meet their MDGs, the focus of many nutrition interventions has turned toward breastfeeding. With the emphasis in public health on the value of breastfeeding to promote positive growth and development outcomes among children, in many cases breastfeeding has become a kind of "silver bullet" solution to the problem of childhood malnutrition, particularly in Vanuatu.

As a potential "solution" and certainly a way to help promote maternal and child health, breastfeeding has many appealing aspects. The biomedical literature clearly points to the health benefits of breastfeeding for infants in terms of building a healthy immune system, providing ideal nutritional balance, and the decreasing of diarrheal diseases (Bartick and Reinhold; Nankunda, et al.; Van Esterik; Victoria, et al.). For example, Borg notes,

Infants that are not breastfed are at least seven times more likely to die from diarrhoea and five times more likely to die from pneumonia than infants that are exclusively breastfed. The Lancet *Child Survival* Series compared breastfeeding with other preventative health interventions and found it was twice as likely to prevent infant deaths as the next most effective intervention (insecticide-treated materials). (23)

For mothers, breastfeeding promotes a healthy bond between the mother and child. It is a way to provide infants with food that needs no additional preparation, comes without the added cost of infant formula milk, is always at the correct temperature, and is safe and clean from the impurities found in some infant formula when prepared with contaminated water supplies or served in bottles that have not been fully sanitized.

From the perspective of development agencies and governmental ministries of health, breastfeeding is particularly appealing because it is an extremely low-cost intervention. It is not a new technology, nor does it involve a lot of expensive equipment that needs to be installed in medical buildings. In many places, including Vanuatu, there is a legacy of breastfeeding among the older generations who can now serve as an incredible support system for their daughters and daughters-in-law when problems with breastfeeding arise (Aubel, "Grandmothers Promote"; "Elders"). This is another real advantage to the promotion of breastfeeding as a nutrition intervention in Vanuatu, and many other countries around the world, because there is already a support network, often times kin based, for many mothers (Burton, Nero, and Egan; Douglass and McGadney-Douglass; Moestue, et al.; Speirs et al.; Widmer), although it should be noted that the positive effects of a kin based support network are also influenced by household wealth (Hadley). In addition, the presence of kin does not always lead to positive infant-feeding outcomes, and there are examples from Vanuatu and around the world that indicate kin can have a negative impact on breastfeeding practices (Sear; Sharma and Kanani; Wentworth, *The Influence of Kin Networks*). Nevertheless, recognizing these biomedical benefits, the WHO and UNICEF partner to promote the MBFHI by regularly working with the governments of developed and developing countries to certify their hospitals. Concepts of breastfeeding represent a cosmopolitan medicine (Lock and Nguyen; McPherson, this volume), which links biomedical intervention promoting scientific research that demonstrates the health benefits of breast milk with the "natural" practice of breastfeeding.

Although the policies and tips promoted in the BFHI program do include steps to teach women about breastfeeding management and do call for support even after the mother and baby have been discharged from the hospital, the various parts of the policy are not uniformly implemented (see Table 2 for an outline of the steps promoted and commonly referred to in the hospital in Vanuatu). The majority of the steps for successful breastfeeding are focused on the initial period right after birth, and they are universally implemented without any real room for cultural variation. Because some steps are easier to implement than others, health care practitioners can attempt to draw on their strengths and capabilities both professionally and in terms of what resources they have available. For example, promoting cosmopolitan medicine (Jordan; Pollock, this volume) by telling mothers about the biomedical benefits of breastfeeding, per step three, and not permitting any other food or drink besides breast milk, as stated in step six, are much easier to implement regularly than to ensure mothers know how to maintain lactation throughout their child's first two years, as outlined in step five. In the context of the developing world struggling to achieve the MDGs, where resources are already scarce, health care practitioners do their best within the framework and resources in which they operate.

Nevertheless, in analyzing the advantages of breastfeeding, a discourse laden with ideas of "natural" behaviours and the "natural" ways women should breastfeed with ease is revealed. The biomedical benefits of breastfeeding have been clearly defined in medical practice for decades, and the relatively low-cost of promoting breastfeeding as a nutritional intervention, when compared to other health care interventions, has led health care practitioners and some women themselves to believe it is the easy, cost-effective way to promote infant health. Indeed, for some women this may be the case.

Table 2: The Ten Steps of Successful Breastfeeding with the Baby Friendly Hospital Initiative (United Nations Children's Fund)

1.	Have a written breastfeeding policy that is routinely communicated to all health care staff.
2.	Train all health care staff in the skills necessary to implement this policy.
3.	Inform all pregnant women about the benefits and management of breastfeeding.
4.	Help mothers initiate breastfeeding within one half hour of birth.
5.	Show mothers how to breastfeed and maintain lactation, even if they should be separated from their infants.
6.	Give newborn infants no food or drink other than breast milk, unless medically indicated.
7.	Practice rooming in—that is, allow mothers and infants to remain together twenty-four hours a day.
8.	Encourage breastfeeding on demand.
9.	Give no artificial teats or pacifiers (also called dummies or soothers) to infants.
10.	Foster the establishment of breastfeeding support groups and refer mothers to them on discharge from the hospital or clinic.

However, many women experience difficulty breastfeeding, even when their desire to exclusively breastfeed is sincere, and they work extremely hard in their attempts to be the sole source of their child's nutrition. Many women feel frustration when they experience difficulties because of cultural discourses that suggest if breastfeeding is "natural," it should be easy. Therefore, women who experience problems with breastfeeding are somehow inferior, "unnatural" mothers. Presented with a litany of benefits, mothers are taught that this substance they produce is the key to their child's health. Often the discourse of breastfeeding promotion is intimately linked with images of happy, healthy women nursing their infants—"good" mothers on display in posters and informational brochures (Rudzik). These images and discourses serve to prioritize the biomedical model that promotes breastfeeding as the "natural" choice, good for mothers and babies, without any real discussion of a range of choices that are actually available or of the reality that many women need coaching and help throughout the breastfeeding process.

During this fieldwork, women in Vanuatu described feeling pressure to breastfeed, even if they had reservations or concerns. In this research, there was not a single participant who was told by a health care practitioner that it was "normal" to need help and that there was support or help available for women should they encounter any problems. In reality, mothers were told to breastfeed at the birth of their child, encouraged in the maternity ward, and possibly offered some limited help during the approximately twenty-four hour period mother and infant spend in the hospital for a full term baby with no complications. Then, they are sent home to continue this practice. It was assumed that mothers should intuitively be able to move through the process without any supplemental outside advice or aid. The reality is that many women need additional support throughout the duration of time they breastfeed their children.

Castro and Marchand-Lucas examine the ways women are educated about breastfeeding and infant-feeding options, to expose the positivist and materialist authoritative knowledge that is present in discourses of infant and young child-feeding practices. In both developed and developing countries, they question whether women and their families are truly informed about their feeding practices, which can be indicative of larger problems. As the authors state, "the lack of informed choice raises the question of whether there is a level playing field in the way women and their partners, as well as the whole society, are given appropriate information" (234). The processes mothers engage in when learning about infant feeding have become increasingly medicalized, presented in the context of biomedical benefits and the prevention of health problems. However, there are cultural values embedded in infant-feeding practice that are often ignored when the biomedical model is the sole authority. Biomedical knowledge is the primary means of educating mothers about infant feeding, which, in part, makes sense, as it is the method used for the education of health care practitioners. To truly understand the issue of maternal choice in infant-feeding practice a more comprehensive approach is needed, which includes analyzing the political arena, the lives of individual women, private sector health workers, public health professionals, and the cultural perceptions of breastfeeding (Castro and Marchand-Lucas 258). Thus a holistic approach is necessary to understand how these global programs, certifications, and lessons regarding breastfeeding are accessed and interpreted by mothers in local and cultural contexts.

Ultimately, there can be such a focus on the biomedical aspects that the complexities of mothers' lived experiences are lost. For example, as reported in Vanuatu's 2007 nutrition survey:

> The main problem with infant and young children practices in Vanuatu is that many caregivers introduce other milk and non-milk liquids or formula and then semi-solid and solid foods, too early and the majority of mothers stop breastfeeding by around 17 months. These practices can contribute to susceptibility to infection, micronutrient deficiencies and imbalanced growth. The sharp increase in underweight and stunting from 6-11 months and 12-23 months of age most probably reflects the above inappropriate practices together with the fact that the choice of complementary foods may not be in line with WHO/UNICEF recommandations. (Knowles 42-43)

My interviews and participant observation revealed that mothers often stray from the WHO/UNICEF guidelines; however, the multiple realities of work, financial obligations, familial pressures, and ease of breastfeeding practice all contribute to the reasons why breastfeeding was not a feasible situation for that family at the time. The emphasis of the biomedical model overshadows any other cultural context that is critical to understanding health behaviour.

Anthropologists can supplement biomedical understandings of the importance of breastfeeding by offering broader questions about the cultural constructions of breastfeeding and motherhood and the factors that affect choice of infant-feeding methods (van Esterik). This is particularly important as many of the disciplines that research breastfeeding, such as public health, nursing, and pediatrics, have not relied heavily on qualitative research. Van

Esterik states that "as a result, breastfeeding has not always been seen as a complex process shaped by social and cultural forces interacting with local environmental and political conditions" (258). The ethnographic data presented in this case study will help highlight voices and processes of infant-feeding practice not often present in the biomedical discourses.

PERSPECTIVES OF HEALTH CARE PRACTITIONERS

As part of the visual-cognitive elicitation methodology (Wentworth, *Feasting and Food Security*) used in this research, I distributed inexpensive digital cameras to groups of three to five individuals. I requested that participants use the cameras to photograph scenes or items they could use to teach me about child feeding. I intentionally left the topic very broad to encourage participants to photograph what they felt was most important and most relevant rather than what I as a researcher thought they should photograph. Although many people were uncomfortable at first with the broad topic, expressing concern that they might not take the "right" pictures, after reassurances, the majority of participants really enjoyed the project. They kept the cameras and took pictures of their experiences and perspectives of child feeding for one week. Then I collected the cameras, developed the photographs, numbered the backs, and returned the printed photos to the participants with captioning worksheets. On the worksheet, I asked each participant to caption every photograph they took, describing where the photograph was taken and what specifically it depicted. I found that with lots of pictures of cooked foods it was helpful to clarify exactly what was on display in the photo. I also asked the participants to write down why they took that photograph—to write a caption relating what the photograph means to them or serves to teach me, the researcher who is interested in child-feeding patterns. After collecting the completed captioning worksheets, the participants met for a discussion group. During this small group meeting, participants looked at one another's photographs, discussed the photos as a whole, and participated in pile-sorting activities with the photos.

One set of visual-cognitive elicitation data came from a group of nurses from a variety of different wards at Vila Central Hospital.

Because breastfeeding is promoted so heavily at the hospital as a result of the MBFHI, photographs and discussion about breastfeeding were common. Figure 1 shows a mother bottle feeding her child. The nurse wrote, "I want to show that bottle-feeding is not safe for children." Another nurse took a photograph of a newborn baby breastfeeding for the first time, shown in Figure 2. She articulated that it is important for the baby to "breastfeed within the first hour after he is born."

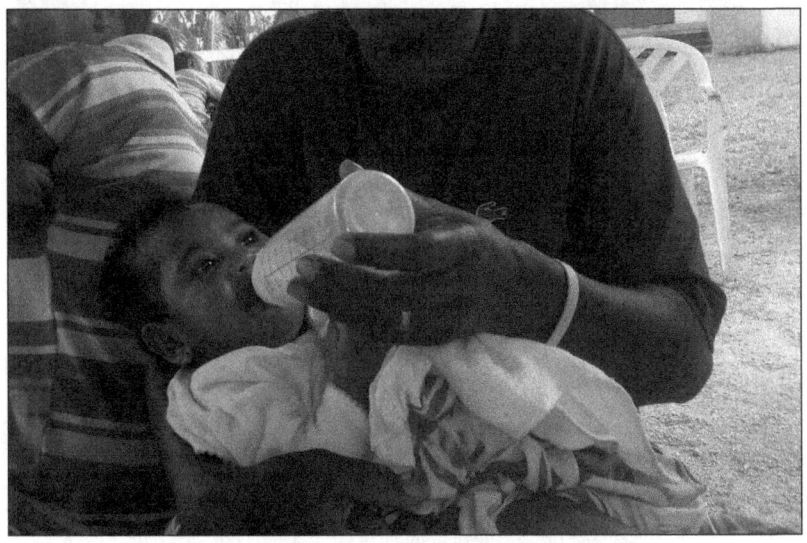

Fig. 1: Infant and mother attend a well-baby check-up.
Photo taken by Visual-Cognitive Elicitation Participant © Chelsea Wentworth, 2012.

It is interesting to note that the perspectives of each of these health care practitioners reflect the biomedical discourses of the importance of breastfeeding and both the positive and negative perspectives of maternal behaviour. Health care practitioners receive basic training on the MBFHI policies and learn about the biomedical benefits of breastfeeding. However, in practice, they often relate essentialized versions of those policies. The MBFHI steps to success state, "Give newborn infants no food or drink other than breast milk, unless medically indicated" (United Nations Children's Fund). Many health care practitioners interpret this MBFHI recommendation within the context of their biomedical training, reflecting on the high rates of diarrheal diseases and illness associated with bottle feeding in areas where it is extremely difficult to access clean water and sterilize bottles. Thus, the message from health care practitioners becomes bottle feeding is unsafe—a broad statement that does not leave room for women to learn safe and sometimes necessary bottle-feeding practices.

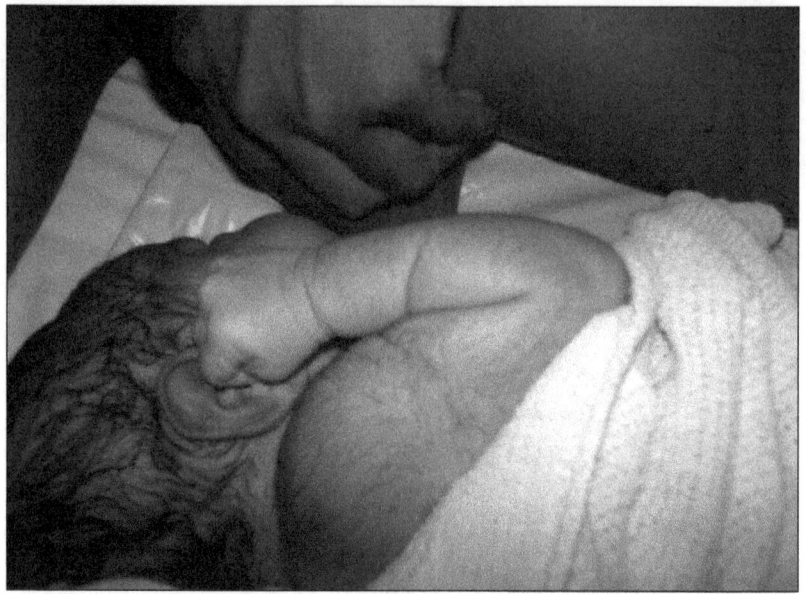

Fig. 2: Mother breastfeeds her infant within the first hour after birth.
Photo taken by Visual-Cognitive Elicitation Participant © Chelsea Wentworth, 2012.

Given that breastfeeding is the optimal feeding behaviour and bottle feeding is "unsafe," any outreach or questioning to reveal mothers' hidden problems or fears associated with breastfeeding is absent from routine medical care or check-ups for either the infant or the mother. Many health care practitioners cannot understand why mothers would not comply with their recommendations. In my conversations with health care practitioners, I repeatedly heard that mothers were "lazy" and "ignorant" when they did not follow the guidelines for breastfeeding. Even mothers who breastfed with ease related stories of other mothers who opted out of the practice, describing them as "lazy." This type of general dismissal is largely a product of the dominant discourse that situates breastfeeding as the *only* valid option for mothers, regardless of other circumstances, and as a requirement for "good" mothering.

Nevertheless, it is critical to note that the health care practitioners I interviewed and observed for this research are compassionate and work tirelessly with very limited resources. Based on my observations in Vanuatu, the nurse to patient ratio in well-baby clinics is high—often two or three nurses with the help of two nursing students or nurse aides need to weigh, vaccinate, and advise up to 219 mothers in a four hour period. Nursing students need help and direction themselves, and nurse aides can begin work with as little as three weeks of training; thus, although these staff members can be helpful, they often do not have the training to talk mothers through complications with breastfeeding. Clearly, there is inadequate staffing to answer questions and provide lactation support for mothers who have questions or are struggling with breastfeeding, particularly after they leave the labor and delivery ward. This is a reflection of the larger international health care system that promotes BFHI policies without contextualizing the lived realities of mothers, their families, and the health care practitioners they are responsible for training. Without the resources to analyze and adapt to the various needs of those they serve, health care practitioners are understandably frustrated with those mothers who seem to never follow their advice. In this situational context, it becomes easy to continue with the discourse of cosmopolitan medicine in which they were trained, a discourse that too often places blame with the mothers.

PERSPECTIVES OF MOTHERS

Mothers predominantly support the value of breastfeeding and want to breastfeed their children. However, they lack the framework to deal with unanticipated problems. One participant explained, "My son breastfed on just one of my breasts. My other breast was only producing a small amount of milk, so I could just use one side. I wanted him to be fat and healthy, but the one side wasn't enough ... He was eight months when he stopped breastfeeding entirely, and then he drank Sunshine milk [a brand of powdered whole milk]." She described how, beginning at around three or four months, she fed the child fresh fruits like papaya, the juice from oranges, and the water used to boil vegetables and meat for the family's dinner to supplement her lower milk supply. These were decisions that she made on her own, with the consultation of her family and friends, and after talking with and observing what other mothers feed their children. She never discussed these feeding practices with a health care practitioner, nor did she receive help or advice on her problem with low-milk supply on one breast.

In the presence of hospital nurses, many mothers who struggled with breastfeeding felt that their concerns were not heard and that they truly feared for the health of their infants. Reflecting with furled brow on the birth of her third child, a mother explained how hard it was to be in the hospital while having problems breastfeeding. She delivered all three of her children at Vila Central Hospital, but her most trying experience came with the birth of her third child, and only son, who was born prematurely. After a difficult pregnancy, she went into labour about two months early and was admitted to the maternity ward where she delivered a couple of days later. Her son was very small, under two kilograms in weight, and she knew that she needed to feed him to increase his weight. She produced no colostrum or milk for nearly two days. Visits from the nurse were stressful, and the nurse attempted to reassure her that the milk would come and, in the meantime, her son would be fine without food. After inquiring about infant formula, she was told that infant formula is bad for babies and that they do not allow it in the hospital. "He was so small, and he was starving!" she exclaimed, still in disbelief that the nurse could approach her concerns so callously. "But fortunately, my cousin had delivered around the same time, so she came down and nursed my baby," she quietly explained, as though this cross-nursing practice still needed to remain hidden.

Nurses do not permit babies to breastfeed from women who are not their biological mothers because of fears of HIV/AIDS transmission, even though the disease is very rare in Vanuatu, and research shows that HIV-positive women can breastfeed without spreading the disease to nursing infants (Nduati et al.; Coovadia et al.). The mother relayed her story involving a network of female relatives working together to help her feed her tiny infant son. Some female relatives would keep watch for the location of the nurses while her cousin would sneak in and quickly breastfeed the baby when the nurses were not looking. When her own milk came in, she breastfed as much as possible and tried hard to increase her child's weight. Hospital policy requires mothers and infants to stay until the child reaches 2.5 kilograms, which took her son slightly over one month. During this time, she feared she did not have enough milk to support her son. So her cousin would come down to visit her at the hospital and secretly nurse the small boy, supplementing his diet until he gained enough weight to come home. "We would have had to stay longer if we didn't have this help," she assured me, convinced that their hospital stay would have been extended if she had been unable to have the supplemental breast milk provided to her infant by her cousin.

Participant observation and interviews revealed that the MBFHI policies associated with infant feeding, including no infant formula and no breastfeeding children that you did not birth, were regularly violated. Numerous mothers related stories of sneaking around nurses, employing friends, and relatives to keep watch for nurses while they fed their babies in ways that violated hospital policy. Using female relatives who were also lactating to supplement infant diets through cross-nursing was the most common practice. In my interviews, I talked with mothers who recounted using the support of female relatives in breastfeeding their children and also those who reported helping female relatives by feeding other children. However, several mothers also explained how family members smuggled in infant formula and bottles—items not permitted in the maternity or pediatrics wards.

Not limited to mothers whose infants were premature, several mothers explained problems with lactation where they felt they required supplemental milk for their infants who were otherwise born at a healthy weight. Years before her pregnancy, another mother had undergone surgery on one of her breasts, which she explained prevented her from producing milk in that breast upon the birth of her child. Anticipating this problem—as her doctor had warned her that his could be the case at the time of her surgery—she brought infant formula and bottles with her to the hospital. But the bottle and can of formula were taken away from her when a nurse spotted her bottle feeding her newborn. Horrified at her treatment by the nurse and fearful that her new baby, her first child, would go hungry without supplemental infant formula, she sent her husband out to replace the bottle and can of formula. She supplemented her child's diet with infant formula secretly, away from view of the nurses for the remainder of her hospital stay.

As these were all retrospective stories from women who have no medical records to indicate biomedical problems with breastfeeding, there is no clear way to tell exactly what type of biomedical support these mothers needed specifically. However, the regular services of an internationally board certified lactation consultant (IBCLC) would clearly be beneficial, as during interviews, several women reported having difficulties breastfeeding. What is particularly noteworthy in the context of achieving the MDGs, however, is that these hospital policies did not seem to change the practice of supplemental infant feeding; rather, mothers employed elaborate covert methods for supplementing their child's diet. This fostered a relationship of distrust and secrecy between mothers and nurses at the very beginning of a child's life.

While in their presence, mothers consider the nurses to be authoritative figures and defer to their requests; however, once outside of the nurses' gaze, mothers largely consider nurses' recommendations as advice that should be evaluated alongside other advice and information that they receive from kin and friends (Wentworth, *Feasting and Food Security*). The ethnographic data presented here indicate that early interaction between nurses and mothers is fraught with distrust, so it is not surprising to learn that subsequent patient-provider interactions reflect a disingenuous relationship. Well-baby visits begin at two weeks of age and should continue monthly until the child reaches one year of age, and ideally for the first two years. Well-baby visits take place at Maternal and Child Health (MCH) clinics; however, I never observed any maternal health care services provided at these clinics, nor did I see health care practitioners asking about the health and well-being of the mother. In this way, the mother was marginalized, her health clearly second to the health of her child. MCH clinic health care providers have an enormous task in Port Vila as well as in the peri-urban and rural areas that they serve on the southern half of the island of Efate, where this research took place. Charged with conducting visits on a strenuous time schedule, in some locations MCH staff will serve well over two hundred children in four hours, and over the years of this research, the number of children served only continues to grow. The high number of children who attend the MCH clinic for examination limits the time that nursing staff are able to spend with each individual mother and child and, thus, the amount of educational and health information they are able to provide. With directives to prioritize immunizations and the weighing of children, MCH staff members focus on that work, since it is not possible to provide all the services necessary in the time allotted.

Occasionally, mothers find it hard to prioritize the information garnered in these extremely brief conversations with health care practitioners. The number of children who are brought to a health clinic on a given day, the weather (because many are outdoor clinics), the nurses, and the nurse aides' visual evaluation of individual children all contributed to the length of time a child spent being evaluated by a health care practitioner. Participant observation demonstrated that these visits could consist of anywhere from five to ten minutes of non-contiguous involvement with the health care provider, despite the fact that many women wait more than three hours for their child to be seen by the provider. Some mothers commented on their brief interaction with a nurse or nurse aide, who spent most of her time writing notes rather than examining the child. One mother exclaimed, "She didn't really look at [my baby], so how can she know?" This distance and lack of deeply attentive care from nurses and nurse aides is evaluated in the context of the time consuming and loving care provided by grandmothers and other lay practitioners who "know" the child better than the biomedical health care providers. Both formal training in cosmopolitan medicine and time spent interacting with the child are valued, but since mothers often do not perceive that they are receiving both of these at the MCH clinics, the advice is re-evaluated within the larger contextual framework.

Nevertheless, the vast majority of mothers in this research believed breast milk was the best food for their child. Nearly every mother had breastfed her children initially, and many indicated that they valued breast milk over infant formula, powdered milk, and juices made of local fruits. They realized and agreed with many of the benefits of breastfeeding as presented by health care practitioners, including that breast milk is free, clean, and always ready. However, due to the narrow constraints of the MBFHI as implemented in Vanuatu, health care practitioners lack the tools necessary to educate and support mothers as they encounter problems with breastfeeding or with the ability to work within mothers' social, economic, and familial environment to modify their breastfeeding practices so they can be beneficial to both the mother and the child.

THE USE OF INFANT FORMULA AND POWDERED MILK IN VANUATU

Although the national nutrition survey data revealed high initial rates of breastfeeding, the numbers of women who continue to breastfeed exclusively for the first six months are low, especially considering these high initial rates. Furthermore, my research suggests that these percentages may be over reported. Almost all of the women I interviewed initially stated that they breastfed exclusively for their child's first six months of life. However, later during our interviews, they revealed that, in fact, they often provided a number of different beverages and foods to their infants, typically beginning between the ages of two and three months. Common examples of these supplemental foods included papaya juice, tea made from lemon or orange leaves, powdered milk, and infant formula. When asked by a health practitioner if they are breastfeeding currently or if they breastfed exclusively for six months, mothers often replied "yes." In general, mothers wanted to respond to questions according to what they thought health care workers wanted to hear. Mothers believed that this would provide good help with research, and avoid conflict with health care practitioners. A response that would avoid conflict or a health care worker challenging the behaviours of mothers must be analyzed in the context of the mistrust fostered at the hospital through the promotion of MBFHI behaviours. Remembering their initial conflicts with health care workers that required mothers to hide infant formula or covertly find female relatives to breastfeed their newborns, mothers responded to nurse questioning by furnishing the answers that they think nurses want to receive. Mothers do not want to hear that they are not "good" mothers because they are not breastfeeding "properly," according to the MBFHI guidelines. This finding demonstrates that in-depth interviews, participant observation, and long-term anthropological research can provide data not accessible via short surveys and some quantitative methods of data collection, which do not account for these patterns and cultural nuances.

In addition, my participant observation showed that mothers are generally passive in the presence of health care practitioners, deferring to their advice and always verbally agreeing and acknowledging their recommendations. However, that is not an accurate indicator of whether or not those mothers agree with or will follow through with that advice. Beyond the distrusting relationships that mothers experience with nurses and health care workers early in their child's life, other situations necessitated supplemental child feeding. Most often one of two reasons was provided. First, the mother was returning to work and could not exclusively breastfeed anymore or, second, the mother was having problems with her milk supply and was not able to provide enough food for her child.

Participants explained to me that they stopped breastfeeding when they returned to work. This is often when the child is three months old because national law permits three months of paid maternity leave. However, in practice, this depends on the mothers' employer much more than laws governing maternity leave, as many women reported their employers refused the paid maternity leave, requiring them to return to work shortly after the birth of the child. Some employers forced mothers to take some of the maternity leave early, before the birth of the child, and provided three months total paid leave. This results in some women taking six weeks before birth, leaving them only six weeks maternity after the birth of their child. Many women switch to breast milk substitutes like infant formula, although it is also common to see soft foods like papaya and sweet potatoes and powdered milk fed to infants when breastfeeding ceases. In addition, many women reported that they did not receive information about weaning infants, so frequently they stopped breastfeeding abruptly, completely switching to other foods and infant formula. Therefore, babies regularly move from exclusive breastfeeding to exclusively receiving formula and soft foods, a sharp transition that can be problematic for some infants.

After only receiving information about exclusive breastfeeding, attempting to navigate infant-feeding options is a challenge for any mother. One participant emphasized that, "Many women *try* to bottle feed during maternity leave. They want them [their babies] to be used to the bottle before maternity leave is over, even when they think that breastfeeding is best." This participant's sentiment was echoed by others who sincerely worried that if they exclusively breastfed for three months of maternity leave and then abruptly switched to infant formula upon returning to work, their babies would not make a smooth transition. In fact, many mothers recalled anecdotes from their friends, relatives, or previous children who had not transitioned well and would not eat the other foods. Mothers feared that their child would go hungry all day while they were at work, causing the child to get sick. They viewed supplementing infant formula with breast milk from the beginning of the child's life as the best way to prepare the child for the realities of a working mother—a problem particularly prevalent in urban areas, as there are significantly fewer opportunities for women to engage in the wage economy in rural areas. One working mother lamented, "I feel pressure to buy formula milk because my work demands a lot of my time." Purchasing infant formula is not a decision that is made lightly.

In addition, infant formula is extremely expensive. I conducted a survey of formula availability and cost in downtown Port Vila and some stores in the surrounding areas. I inspected the inventory of twenty-four stores and found formula available that ranged in price from VT 1,490 to 4,850 (USD 16-53) per 900 gram can. SMA brand was the most commonly used by mothers interviewed for this research because, reportedly, it was the least expensive brand. I found that this brand ranged in price from VT 1,490 to 1,900 (USD 16-20) depending on the store. Mothers reported their infants typically consume approximately one 900 gram can per week, and the monthly minimum wage[2] is VT 30,000 (USD 325). This demonstrates that when women feel compelled to use infant formula, they are doing so in the face of huge economic losses, as the cost of formula can easily account for 20 percent to 25 percent of a mothers' monthly salary. In some cases, this leads mothers to opt for powdered whole milk instead of infant formula because it is significantly less expensive. Without any education on the use of infant formula, many mothers cannot explain differences between powdered whole milk and infant formula. Additionally, the high cost of formula leads some mothers to water down the milk, which diminishes the nutritional benefit of the milk that children are receiving. When a child is only consuming infant formula made according to the directions on the can, the child will often consume one can or more per week. Understanding the price of the formula is critical to understanding the factors women negotiate when making infant-feeding decisions. This is clearly not a case of laziness or thoughtlessness. One participant explained, "Nutrition, family, *pikinini* ["baby" or "child"], it's the mother's duty." However, the feeding practices women enact do not always match the choices they wish that they could make.

CONCLUSIONS AND STEPS FORWARD

Effective nutrition education and breastfeeding policies can provide a significant boost to maternal and child health, and the Mother and Baby Friendly Hospital Initiative's attempt to achieve higher rates of breastfeeding could be very beneficial to mothers and children in Vanuatu. Lowering rates of infant illness and fostering close loving relationships between mothers and their children are achieved through the process of breastfeeding and should be promoted by health workers and through international programs, such as the MBFHI. The recent renaming to add 'Mother' into the title of the program indicates the broad benefits that a program like the MBFHI can have on both maternal and child health indicators, including those of the MDGs. However, these changes are seemingly in name only, as there is still much work to be done to enhance the care and support provided specifically to mothers. This case study from Vanuatu illustrates a problem with implementation and execution of the program, in that it ultimately ends with alienating some of the mothers whom the program attempts to serve. Early negative experiences in the hospital setting may affect the confidence and ability of mothers to make healthy choices for their infants upon leaving the hospital. This situation fosters distrust between mothers and health care providers that can affect the variety and scope of health issues for which mothers will subsequently seek biomedical advice.

Planting the seeds of distrust can lead to negative health outcomes for other MDGs, as mothers exit the health care system with feelings of distrust and inadequacy. Mothers report not feeling confident that health care practitioners can adequately serve them and their families in times of need. Other studies have shown that decreased self-efficacy can have long-term negative nutritional health outcomes (McGarvey; Worsley). If women have negative experiences with the MBFHI and are marginalized in the health care system at early stages in their lives, the potential long-term consequences could be severe for both the mother and the child, in addition to subsequent children. However, the research findings presented here do not indicate that the system should be entirely eliminated but rather the implementation process needs to be changed to accept mothers who struggle with breastfeeding and to provide compassionate and specific advice to individual mothers and their infants.

Promoting maternal and child health through breastfeeding is important and has been demonstrated to yield positive health outcomes, which indicates that there is something here worth saving. Rather than throwing the mother out with the bathwater, MBFHI implementation should change to support mothers by creating a safe and trusting relationship between mothers and health care providers, which will ultimately lead to continued support and interaction between mothers, children, and health care workers throughout a child's life. The research results indicate that the authoritative biomedical discourse, which separates the individual mothers from the realities of their lived experience, perpetuates a system where cultural context is overlooked in favour of one-size-fits-all health recommendations. Providing lactation consultations and support as well as recognizing that not all mothers "naturally" breastfeed without any complications will improve communication between mothers and health care practitioners. Social and family organization, socio-economic status, the type of wage labour a mother engages in, and food beliefs and preferences all influence the infant- and child-feeding practices mothers employ. Providing health care practitioners with the resources and skills to acknowledge and work within those social and cultural structures and to encourage and support mothers through the breastfeeding process will strengthen the MBFHI. These changes can reshape the discourse of breastfeeding and foster a relationship of trust rather than secrecy and shame between mothers and health care practitioners, which will, ultimately, improve health care interactions for both mothers and children for decades to come.

ENDNOTES

[1] All child growth statistics used in this paper follow the WHO 2005 growth standard. However, the MICS also reports statistics using the National Center for Health Statistics (NCHS) growth reference for the purposes of comparison with earlier studies.

[2] In September 2012, during the middle of this fieldwork, the monthly minimum wage was raised from VT 26,000 (USD 280) per month to VT 30,000 (USD 325) per month. Only women with great educational success enjoy wages that are much higher than the national minimum wage.

WORKS CITED

Aubel, Judi. "Grandmothers Promote Maternal and Child Health: The Role of Indigenous Knowledge Systems Managers." *IK Notes: The World Bank* 89 (2006): 1-6. Web. 26 Oct. 2015.

Aubel, Judi. "Elders: A Cultural Resource for Promoting Sustainable Development." *The World Watch Institute* (2010): 41-46. Web. Last accessed 26 October 2015.

Bartick, Melissa, and Arnold Reinhold. "The Burden of Suboptimal Breastfeeding in the United States: A Pediatric Cost Analysis." *Pediatrics.* (2010): e1048-e1056. Web. 11 Oct. 2015.

Black, Robert E., Lindsay H Allen, Zulfiqar A Bhutta, Laura E Caulfield, Mercedes de Onis, Majid Ezzati, Colin Mathers, Juan Rivera, for the Maternal and Child Undernutrition Study Group. "Maternal and Child Undernutrition: Global and Regional Exposures and Health Consequences." *Lancet* 371 (2008): 243-260. Web. 27 Oct. 2015.

Borg, Bindi. "Development for Babies. Just Change: Critical Thinking on Global Issues." *Dev-Zone* 14 (2009): 23-46. Web. Last accessed 11 Oct. 2015.

Burton, Michael L., Karen L. Nero, and James A. Egan. "The Circulation of Children through Households in Yap and Kosrae." *Ethos* 29.3 (2001): 329-356. Print.

Castro, Arachu, and Laure Marchand-Lucas. "Does Authoritative Knowledge in Infant Nutrition Lead to Successful Breastfeeding? A Critical Perspective." *Global Health Policy, Local Realities: The Fallacy of the Level Playing Field*. Eds. Lenore Manderson and Linda Whiteford. Boulder: Lynne Rienner Publishers, 2000. 233-263. Print.

Coovadia, Hoosen M., Nigel C. Rollins, Ruth M. Bland, Kirsty Little, Anna Coutsoudis, Michael L. Bennish, and Marie-Louise Newell. "Mother-to-Child Transmission of HIV-1 Infection during Exclusive Breastfeeding in the First 6 Months of Life: An Intervention Cohort Study." *Lancet* 369 (2007): 1107-16. Web. 11 Oct. 2015.

de Onis, Mercedes, David Brown, Monika Blössner, and Elaine Borghi. *Levels and Trends in Child Malnutrition: UNICEF-WHO-The World Bank Joint Child Malnutrition Estimates*. UNICEF New York; WHO, Geneva; The World Bank, Washington, DC. 2012. Print.

Douglas, Richard L., and Brenda F. McGadney-Douglass. "The Role of Grandmothers and Older Women in the Survival of Children with Kwashiorkor in Urban Accra, Ghana." *Research in Human Development* 5.1 (2008): 26-43. Web. 11 Oct. 2015.

Hadley, Craig. "The Costs and Benefits of Kin: Kin Networks and Children's Health among the Pimbwe of Tanzania." *Human Nature* 15.4 (2004): 377-395. Print

Jordan, Brigitte. "Cosmopolitical Obstetrics: Some Insights from the Training of Traditional Midwives." *Social Science and Medicine* 28.9 (1989): 925-944. Print

Knowles, Jacqueline. *Vanuatu Nutrition Survey 2007*. UNICEF, 2007. Web. 11 Oct. 2015.

Labbok, Miriam, and Katherine Krasovec. "Toward Consistency

in Breastfeeding Definitions. Studies in Family Planning" 21.4 (1990): 226-230. Web. 11 Oct. 2015.

Lock, Margaret, and Nguyen Vinh-Kim. *An Anthropology of Biomedicine.* West Sussex: Wiley-Blackwell, 2010. Print.

McGarvey, Stephen T. "Interdisciplinary Translational Research in Anthropology, Nutrition and Public Health." *Annual Review of Anthropology* 38 (2009): 233-249. Print.

Moestue, Hellen, Sharon Huttly, Lydia Sarella, and Shaik Galab. "'The Bigger the Better:' Mothers' Social Networks and Child Nutrition in Andhra Pradesh. *Public Health Nutrition* 10.11 (2007): 1274-1282. Web. 27 Oct. 2015.

Nankunda, Jolly, Thorkild Tylleskär, Grace Ndeezi, Nulu Semiyaga, and James Tumwine. "Establishing Individual Peer Counselling for Exclusive Breastfeeding in Uganda: Implications for Scaling-Up." *Maternal and Child Nutrition* 6. (2010): 53-66. Web. 27 Oct. 2015.

Nduati, Ruth, Grace John, Dorothy Mbori-Ngacha, Barbra Richardson, Julie Overbaugh, Anthony Mwatha, Jeckoniah Ndinya-Achola, Job Bwayo, Francis E. Onyango, James Hughes, and Joan Kreiss. "Effect of Breastfeeding and Formula Feeding on Transmission of HIV-1: A Randomized Clinical Trial." *JAMA* 284.9 (2000): 1167-1174. Web. 27 Oct. 2015.

Pérez-Escamilla, Rafael. "Evidence Based Breast-Feeding Promotion: The Baby-Friendly Hospital Initiative." *The Journal of Nutrition* 137 (2007): 484-487. Print.

Rodman, Margaret C. *Houses Far From Home: British Colonial Space in the New Hebrides.* Honolulu: University of Hawaii Press. 2001. Print.

Rudzik, Alanna E. F. "Breastfeeding and the Good Mother Ideal." *An Anthropology of Mothering.* Eds. Michelle Walks and Naomi McPherson. Bradford, Ontario: Demeter Press, 2011. 159-171. Print.

Sear, Rebecca. "Kin and Child Survival in Rural Malawi: Are Matrilineal Kin Always Beneficial in a Matrilineal Society?" *Human Nature* 19 (2008): 277-293. Print.

Sharma, Minal and Shubhada Kanani. "Grandmothers' Influence on Child Care." *Indian Journal of Pediatrics* 73 (2006): 295-298. Web. 11 Oct. 2015

Sheeran, Josete. "The Challenge of Hunger." *Lancet* 371 (2008): 180-181. Web. 11 Oct. 2015.

Shuaib, Muhammad and Md. Mokhlesur Rahman. *Monitoring the Situation of Children and Women: Vanuatu Multiple Indicator Cluster Survey 2007*. Port Vila: Vanuatu Ministry of Health, United Nations Children's Fund and The Global Fund. 2008. Print.

Speirs, Katherine E., Bonnie Braun, Virginie Zoumenou, Elaine A. Anderson, and Nicole Finkbeiner. "Grandmothers' Involvement in Preschool-Aged Children's Consumption of Fruits and Vegetables: Exploratory Study." *Infant, Child, and Adolescent Nutrition* 1.6 (2009): 332-337. Web. 11 Oct. 2015.

United Nations Children's Fund. *The 10 Steps of Successful Breastfeeding with the Baby Friendly Hospital Initiative*. UNICEF, 2014. Web. 20 July 2014.

van Esterik, Penny. "Contemporary Trends in Infant Feeding Research." *Annual Review of Anthropology* 31 (2002): 257-78. Web. 11 Oct. 2015.

Vanuatu Ministry of Health. *Master Health Services Plan. World Health Organization: Western Pacific Region*. WHO, 2004. Web. 11 Oct. 2015.

Vanuatu Young People's Project. *Young People Speak 2: A Study of the Lives of Ni-Vanuatu Urban Youth and the Issues Affecting Them in Port Vila. AP Youthnet: Asia Pacific Youth Employment Network*. ILO, 2008. Web. 11 Oct. 2015.

Victoria, Ceasar G., Linda Adair, Caroline Fall, Pedro C. Hallal, Reynaldo Martorell, Linda Richter, amd Harshpal Singh Sachdev. "Maternal and Child Undernutrition: Consequences for Adult Health and Human Capital." *Lancet* 371 (2008): 340-57. Web. 11 Oct. 2015.

Wentworth, Chelsea. *Feasting and Food Security: Negotiating Infant and Young Child Feeding in Urban and Peri-urban Vanuatu*. Diss. University of Pittsburgh. 2014. Print.

Wentworth, Chelsea. *The Influence of Kin Networks on Food Choice in Vanuatu*. Master of Public Health Essay. University of Pittsburgh. 2014. Print.

Wentworth Chelsea. "Public Eating, Private Pain: Children, Feasting, and Food Security in Vanuatu." *Food and Foodways*. Forthcoming.

Widmer, Alexandra. "Making Mothers: Birth and Changing Relationships of Mothering in Pangolin Village, Vanuatu." *An Anthropology of Mothering*. Eds. Michelle Walks and Naomi McPherson. Bradford: Demeter Press, 2011. 102-114. Print.

Worsley, Anthony. "Nutrition Knowledge and Food Consumption: Can Nutrition Knowledge Change Food Behavior?" *Asia Pacific Journal of Clinical Nutrition*. 11, Supplement (2002): S579-S585. Web. 11 Oct. 2015.

9.
Reproductive Anomalies in the Marshall Islands

NANCY J. POLLOCK

RONGELAP WOMEN'S REPRODUCTIVE HEALTH has suffered as a result of radioactive fallout on their atoll (homeland residence) from U.S. atomic bomb test, Bravo, in March 1954 in the northern Marshall Islands (Pollock, "Marshall Islands Women's Health"). To understand those women's concerns about failed pregnancies, I offer an examination of Marshallese beliefs about reproduction and their concern for explanations about the "jelly babies" that they were expelling from their bodies. Follow-on effects for the whole Marshallese population include reluctance to comply with international pressures for birth control measures to reduce the number of pregnancies, attitudes to teenage pregnancies, and associated maternal health concerns. Ethnographic data can explain the Marshallese position with regard to Millennium Development Goals 4 and 5.

In this chapter, I discuss a major disjuncture between local views of the place of reproduction in Marshallese society and outsiders' assessments of reproduction. Successive generations of Marshallese women have lost trust in outside agencies, which have failed to acknowledge their suffering with reproductive abnormalities after the U.S. nuclear testing program. The pressure put on the Republic of Marshall Islands Department of Health by WHO, UNFPA, and other agencies to reduce the number of pregnancies fails to recognize women's contributions of healthy children to future generations of Marshallese. The health transition between Marshallese views of maternal health and those of outside agencies is occurring, slowly.

NUCLEAR TESTS IN THE PACIFIC

The Marshall Islands lie south and west of Hawai'i. They comprise twenty-six coral atolls and low islands—with a maximum height of only three metres above sea level—scattered over an area of the central Pacific Ocean referred to as Micronesia. Rongelap atoll, in the north of the chain of atolls, lies two hundred miles to the east of Bikini, where the Bravo bomb was exploded in March 1954. A massive hydrogen bomb, Bravo was one of fifty-eight atmospheric tests that the U.S. conducted in the northern Marshalls between 1946 and 1958, with consequent nuclear fallout on other atolls. The mid-Pacific position of these atolls made them an ideal U.S. nuclear testing location, that is, far from the U.S. mainland.

Marshallese women's search for explanations for the sudden change in their reproductive health after 1954 failed to receive either clarification or support from Atomic Energy Commission medical teams. The women's reports of reproductive anomalies were deemed a figment of their imagination. Forty years later, declassified papers reveal that those pregnancy anomalies were part of Project 4.1, a deliberate U.S. experimental plan to gain information on the effects of nuclear radiation substances on human bodies, such as reproduction (Welsome). Women's failed pregnancies are part of this ongoing legacy.

These disrupted pregnancies must be considered within the context of Marshallese beliefs and practices about reproduction, as these are targeted by outsiders' demands for statistics on reproduction that place modern-day pressures on government departments, such as the Marshall Islands Department of Health. I discuss here a major disjuncture between Marshallese views of the place of reproduction in their society and international assessments of reproductive health, including birth control to reduce population size. People of the Marshalls hold unique beliefs about bodies as the place where reproduction occurs, with women's bodies being considered particularly special. Reproduction is managed by practices that have been developed over many years and which differ from other peoples' views of reproduction.

International programes to reduce the numbers of conceptions, to increase use of contraceptive methods, and to reduce teenage pregnancies are contrary to Marshallese beliefs that women should reproduce every two years. Reproduction rates are too high, according to the ideals of the World Health Organization (WHO) and of the United Nations Population Fund (UNFPA). These organizations claim that for Pacific island nations, according to their statistical standards, the total fertility rate is not decreasing fast enough, nor is the rate of contraception uptake increasing fast enough. Consequently, "the Pacific region is not likely to achieve [MDG] targets 4 and 5; there is a need to analyse reasons for slow improvement" (WHO).

To consider the opposing views of the Marshallese and the WHO, the concept of "disjuncture" may be used to highlight the gaps between global demands of modernity for reduced reproduction, expressed in statistical returns, and descriptions of local values and experiences. As Appadurai has noted, such disjunctures can be captured in the construct of various "ethnoscapes," which are descriptions of local social backgrounds that link what he terms "imaginations" through modern-day media use of statistical returns. He suggests that "Electronic mediation is a technically new force that impels (and compels)" the work of the imagination. This new force is itself "a space of contestation in which individuals and groups seek to annex the global into their own practices of the modern" (4). For example, each nation state around the world will gather and file statistics on family planning practices in order to meet the demands for this information from international bodies, such as the WHO. Local health department officials must complete forms with pre-set categories that allow no room for variations in the local record. The "space of contestation" between numbers and practices can best be revealed by an ethnographic description of the values behind successful reproduction as a key element of maternal health.

MARSHALLESE CONCEPTS OF MATERNITY AND REPRODUCTION

My consideration of Marshallese beliefs and practices surrounding reproduction is based on ethnographic data from several visits to different Marshall Islands over more than three decades, data that provide background information to assist in understanding Marshallese resistance to international calls for birth control. Since 1954, Rongelap and other Marshallese women's experiences of reproductive failures, such as stillbirths and malformed fetuses, have contributed to their resistance to birth control. The women attribute these reproductive failures to their exposure to radioactive substances both in the environment of their atoll and in the foods that they eat. Their distrust of outside agencies, stemming from the history of nuclear testing, has been extended to include other agencies that are now promoting birth control to reduce population size. Millennium Development Goal 5, to reduce populations worldwide by providing access to contraceptive devices and information, is far removed from, even considered alien to, women's own reproductive beliefs. These disjunctures— including Marshallese cultural beliefs in women's social contribution of new members of society and their history of experiencing reproductive failures due to exposure to radioactive substances from U.S. nuclear testing—have led to rejection of birth control practices.

MARSHALLESE REPRODUCTIVE BELIEFS AND PRACTICES

Marshallese women's bodies not only produce new life, they also reproduce the well-being of their society. Successful pregnancies are a tangible expression of women's contributions to their lineages and clans as well as to the wider Marshallese community. Each Marshallese newborn belongs to the lineage of its mother. Children are actively part of their matrilineage, with whom they live, and are cared for by any of the mother's siblings or their offspring, the infant's maternal cousins. In large households, there is always someone around—not necessarily the biological mother—to pick up a baby and attend to its needs.

Marriage in this society is complex, consisting of four stages of "being together" [*koba bajjik*], only the last of which is considered "marriage" in the Christian-Western sense (Pollock, "Birthing Practices"). The Congregational church, the dominant Christian mission in the Marshalls until the 1990s, has had marginal influence on birth within a "marriage" context. Young people engage in sexual relations, sometimes before the girl has started menstruating, and girls may have several sexual liaisons. Marriage in church is likely to occur after several children have been born or even when the woman is past reproductive age.

Children are born into their mother's lineage and welcomed throughout the whole atoll community, with only peripheral consideration of the mother's relationship to the biological father. The role of the father in such relationships is less important than a man's relationship to his own mother and siblings, particularly his sisters. He should make his contributions by fishing and making copra (dried coconut for sale), first for his mother's household and secondarily for the household in which he has fathered children. All children are born belonging to their mother's matrilineage, and the role of a child's father is to help the mother's lineage and/or household by providing them with breadfruit and coconuts, including using coconuts to produce copra for the household's cash income. These "marriage" rules have strong local significance but differ markedly from European or North American principles of "legal marriage," sanctioned by a church or a civil union. Instead, these rules reflect local beliefs about the ongoing maintenance of the well-being of society, both for women and children as well as for men.

A paramount chief derives his power, in part, from the vitality of his several lineages, each of whom owes allegiance to a chief. In the past, when atoll life was fragile, the survival of lineages through mutual support was vital; the paramount chief relied on these major supporters, and he (or she) acknowledged their contributions to maintaining society. Marshallese custom [*manit in majol*) was maintained by these mutual-support mechanisms, including for new members of lineages. Marshallese heritage is the legacy of many generations of newcomers to the lineages.

Key factors in understanding Marshallese maternal health beliefs include women's expectations of regular reproductive success, usually at two year intervals, and the high value placed on adding to and reproducing the lineage and the community. Starting after their first or second menstruation, women expect to be pregnant or lactating for most of their lives. Disruptions to this pattern of reproduction are a matter of major concern, particularly for the woman but also for her male partner. Any suggestion that women should reduce that pregnancy rate, and thus family size, threatens women's own feeling of well-being as well as their contribution to social well-being.

In the past, and continuing today, large sibling sets cluster around the mother and her siblings. They may share one large house and those living elsewhere are still expected to maintain their responsibilities to support their mother and their sisters. Women, thus, have large support networks. Men are also expected to support their mother's matrilineage networks as well as to contribute to their partner's household. New additions are welcomed, but the realities of surviving in an atoll environment lead to formal social acknowledgment of belonging being deferred until the baby is one year old, when a *kemeem*, or first birthday celebration, is held. In this context, birth control is not widely accepted, as it intervenes in the vital ways that new life supports lineages, clans, and the whole community. Even during my field research in 1967, I noted that fear of their population dying out has pervaded atoll communities in the past.

COMMUNITY EXPERIENCES

This ethnographic description of reproductive beliefs and practices is constructed from my censuses, genealogies, and discussions with residents on several atolls in the Marshall Islands in the course of several research exercises between 1966 and 2004. Most of my discussions were with women, since a woman speaking to men about reproduction is not appropriate. In the course of these discussions, I became aware of several reproductive factors that were unusual in my (European) experience. From household censuses, I have conducted since the 1960s, and which go back six generations, I learned that in past generations, a woman would bear six, eight, or more children but not all of them lived to reproductive age. These births occurred at two year intervals according to the expectations of both the woman and the man and other members of the community.

I also learned about several different modes of prenatal care given by local midwives and about discussions of the distance, both physical and spiritual, between local management procedures and hospital services (Majuro Health Department) and women's needs. The Marshallese population, which is spread over twenty-six atolls, has accommodated its attitudes to reproduction to the many eventualities that can arise around the time of a birth.

As I was living in a household of eleven adult women and their children, I was privy to frequent discussions of "women's matters." Three of the adult women in the household had male partners, but only one pair was married. All of them were daughters of a woman who herself had twelve siblings. Talk frequently turned to matters of reproduction, either about themselves or about women in other households. One woman in her forties, who had not borne any children, sought outside advice about her infertility. She had adopted a son born to her sister, the same sister who produced another baby boy, her seventh, during my stay. Two young women in the household, aged fifteen and sixteen, also produced their first babies during my stay, but both babies lived for less than a month—starving to death because the young mothers had no breast milk, and wet nursing is not common practice (see Pollock, "Birthing Practices").

Jera, one of the sisters in the household, was pregnant with her seventh child during most of my stay. Her pregnancy highlighted for me how her siblings helped her, particularly her mother's sister, both during the pregnancy and afterwards. She was attended by a local midwife who provided prenatal care, which included local potions (Kabua and Tafaki) and body massage, beginning some two months before the expected delivery date and through to her postnatal care. Jera was not allowed to eat certain foods, such as shark or young coconut inflorescence, which might harm her baby. Her diet, as for everyone on that atoll, was very limited, simply due to the few food plants available (Pollock, "These Roots Remain"). After her delivery, which most of the senior women of the community attended, Jera was confined to the woman's hut for a month, while she underwent procedures for "drying her womb." The baby was watched over by one of its many siblings and brought to her to be breastfed when he cried (see Pollock, "Birthing Practices").

Local midwives, who are a vital part of community structure

but outside the aegis of the government health department, still bear the major responsibility for prenatal care of women in outer island communities. The local health aides employed locally by the Ministry of Health in Majuro —all men appointed and paid by the central Hospital board—cannot assist in any way because according to Marshallese custom, no man should view or touch a woman's body other than that of his wife. The health aide can only offer an analgesic, such as Nurofen, if the woman asks for pain relief. One woman told me of her "difficulties" with each of her seven births that necessitated a long trip from her home atoll to Majuro hospital as part of her prenatal planning. Before her expected delivery, she waited some three months for a ship—shipping is highly erratic among the outer islands and even the plane service is not a great improvement. After delivery, she had to await a ship to take her back to her home atoll. Thus, she expected to be away from her other children for eight months or more for each delivery, leaving older children to look after their younger siblings. A recent recommendation in the 2011 Marshall Islands MDG report underlines the need for the Health Department to post women health aides on outer islands, which is long overdue. The responsibilities and knowledge held by local midwives also needs far greater recognition. But such recognition of local midwives is still largely suppressed due to a Marshallese custom that forbids interventions, either verbal or physical, between women and men regarding women's bodies and associated reproductive matters at all levels. Attempts by women nurses to change the Health Department policies regarding the appointment of women as health aides on outer islands have only recently been recognized.

Thus, complications both before a birth or postpartum have long been dealt with on outer islands by women midwives, based on their knowledge and previous experiences. Breech births or bleeding during pregnancy had been treated with local medicines and massage. Postnatal care, including failure of the baby to thrive or other abnormalities, is discussed by the midwife with other women of the household. Most women lactate abundantly, providing a healthy start for the newborn. Lack of breastmilk by teenage mothers is more or less accepted with no locally approved solutions; wet nursing is not practised, so if their babies failed to thrive, their deaths were accepted.

Women expect to lactate freely, a point that came up often in women's discussions. One woman who was still breastfeeding both a four-year-old boy and a one-year-old faced the disapproval of other women, as it was not usual practice. In remote communities, such as outer island atolls, such prolific milk production was life saving for newborns. Yet shortage of breast milk experienced by teenage mothers (aged sixteen or seventeen years) is a major contributor to infant mortality, as wet nursing is rarely practised, but adoptions are common. Weaning food, given after about eight months, consisted of warm rice steeped in sweet tea, perhaps with a small piece of fish once or twice a week (Pollock, "These Roots Remain"). The association between lactation and delayed pregnancies could not be explained by medical personnel whom I consulted. It was only clarified by local expectations of two-year intervals between births. Both men and women expected a new baby every two years. Marital status was not an issue, as the baby was born into and belonged to its mother's lineage.

The regularity of two-year intervals between births was later explained to me in several local contexts. A young woman, aged sixteen, conceived after she had her first or second menstrual period. She expected to conceive again, about a year after the first child was weaned. Thus, Marshallese women expect to spend most of their lives either pregnant or breast-feeding. Men also expected their partners to bear a child every two years. As women are now living longer, so their reproductive capacities are extending. One woman told me that she was the eldest of the twenty-one children (including two sets of twins) that her mother had borne; she had raised her siblings, taking each newborn as it came along. Working as a nurse and becoming a mother herself, she considered her own three children to be an adequate fulfilment of her responsibility to Marshallese society.

My research interest in 2004 explored how these beliefs affect the incidence of menopause, since women are living longer, but satisfactory data proved elusive. But it did, however, give me further insights into the strength of Marshallese reproductive beliefs. Discussions with two nurses revealed major difficulties in access to data because much of this traditional knowledge remains covert, coded in traditional language, and rarely discussed even between women. The degree to which those old beliefs are dying out is an open question, since any discussion between men and women of matters associated with women's bodies violates Marshallese custom. Statistical data on menopause is not available, as I quickly discovered (Lock, "Encounters with Aging").

Ethnographic records underline how Marshall Islands women expect to be pregnant most of their adult lives. Women who mourned their inability to bear children are seen as a failure in their own and others' eyes. The occurrence of one such infertile woman in each of the ten large sibling sets (ten or more births for one woman) that I recorded, fell outside my usual experience, but I can gain no explanations from Western "experts," since contemporary gynaecologists and obstetricians rarely encounter women who have borne ten or more children in their European and/or American practices. The births, and birth order of named children, as written in the front of a woman's Bible, provide a major ethnographic source of data but are difficult to align for statistical purposes.

STATISTICAL RETURNS

The two hospitals in the major population centres, one in Majuro and the other in Ebeye, keep statistical records of reproductive activities for the Marshall Islands Health Department but only for the past twenty years. These include the numbers of women admitted for antenatal care, numbers of births, as well as other gynaecological and obstetric admissions. Data pertaining to reproductive activities for the other twenty-four islands of the Marshalls are uneven. Male health aides on outer islands are expected to provide such returns monthly, but due to communication difficulties, such returns may not reach the Health Department. Record keeping is fraught with difficulties.

Ten children per woman, as I found in my ethnographic data collection, is not far in excess of the average national statistic, recorded in 1973, of 8.4 lifetime births per woman (Republic of Marshall Islands Dept. of Health Services). Outer island data is subject to irregularities, and statistics on reproductive rates do not account for all births or all infant deaths that occurred over the last thirty years. On one of my visits to the Health Department in Majuro in 1969, the department head expressed surprise when I told her about three teenage mothers on an outer island who had lost their babies in the previous six months. Still births and miscarriages may be recorded for urban women who (nowadays) attend the hospitals in Majuro or Ebeye. But on outer islands, such deaths are unlikely to be reported by the local (male) health aide. Attempts to improve record keeping are being addressed by the South Pacific Secretariat as part of the requirements for MDG statistical returns.

RONGELAP WOMEN'S REPRODUCTIVE CONCERNS

The women of Rongelap atoll have experienced many reproductive failures since 1954, which they attribute to exposure to radioactive substances (Pollock, "Radioactive Contamination of Food"). On 1 March 1954, the mushroom-shaped cloud that emanated from the U.S. atomic explosion over Bikini atoll, deposited a white ash, on Rongelap atoll some two hundred miles away, which Marshallese refer to as *schnow*. They later learned that this ash was a radioactive deposit, fallout from the Bikini nuclear explosion. Subsequently, Rongelap people noted many changes in their environment, their foods, and their bodies, changes that they attributed to that radioactive fallout. They still refer to that fallout across the Marshall Islands as *paisin* or "poison." In addition to goitre problems and other health issues affecting the whole community, women have experienced several stillbirths and malformed fetuses, or what they call "jelly babies," which they spontaneously excreted (Johnston and Barker). These lost babies, counted as interruptions to their usual pattern of giving birth every two years, caused families great distress.

The deformed fetuses were not even considered by the U.S. Brookhaven Medical team during their annual health check-ups of the Rongelap population between 1957 and 1978. Forty years later, in 1997, one of the leaders of the Brookhaven medical team reported that "there was an increase in miscarriages and stillbirths in the exposed Rongelap women but the numbers were small and it is uncertain if this increase was related to radiation effects" (Cronkite and Bond 185). But these still births and miscarriages were not reported at the time. The male health physicists referred to these events as, in their terminology, "hydatidiform cysts." They insisted that the women had "imagined" these "cysts" because they could not provide evidence that they had discharged them from their bodies. I witnessed one such fetus—a horrific reminder of women's sufferings—preserved in a large jar that sat on a shelf in the Rongelap atoll office in Majuro. There was a major disjuncture between what the Atomic Energy Commission (AEC) nuclear physicists dismissed as "imagination" and Marshallese women's concerns about the "poison" that affected their reproduction and their atoll environment.

The AEC team of nuclear physicists failed to consider Marshallese reproductive beliefs in their annual assessments of Rongelap residents' health. As Cronkite and Bond (185) noted in 1997, the numbers were "too small" to be considered significant by statistical standards. But these male outsiders did not understand the women's widespread distress that their reproductive beliefs were not even being considered by so-called experts and were not being taken seriously. Women's general well-being was deeply implicated in these reproductive failures, which added to all the other traumas the community has suffered in association with nuclear fallout. The recent declassification and release of documents about Project 4.1, as a U.S. designed experiment on the effects of radiation on human bodies, has further exacerbated Marshallese (and others') concerns (Welcome). Today, such experimentation on human subjects would be subject to severe international sanctions.

Documents declassified under President Clinton's authorization have confirmed Marshallese suspicions that AEC medical authorities knew about the levels of radiation exposure in the 1960s but did not intervene. Rongelap peoples' ongoing requests to U.S. officials to move them from their contaminated atoll went unheeded until community members took matters into their own hands in 1985 and with assistance from Greenpeace, moved to a nearby islet in Kwajalein atoll that had not been contaminated (Pollock, "Nuclear Contamination of Food"). Thirty years later in 2015, the Rongelap people are still awaiting assurance that their home atoll is no longer contaminated and that it has been cleaned of *paisin*, so that they can safely resume their lives there.

Fears that reproductive anomalies will recur if irradiated soil is not thoroughly removed from their land are prevalent. The Rongelap community has been told that when they return, they must limit their use of local foods, such as breadfruit and coconuts, to only 25 percent of their diet; the balance will come from imported foods (with all the health hazards associated with such an obesogenic diet). But calculating such a dietary split is hard to contemplate (Pollock, "Nuclear Contamination of Food").

Discrepancies in the language used to address reproductive matters have added to the confusion. Marshallese described their failed pregnancies in language other than that which the Brookhaven medical team used. Women referred to these malformed fetuses as "jelly babies" (Darlene Keju Johnson). They were the outcome of incomplete pregnancies and were not quite babies but very much like them, as Darlene Keju Johnson described them. But for the nuclear physics team, these were described as "hydatidiform cysts" or "events," not even considered as having had life. Reluctantly, the nuclear physicists later suggested that the "cysts" may have been associated with intake of radioisotopes from nuclear fallout. In their 1997 report, the AEC team noted that "some of the problems affecting the [annual] examinations included a language barrier and cultural differences left a fear of the 'poisonous powder'" (Cronkite and Bond 183). This report was published in the *Health Physics* journal, a source not readily available to Marshallese readers. None of the Brookhaven team or other AEC appointed health physicists approached local people for cultural assistance, nor did they approach for advice from those of us who had lived and worked in the Marshall Islands for long periods. The resulting misunderstanding of reproductive concerns persists in Rongelap peoples' fear of returning to an atoll where some "poison" may linger.

Only recently has it been acknowledged in some quarters that a major secret U.S. experiment had been initiated by the Atomic Energy Commission before the Bravo test in 1954 (see Horowitz film, Nuclear Savage). Information in the four-hundred page Advisory Committee Report on Human Radiation Experiments (ACHRE), released for general perusal by President Clinton in 1996 (Welsome), provided details of Project 4.1. The author of that report noted that "[President Bill] Clinton directed us to uncover the history of human radiation experiments and intentional environment releases of radiation in order to identify ethical and scientific standards for evaluating these events and to ensure wrong doing cannot be repeated" (21).

Failure by the AEC teams to make the link between ingested radiation from eating local foods and Rongelap people's health issues is another concern for Marshallese people (Pollock, "Nuclear Contamination of Food"). Nuclear physicists, including the Brookhaven medical team, continued to report annually (from 1957) that Rongelap people's health was "good," but they had not examined the diets in detail and provided no personal or individual reports to the people. The 1996 ACHRE report revealed that the limited food data that the AEC team had collected was not considered as a serious health hazard.

Rongelap community members themselves have observed that over some thirty years, their sicknesses were probably directly linked to eating local foods, such as breadfruit, pandanus, coconuts, and fish, their only food sources. Those observations, though not confirmed by the AEC 'expert' teams, drove them to move from their atoll.

After 1996, Marshallese people and the wider world learned that the U.S. had deliberately exposed Marshall Islands people to radiation in order to track its effects on human bodies, as set out in Project 4.1 in 1953. Women's bodies were thus integral to this human experiment, including the failed pregnancies and "jelly babies" that Marshallese women had been enduring. But the U.S. has failed to pay full compensation claims for hardship and mental distress, despite these years of suffering (Pollock, Nuclear Contamination of Food).

Health physicists involved in these medical experiments still vary in their opinions on what constitutes a safe dose of radiation as well as on the health outcomes of exposure to radioactive isotopes. *Cesium* 137 and *Strontium* 90 both damage human tissue and bone, whereas high doses of *Iodine* 131 disrupt the function of the thyroid (Bertell; Sublette). Many cancers are implicated, with nodules on the thyroid being the most widely reported health problem for many Marshallese, both female and male. People received background radiation while living amid the heavily contaminated environment, from performing daily practices. These included preparing food, washing clothes, and squatting on the ground when working, which directly exposes female and male genitalia—covered only by thin cloth—to radioactive substances in the soil. In addition, women fed their families contaminated foods for twenty-eight years while also experiencing reproductive failures and other negative health outcomes (Pollock, "Nuclear Contaminated Food").

Claims for compensation for "hardship," as the Nuclear Claims Tribunal labelled the medical claims by Rongelap and other women exposed to radiation, included cultural loss and disruptions to their lives. The people of the four northern atolls—Enewetak, Bikini, Rongelap and Utrik—were awarded various sums of compensation following their individual claims at the 2001–2004 Nuclear Claims Tribunal hearings in Majuro (Plasman and Danz). But those awards have only been partially paid, and many claimants have since died without receiving the compensation payments they were due.

CONTRACEPTION

Attempts to introduce contraceptive devices to Marshall Islands women began at the height of the worldwide birth control movement in the 1960s. Birth control pills were dispensed to all of the atoll communities. The outer island women, with whom I was working, were not impressed about the suitability or the necessity for contraceptives. Nevertheless, they accepted the pills that the Health Aide handed out to them and left them, forgotten, on a ledge in the house or they took them only intermittently. In my 1966–1967 field notes, I recorded that pregnancies occurred despite the pills. Talk of contraception continues into the new millennium through messages from the Department of Health, but practices are little changed.

Marshall Islands women see contraceptive usage as an interruption to their customary way of life; besides, women with few or no children are considered socially unsuccessful. Women hear the message about birth control methods, but do not see such messages as relevant to their lives and well-being. Young people are more receptive when the message of contraception is delivered by one of their own, such as Darlene Keju Johnson's "Youth to Youth in Health" program. Although this program did not overtly target contraceptive use, it introduced transitional values associated with reduced reproduction and teenage pregnancies within new socio-cultural settings (Johnson).

A 1994 UNFPA report castigated the Marshall Islands for its lack of clear family planning goals, citing "the health benefits of child spacing" among its purported attributes. But Marshallese have long practised child spacing. The agency's proposed Target Model bears little relationship to Marshallese practices, as it fails to understand cultural values behind the rejection of contraception ideas. Considerations of the number of condoms distributed and verbal responses to questions about contraception usage that target an outsider concept of "married" women , neither add up to nor represent "birth control" practices in the Marshalls.

In 2011, both the WHO and the UNFPA listed the low levels of "success" in increasing contraceptive use in Pacific nations (47 percent in the Marshall Islands). For urban populations in the Marshall Islands (67 percent of total population), contraceptives are readily accessible from urban hospitals. But on outer islands, condom distribution and their use are not directly recorded. Condoms distributed since the 1970s have many uses, not necessarily as a contraceptive. Reports to WHO and other agencies (Levy et al.; UNFPA), note that contraceptive practices include long-term methods—female sterilization, subdermal implants (Norplant) and injectable hormones—as the most acceptable, compared to sterilization (41 percent), pills, and IUDs. Male contraceptive methods are not recorded.

It is not surprising that a 2010 UNFPA report referred to a "stalled fertility transition" in the Marshall Islands, where "contraceptive use is generally low," even though as the report noted, contraceptives are readily accessible in urban areas. The report found that both women and men are "unwilling rather than unable" to use contraceptives and that they lack confidence about their use. The UNFPA report authors recommended another survey to uncover the reasons for and the bases of opposition to contraceptives use. Such a survey must include an in-depth appreciation of philosophies and practices related to reproduction, as I have noted above, from both Marshallese women and men.

TEENAGE PREGNANCIES

Teenage pregnancies have become a matter of major concern across the Pacific, both for local communities and for external agencies. The Marshall Islands is reported to have the highest rate of teenage fertility in the region, with a birth rate of 67 per 1000 (RMI DHS Survey), although these figures must be a "guesstimate." These rates are of particular concern to public health and social authorities in the two high density urban atolls of Majuro and Ebeye. Darlene Keju Johnson's "Youth to Youth Program," (YTYH) initiated in Majuro in the 1990s, consisted of a few young women and men raising young peoples' awareness of the consequences of pregnancies. Keju Johnson promoted the idea that pregnancies were not the only contribution young people could make to Marshallese life. By drawing in talented singers, musicians, and those who enjoyed expressing themselves in drama, she encouraged young people to think about sharing their new thoughts about reproduction as it affected their lives. For example, one skit portrayed a young household with the pregnant male (with a large "baby bump") staggering around the stage doing female tasks while a group of young women sat around chatting and laughing. The skit, which I saw in 1993, was received by the public with much hilarity and prolonged clapping. This mode of message delivery was a potent means for exposure to reproductive education and an effective alternative to forms of delivery used elsewhere. Unfortunately, YTYH has become marginalized without Darlene's voice to bridge the discourse. The RMI Ministry of Health has separated YTYH from Family Planning activities. In 2014, Giff Johnson (Personal interview.) advised me that planning activities had reverted to a "clinical" approach rather than an outreach approach to involve young people within their communities. Yet the UNFPA remains concerned about reducing adolescent pregnancies.

It is ironic that many of the parents of these young people have followed Marshallese custom of regular pregnancies, resulting in large families. Transition from those earlier reproductive expectations to new policies—as introduced by the UNFPA, WHO, and the Secretariat of the Pacific Community—is successful when it is delivered in a locally acceptable format, as Darlene Johnson established. Drawing on her experience in public health studies, she "translated" what she considered to be the essence of "foreign" messages into Marshallese thinking. Since her death, YTYH is even more necessary as an alternative approach to "education about birth control." The disjuncture is an example of Lock's "cosmopolitan medicine," which encompasses both traditional medical systems within modern medical practices, as assessed within cultural, historical, and environmental settings. The message in Darlene Johnson's biography, *Don't Ever Whisper*, spreads the word in a Marshallese (and Pacific) way, which is ever more vital in times of health transitions between two very disparate approaches to reproduction.

OTHER MATERNAL HEALTH ISSUES

Support for women's maternal health and other physical concerns has largely been overlooked by central health authorities in the Marshall Islands, as noted in the 2011 RMI MDG report. Women's health concerns, particularly back pain after deliveries, were noted in a South Pacific Communities (SPC) report in 1987, but remedial actions are difficult to establish in far-flung islands. Night blindness is well known, but remedial care—apart from recommendations that pregnant women eat plenty of papaya, culturally considered a pig food—has been difficult where diets are limited in terms of local foods.

Night blindness has been a particular health concern for pregnant women in the Pacific, along with anaemia (Levy-SPC 182). Lack of vitamin A can be rectified, if availability of the "super banana," known as *karat* in Pohnpei, can be supported. Research funded by the Bill and Melinda Gates Foundation, and carried out by the late Lois Engleberger in Pohnpei, showed that vitamin A deficiency in pregnant women can be reduced when this locally grown fruit becomes widely accepted and used.

The MDG report for the Marshall Islands recommends that women should be trained for inclusion in the outer island Health Aide program. Hopefully, the many women midwives who have brought numerous Marshallese babies into the world will be included in any reformulated midwifery service. The midwives, mothers who have experienced many births themselves, share a vast range of knowledge and experience that they draw on to handle the range of problems they might encounter, particularly in outer islands. Diets, medicines, and diseases, such as diabetes, together with the vagaries of transportation, whether by sea or air between outer islands and the main centres, continue to create logistic challenges both for midwives and for pregnant women.

The Millennium Development Goals Report for the Marshall Islands (32) set out specific targets to increase the numbers and skills of trained midwives across all the atolls and to increase maternal health care staff at the two urban hospitals (RMI). The need for Pacific Island countries to build on a "continuum of care" model of essential services, from pre-pregnancy to pregnancy delivery and early childhood, as proposed by a 2011 WHO report, suggests a positive step forward. However, the feasibility problems of delivering such a service to all twenty-four outer islands of the Marshall Islands will require not only money but also dedicated administrative attention.

Reproductive tract infections and sexually transmitted infections, including gonorrhoea and syphilis, are high among urban-based adults across the Pacific, according to UNFPA reports. This is not new, although the rate of infection may be under closer scrutiny as Health Departments are required to provide statistics to outside agencies. I recorded three children bearing the names Konorea or "gonorrhoea" in my ethnographic household data from various atolls in the 1960s. Namu women discussed "interactions" with *ri-belle* or "foreign" men while living on Ebeye, near the U.S. Kwajalein missile base in the 1960s. Whether they became infected in these encounters is unknown, as no tests were conducted at the time. Any effects on fertility are not evident in either the ethnographic or statistical records.

CONCLUSIONS

A major disjuncture continues to exist between Marshallese views of reproduction and outsiders' pressures for statistics. Local knowledge of Marshallese beliefs and practices is not easily collated in numerical form. And statistical returns only marginally reflect actual practices and beliefs. Claims that the health transition is slow rest on the gulf between these two views. Marshallese women's beliefs have been impacted negatively by the ongoing outcomes of nuclear testing deposits on human health. Any measures of the health transition need to include past experiences as these inform practice today. So-called low uptake of birth control measures is one example discussed here.

Assessments of health transition or, uptake of "cosmopolitan medicine" in the Marshall Islands, must include regard for new criteria for control of reproduction, as espoused by international family planning and population control agencies, most recently expressed in the Millennium Development Goal Targets 2000–2015. An ethnoscape of reproduction within an assessment of maternal health in the Marshall Islands highlights women's fears of reproductive failure as these are locally perceived. Those fears, are derived from the history of radioactive testing on these islands and peoples. In Giff Johnson's *Don't Ever Whisper*, Darlene Keju Johnson offers an educational solution for the Marshall Islands Health Department to reach young Marshallese women and men in easy to understand and culturally acceptable forms. Fears of further disruptions to Marshallese reproductive cycles, such the jelly babies that resulted from radioactive contamination, lead Marshallese women to continue to ask why they should have to reduce the number of their pregnancies. Modern discourse on reproduction is attempting to bridge concepts of women's bodies as central to social as well as physical well-being. Greater understanding of the social context of reproduction will reduce the disjunctures discussed here between local views and universalized statistical protocols for recording reproductive health anomalies.

WORKS CITED

Advisory Committee on Human Radiation Experiments (ACHRE). *The Human Radiation Experiments.* New York: Oxford University Press, 1996. Print

Appadurai, Arjun. *Modernity at Large: Cultural Dimensions of Globalization.* Minneapolis: University of Minnesota Press, 1996. Print.

Bertell, Rosalie. *No Immediate Danger—Prognosis for a Radioactive Earth.* New York: The Women's Press, 1985. Print.

Cronkite, E. P., and V. P. Bond "Historical Events Associated with Fallout from the Bravo Shot: 25 Years of Medical Findings." *Health Physics* 73.1 (1997): 176-186. Print.

Engleberger, Lois, A. Lorens, A. Levendusky, and J Daniells. "Banana." *Ethnobotany of Pohnpei, Plants, People and Island Culture.* Ed. Michael J. Balick. Honolulu: University of Hawai'i Press, 2009. 89-131. Print.

Hayes, Geoff and Annette Robertson. *Family Planning in the Pacific Islands.* Suva: UNFPA-ICOMP Regional Consultation, Suva. 2010. Print.

Horowitz, Adam Jonas, Director and Writer. Nuclear Savage: The Islands of Secret Project 4.1. Documentary, 60 minutes / 87 minutes. 2011.DVD.

Johnson, Giff. *Don't Ever Whisper. A Biography of Darlene Keju Johnson.* CreateSpace Independent Publishing Platform, 2013. Print.

Johnson, Giff. Personal interview. 2014.

Johnston, Barbara Rose, and Holly Barker. *The Consequential Damages of Nuclear War: The Rongelap Report.* Walnut Creek, CA: Left Coast Press. 2008. Print.

Kabua, Maria and Irene Tafaaki. *Traditional Medicine in the Marshall Islands.* Honolulu: University of. Hawaii Press, 2004. Print.

Levy, S. J., R. Taylor, Ilona Higgins, and Deborah Grafton-Wasserman. "Fertility and Contraception in the Marshall Islands." *Studies in Family Planning* 19.3 (1998): 179-183. Print.

Lock, Margaret. *East Asian Medicine in Urban Japan: Varieties of Medical Experience.* Berkeley: University of California Press. 1984. Print.

Lock, Margaret. *Encounters with Aging: Mythologies of Menopause in Japan and North America*. Berkeley: University of California Press. 1993. Print.

Marshall Islands-UNFPA. *Reproductive Health and Family Planning in the Pacific. Discussion Paper #14.* UN, 1995. Web. Nov. 2013.

Nuclear Claims Tribunal. *Reports*. Majuro: Republic of Marshall Islands, 1990. Print.

Pollock, Nancy J. "Birthing Practices in a Marshall Islands Society." *Newsletter of European Association of Gynaecologists and Obstetrics.* 99 (2000): 5-9. Print.

Pollock, Nancy J. "Marshall Islands Women's Health Issues—Nuclear Fallout" Address to Women's League for Peace and Freedom (WILPF), Asia-Pacific Region. (2004): n.pag. *Highbeam*. Web. 20 Sept. 2015

Pollock, Nancy J. "Nuclear Contamination of Food: Fallout from the U.S. Nuclear Bomb Tests on Hiroshima and the Marshall Islands." *Pacific Ecologist* 22 (2013): 20-29. Print.

Pollock, Nancy J. "Radioactive Contamination of Food: Lessons from Hiroshima and the Marshall Islands," *Food and War in Mid-Twentieth century East Asia*. Ed. Katarzyna Cwiertka. Farnham: Ashgate, 2013. 165-187. Print.

Republic of Marshall Islands (RMI). *National Progress Report—Joint RMI/UNDP*: Suva: UNDP, 2011. Print.

Republic of Marshall Islands (RMI). *Demographic and Health Survey*. Majuro: Department of Health. 2011. Print.

South Pacific Community (SPC). *Marshall Islands Women's Health Issues*. New Caledonia: South Pacific Community, 1987. Print.

UNFPA. *Marshall Islands Report*. UNFPA, 2013. Web. Oct. 2013.

U.S. Committee on Radiological Safety in the Marshall Islands. *Report*. U.S. Scientific Committee on Effects of Atomic Radiation. Washington, DC: U.S. National Research Council, George Washington University, 1994. Print

Welsome, Eileen. *The Plutonium Files: America's Secret Medical Experiments in the Cold War*. New York: Dial Publishing, 1999.

World Health Organization (WHO). *Report on MDGs for Pacific Island Countries. Ninth Meeting of Ministries of Health for Pacific Island Countries. World Health Organization: Western Pacific Region*. WHO, 2011. Web. Oct. 2013.

10.
Examining the Intersections of Gender and Reproduction in Chuuk

Reflections on the Relevance and Utility of MDGs in a Small Island(s) Community

SARAH A. SMITH

THE 2000 MILLENNIUM SUMMIT AND resulting Declaration was an important benchmark for the development world, thought to reform and guide the entire global agenda for development. Although it did render a document that guided a global agenda, the expectations of the products of this Summit were much higher, and there has been a considerable amount of critique of the structure and implementation of the resulting United Nations Millennium Development Goals (MDG) birthed out of this event. As McPherson (this volume) describes, those MDGs that specifically focus on women were particularly disappointing to the feminist activists who, for decades, fought for the inclusion of attention to gender equality in development agendas. The simplification and complete separation of MDG 3 and MDG 5 made their functionality questionable in such diverse global contexts, one of which I will explore in this chapter.

This chapter addresses MDGs 3 and 5 with a particular place in mind: Chuuk, a state in the Federated States of Micronesia (FSM). Chuuk is a state composed of twenty-three inhabited islands, and is, like the rest of the world, a place where gender equality is intimately linked to sexual and reproductive health and rights (SRHR) at the individual, social, and structural levels. In this very gender- and age-stratified community, it is this social context of gender inequality that perpetuates sexual inequality and the absence of universal access to contraceptives for *all* women, of comprehensive reproductive and sexual health care, and of safe and confidential STI and HIV testing. Even those services that are more readily available—very specific to MDG 5—such as prenatal and hospital care, are so lacking in quality that women who can afford to leave Chuuk for care elsewhere do so. Yet because the social determinants of health are much more complex than simple access to a hospital—also including nutrition, bodily stress, gender inequality, and the other diseases of poverty and patriarchy—Chuukese women continue to suffer the poorest outcomes, even when they migrate to nearby places such as Guam, U.S. This chapter will discuss each of these elements affecting women's SRHR, underscoring the importance of gender equality for considering such health and rights. Finally, I connect these findings to the MDG goals and consider some of the critiques leveraged against these two MDGs that are relevant to this context. I draw on these themes to argue not only that MDGs 3 and 5 should be more appropriately linked and considered in the complex ways the two co-exist but also that all of the conditions of these postcolonial, poverty-ridden countries, which MDGs were created for, must be considered together within their unique social and cultural contexts to truly effect change.

The world of international development should (and at times does) take a few pointers from anthropologists and other ethnographers. Gender equality and SRHR are areas in which anthropological work has flourished, and the context described in this chapter is derived from findings from just such work. The insights from this chapter are part of a larger ethnographic project in Chuuk, FSM and in Guam, U.S. that included participant observation and interviews in clinics with health care workers (HCW) and in-depth, life history interviews with Chuukese women. These methods are the hallmark of the field and bring in a depth and richness that capture social life in ways that development specialists must work to include for any comprehensive understanding of the social world in which they intend to work. This chapter focuses primarily on findings from Chuuk.

This was a feminist-inspired project examining the interplay of gender and SRHR, a topic that received considerable attention in anthropology for decades. The "politics of reproduction"—a phrase often cited to discuss anthropology's theories about reproduction—delineates how reproduction is represented and experienced in every aspect of human social and cultural life, primarily because it is responsible for the biological and social reproduction of cultures (Ginsburg and Rapp). Anthropologists have demonstrated reproduction as inevitably linked to an analysis of gendered processes, kinship and the family, medicalization, social hierarchies, and concerns of the control of both the social and individual body (Browner; Ginsburg and Rapp; Scheper-Hughes and Lock). Furthermore, anthropologists have called attention to the social inequalities that not only stratify reproduction but also demonstrate social stratification through looking at a particular community's reproduction (Colen). Thus, a study of SRHR is a study of gender roles, kinship, control of bodies, colonial histories, social inequality, and so much more.

Anthropologists also consider the political economy of health or the adoption of Marxian ideas of capitalism, class struggle, and inequality and their impact on health, including reproductive health (Baer, Singer, and Susser). In this framework, health is considered a great indicator of inequality, and reproduction is a great perspective through which to explore social life. This chapter is a study of a place in which capitalism and its stratifying forces were "introduced" through a long and enduring history of colonialism, which, arguably, still exists today.

Drawing from these perspectives, I address the gender stratification of Chuuk, including the roles of men and women; kinship organization and kinship-based taboos; the ways in which women's bodies are controlled; and the social inequality reflected and perpetuated through reproduction. First, however, the social history of Chuuk's colonial past is important to consider in this holistic portrayal of gender and SRHR.

CHUUK COLONIAL HISTORY

The Pacific region of Micronesia has been the site of numerous colonial projects over centuries, resulting in inconsistent and discontinuous development to the present day. The Caroline Islands encompass what is known as the Federated States of Micronesia (FSM), including Chuuk. The FSM experienced a succession of colonial occupations, beginning in the sixteenth century with Spain, continuing with Germany in 1899, and then Japan, from World

War I (WWI) to World War II (WWII) (Hezel). With the Japanese surrender and American occupation of the islands in WWII, Micronesians found themselves yet again under a new colonizing power (Rogers).

At the end of WWII, the U.S. convinced the United Nations (UN) to allow them control over Micronesia in what was called a "strategic trusteeship," as Micronesia was "developed" (Hezel 256). The entire group of Mariana, Marshall (see Pollock, this volume), and Caroline Islands were broken up into seven districts (Chuuk being one of them) and became known as the Trust Territory of the Pacific Islands (TTPI) administered by the U.S. Navy (Hezel; Rogers). Kiste describes this era as one of "benign neglect" from the U.S. Navy, which denied access to these islands from most of the world and, simultaneously, ignored the islanders' needs (230). This era ended when the UN issued a report condemning the U.S. for the poor state of "development" in the TTPI in 1961, inciting then President Kennedy to pour significant amounts of money to the originally promised build up (Hezel).

The Trust Territories then negotiated independence and eventually became three countries (the FSM being one), each entering into a Compact of Free Association (COFA) agreement with the U.S. The Compact gave each new nation self-governing rights, but the U.S. continued to have the right of denial of foreign entry and military control of waters, while funding education, economic, and political development and health care infrastructure (Hezel). Scholars have criticized these COFAs for several reasons. Hanlon describes them as creating "a constrained, almost neocolonial future through terms and conditions that compromise the autonomy and national integrity in favor of continued financial assistance from the United States" (101). The COFA agreements are considered to be a major contributor to the poor socio-economic situation in these small island nations today (Hanlon). Initially, there was a large cash flow from the Kennedy-era buildup and then COFA implementation; however, this has decreased over time, leaving the country in a "dismal" state (Levin 8).

Chuuk is the most populated state of the FSM, divided into five regions, with thirty-five municipalities in the twenty-three inhabited island units. The central islands of Chuuk lagoon politically and economically dominate the state, and many Chuukese from all over Chuuk state migrate to this central location (Gorenflo and Levin; Levin). Chuuk is also the poorest state of the FSM, with deteriorating education, economic, and health care systems.

CHUUK HEALTH CARE

The FSM health care system is a hospital-based "cosmopolitan" (Jordan) system created by the U.S. The implementation of this type of system has been criticized because of the cost for high-tech supplies and the skilled workforce needed for hospital care, which is beyond what the FSM can afford. Essentially, it is not a sustainable system (Benjamin 22). Furthermore, similar to what Wentworth (this volume) describes in Vanuatu and Pollock (this volume) describes in the Marshall Islands, an estimated 30 percent of FSM residents cannot access hospitals because of the long distances from island to island, an issue that disproportionately affects Chuuk, because of the large number of inhabited islands making up the state (Diaz). For Chuuk, the hospital and primary health care services are all located on one politically and economically central island: Wééné. Built in 1969, Chuuk's hospital is considered to be in "serious disrepair" (Feasley and Lawrence 117) and is known to locals as "the place people go to die" (Dernbach, *Popular Religion*; Moral; Smith). The hospital is in such bad shape that women with whom I interviewed told me stories of requesting to be sent home early—not because of a speedy recovery—but because they did not anticipate getting better in a place infested with rats and cats, and with dirty or no running water. Other health care facilities consist of "public health," a clinic built on hospital grounds that focuses on preventative care, such as immunizations, prenatal care, STI and HIV testing and counselling, and non-communicable disease (NCD) detection. There are also dispensaries on other islands, which range from actual small, clinic-like scenarios with medical aides to a medicine cabinet in someone's home. Supply shortages are common and chronic in all three sectors, a problem noted in all the communities described in this volume.

Those who live on other islands must be able to afford the cost of gas for a boat ride to Wééné to access care, except for the minimal care provided by the small and inconsistently staffed island dispensaries. This is not unique to Chuuk, but is also a major barrier to care in many "developing" nations as writers in this volume delineate. Barlow, Pollock, and Wentworth describe the necessary boat trips to access care throughout the Pacific, and Yakong and McPherson show that similar problems occur where there are limited cars available, such as in northern Ghana, forcing labouring women to endure long walks to the clinic. This lack of access to care—by virtue of boat and fuel costs—as well as minimal personnel and supplies within Wééné leaves many people without access to basic health services, including sexual and reproductive health services. Lack of health care is one of many reasons cited for Chuukese transnational movement to the U.S.

Migration to the U.S. is fostered by the same COFA agreement that determined the relationship between the U.S. and the FSM upon their independence and subsequent development plan. Citizens of COFA nations can travel, live, and work in the U.S. with the status of "non-immigrants" as part of the COFA agreement. These "non-immigrants" began moving into the U.S. rapidly after the COFA agreement was enacted and, as of 2010, approximately one-third of the FSM population is living abroad (Hezel and Levin). Chuuk experiences significant transnational migration to the U.S. for a variety of reasons, including access to education, employment, health care, and adventure. Guam, in particular, is described by several scholars as attractive to Chuukese migrants because of its close proximity to home, allowing for ease of movement between the two locations (Bautista; Gorenflo and Levin; Levin; Marshall). Just a quick flight away, Guam has also become a site for medical tourism for those Chuuk-based residents who wish to avoid Chuuk's deteriorating health care system, and who can afford the plane ticket (Smith).

THE STATE OF SRHR IN CHUUK AND GUAM

Unfortunately, the deteriorating infrastructure in Chuuk and the often "neglected" colonial infrastructure of Guam inhibit regular collection and analysis of standard reproductive and sexual health indicators for Chuukese women, and limited scholarly research exists for this region (Smith). Furthermore, those indicators that are collected, especially in Chuuk, are often considered incomplete because of considerable underreporting. Nancy Pollock (this volume) demonstrates that this underreporting is also present in the Republic of the Marshall Islands; the entire Micronesian region of disbursed islands, in fact, is beset by this paucity of consistent reporting. This is an issue in many underdeveloped countries and an important reason why quantitative indicators alone are problematic as the primary development measurement for poor countries.

The little data available do delineate negative reproductive outcomes faced by Micronesian women. First, the major causes of death in the FSM include prematurity and complications during pregnancy and labour (FSM). In fact, compared to Guam's infant mortality rate (IMR) of 12.7 per 1,000 live births, the rate (IMR) of Chuuk is 22, and this low number is likely due to underreporting issues described by the FSM report (FSM, "FSM Health Progress Report"; GovGuam). Women recognize these risks of birthing in Chuuk and make considerable efforts to access safe health care elsewhere during this time (Smith).

When it comes time for childbirth, older anthropological literature portrayed the importance for women to go home if they were not already living on their family land (Fischer). Childbirth used to involve a midwife and the women of the labouring woman's family, who were her primary support system (Fischer). Now, women leave home for Wééné, Guam, and Hawai'i to give birth in hospitals with only a few, if any, family members present (Bautista; Smith). They travel far for hospital birth. Yet in Guam, Chuukese women are not getting the better health outcomes or health care that they often migrate to receive. Chuukese and other Micronesian women account for a disproportionate number of women who give birth with no prenatal care and experience more births with gestational diabetes, leading to a nearly double rate of Caesarean deliveries, compared to the rest of Guam's residents (Haddock et al.; Alur et al.). Additionally, researchers and HCWs in Guam and Hawai'i have expressed considerable concern for the disproportionately high rates of sexually transmitted infections in this population and the subsequent impact on birth outcomes (Haddock, et al.; Kawamoto; Pobutsky, et al.; Yamada and Pobutsky; Wong and Kawamoto).

These are the outcomes important to consider for Chuuk as well, given the lack of data collection systems in the FSM. Yet these data do not appear when considering MDG progress, since these women are in the U.S. when the outcomes occur.

What other factors contribute to women suffering from these poor sexual and reproductive health outcomes, and why do they continue to do so, even when migrating to a "developed" country? Cultural concepts of gender, reproduction, and sexuality also contribute to the state of SRHR in Chuuk and among Chuukese abroad.

CHUUKESE GENDER ROLES, REPRODUCTION, AND SEXUALITY

Chuukese communities have a clan-based matrilineal structure, in which land is of utmost importance (Moral; Pollock, this volume). Women enhance their status in their family and community by reproducing—a central goal of the entire clan structure—thus, creating the next generation of heirs to the land (Moral). As inheritance is matrilineal, the eldest females of families are in charge of clan land, although they work with the eldest brother who makes the "public" decisions. As the "moral" upholders of their clan, women are expected to be silent and modest at all times. Brothers are the most important men in women's lives, according to custom. Husbands are the most important men in women's lives, according to the church. Describing a parallel scenario in southern Malawi, Hayes (this volume) explores a similar history in which missionaries challenged the matrilineal kin structure and, thereby, challenged the authority of the women's uncles (mother's brothers) as their primary leaders and protectors. This leaves women confused and expected to simply follow all the men's directives in their lives, although at times those directives can conflict (Smith). Women and men alike agree, however, that women are "under" men in Chuuk, and they must "respect" men, regardless of what relationship that man has to the woman. I learned very quickly that the definition of "respect" when used in this particular context was more akin to my definition of "obey."

The entire realm of gender relations and gender inequality has been analyzed as a consequence of a strict incest taboo, bridging gender and sexuality in the context of Chuuk. Beatriz Moral conducted ethnographic work in Chuuk in the 1990s with a focus on Chuukese women's sexuality and her entire analysis centres on the brother-sister incest taboo (including parallel cousins[1]). Moral argues that this taboo structures sexuality in Chuuk, especially women's sexuality and, by extension, gender roles. Men are perceived as unable to control their sexual desires, so it is the responsibility of women to maintain control of sexuality both within and outside of families (Moral). Any discussions of sex should not occur in front of opposite-sex siblings, nor should discussions of a person's sexual behavior occur in the presence of their sibling. In fact, women are generally expected to remain silent about *anything* so as not to demonstrate their sexuality in front of their brothers (Moral). The incest taboo's influence on the construction of male-female relations also structures the public arena, in which women's silence is expected, and the community is very gender-segregated in public (Moral). This structure impedes women's abilities to be public figures and, consequently, inhibits participation in elections, leaving public office largely in the domain of men (Moral). Women still have influence in decision making, given their clan roles in this matrilineal community, but it is silent and strategically yielded (Moral). However, Dernbach (*Enacting Motherhood*) argues that the patriarchal ideology associated with Christianity has weakened the influence women had, although women's church groups have become a stronger venue to assert their power (Marshall and Marshall).

Due to the incest taboo, sex or anything related to sex is not to be discussed or demonstrated publicly when both men and women are present; much of what happens within and outside a marriage is conducted quietly, without any public displays of affection (Caughey; Goodenough, *Property, Kin and Community*; Moral). Women especially are expected to keep their sexual activity and sexuality quiet (Caughey; Smith). A man and woman seen alone together are generally assumed to be in a sexual relationship (Dernbach, *Popular Religion*; Smith). Yet Chuukese sexual "freedom" in adolescence and outside of marriage is a common theme in the *older* anthropological literature (Caughey; Fischer; Goodenough, *Premarital Freedom*; Goodenough, *Property, Kin, and Community*; Moral). What this literature less clearly portrays is the gender-unequal standards in which sexual freedom is set: my findings demonstrate that for women, sex is *not* an accepted part of adolescence or marriage. Yet sexual "freedom" is an accepted part of boys' lives, a contradiction embedded in the same incest taboo that portrays men as unable to control their sexual desires (Smith). Extramarital affairs are very common and expected *of men* but when women are caught or even suspected of having an affair, the consequences are much worse, including suffering physical beatings, isolation in the household, and extremely possessive behaviour for years afterward (Dernbach, *Popular Religion*; Goodenough, "Premarital Freedom"). Women, thus, are held responsible for all sexual activity—whether desired, legitimate, or not—in a community in which even legitimate sexual activity must be hidden (Smith). Conversely, men are expected to be sexually "wild" as part of their youth and to pursue as many sexual partners as possible before and after marriage. This requirement for masculinity creates an environment in which men feel compelled to compete for sexual partners, whereas women work hard to hide any "inappropriate" sexual activity in which they do engage.

Women's responsibility for all sexual transgressions also creates a scenario in which there is no word for rape, and instead elder women use euphemisms such as "getting stepped on," to warn girls about the perils of unwanted sexual encounters that may occur if they leave the house at night or walk alone. When girls are warned about these possibilities, it is made clear if they do leave the house at night, for example, they are responsible for what happens to them. When a girl is sexually assaulted, silence is often her best strategy because if she were to report the assault, she will be perceived as having done something to provoke the sexually uncontrolled male, and this "behaviour" will bring shame on her clan. Given that all women are expected to obey men, it is assumed that if she is caught alone with a man, she is likely to succumb to his desires out of "respect." Some girls do fight back, but the social context is one in which silence is the most common response to assault. Women, thus, work very hard not only to hide any evidence of sexual activity or their sexual attractiveness but also to avoid being alone with men, at all times, unless they desire to have sex. The responsibility in this gender unequal environment follows the same "blame the victim" pattern that is found in the context of violence against women worldwide. Of course, as with any culturally embedded norm, it is not a context in which "men are evil;" men and women alike continue to perpetuate these ideas of female modesty and responsibility for all sexuality, of male dominance and sexual prowess and of, subsequently, victim-blaming sexual assault. Yet gender-based violence did not make the "cut" for targets connected to gender equality for the MDGs.

Furthermore, the social expectation that women remain faithful to husbands, with the simultaneous expectation that "boys will be (philandering) boys," creates a scenario in which women are upheld to unfair standards and subject to abuse when they are caught breaking those standards. This also means that women's primary risk for STIs and HIV is most often at home with their husbands. Hirsch et al. and Hammar write extensively about the HIV transmission risk to married women in the Pacific and in Africa (see also Hayes, this volume); Chuuk fits this same profile. Similarly, condom negotiation would bring shame, mistrust and possible beatings resulting from suspected infidelity of the woman asking to use condoms with a spouse, much like Hayes (this volume) describes in southern Malawi. Yet because the social context of gender roles makes women responsible for sexual morality, STIs or HIV discovered will likely bring much more shame to a woman than her male partner, who often exposed her to the infections. A similar shameful fate rests with unmarried women or those who had sex outside their marriage—or—those women who were sexually assaulted. Essentially, women are responsible for sex and, therefore, those infections that arise from sex.

SRH services are not widely sought because a woman seeking such services is publicly demonstrating that she is, indeed, sexually active. This is an especially difficult situation for unmarried women and girls, since they are displaying not only sexual activity by seeking these services but also a sexual activity that should not be happening and that can shame her family. This sexual regulation of women, thus, inhibits access to STI/HIV testing and counselling, contraceptives, prenatal care for unwed women, and other reproductive services.

STI/HIV COUNSELLING AND TESTING

STI/HIV counselling in Chuuk is available for free to anyone who seeks it, as is prenatal care or contraceptives. Yet STI/HIV counsellors informed me that they were lucky to get ten volunteer patients per month, all of whom are usually male. Working around the clear lack of desire to pursue voluntary testing, all pregnant women seeking prenatal care, as well as all people seeking health clearance certificates to work, are required to get STI/HIV testing and counselling. Yet, again, because of the lack of funding and bodies to provide services, not all STIs are tested. Patients are tested for syphilis, hepatitis B, and HIV and presumptively treated for chlamydia—thought to be the most endemic STI in the community—although without recent testing, it is hard to officially declare that is still the case. Those exhibiting symptoms that do not go away with chlamydia treatment are tested for gonorrhea, trichomoniasis. and other infections present in Chuuk. The prenatal care provider estimates that 80 percent of her patients have cervicitis, an infection of the cervix usually caused by STIs, such as chlamydia. Thus, chlamydia is likely still very prevalent but is treated, for those women who seek prenatal care. Those women without access risk poor pregnancy outcomes (or infertility). Furthermore, if women do seek services, they risk their confidential information being leaked—a serious barrier to care in an environment where sex and diseases are both taboo individually and connote moral transgressions. Diseases associated with sex are, thus, *very* taboo (Smith).

PREGNANCY CARE AND EXPERIENCES

These expectations shape pregnancy experiences and the value of reproduction as well. Motherhood is usually perceived as synonymous with becoming a woman (Flinn); it also increases women's power over time (Smith). Similarly, in southern Malawi (Hayes, this volume) and the Marshall Islands (Pollock, this volume), to become a mother is a necessary step to becoming a woman in the eyes of their communities, regardless of the woman's other achievements. It is a common perspective that all women of Chuuk desire children, except those who have several children already (Fischer;

Moral). Given the value of reproduction, it is no surprise that pregnancy is considered the ultimate pampering time for women (Fischer; Moral). Husbands and other family members make considerable efforts to get special foods for the pregnant woman, and her workload is often less (Fischer). Fischer describes this as the time in a woman's life when she becomes "served rather than servant" (535). Yet these descriptions are only for those with socially acceptable "married" pregnancies; young unmarried women who find themselves pregnant—very common occurrences—bring shame and varying levels of anger to their families. This shame is another important aspect of the regulation of women's bodies, lives, and sexuality in Chuuk.

With unmarried women often hiding their pregnancies and all women living outside of Wééné having minimal access to health care services overall, prenatal care is reserved for women who live in Wééné or can overcome these obstacles. I witnessed nearly one hundred women accessing care every week, meaning that many women *do* overcome obstacles to care. Yet prenatal care is provided for a population of fifty thousand by one provider with the (very) occasional assistance of two other providers who work in the hospital. This provider is inundated with patients; thus, even if more women could access services, there are no resources, funding, or bodies to provide those services to more women. The lack of skilled staff, supplies, and space to provide care is pervasive throughout the system.

CONTRACEPTION

Contraceptive prevalence—if defined as women "legitimately" in need of contraceptives (i.e. married women spacing pregnancy with their husband's support)—is actually quite high in Chuuk. Contraceptives are increasing in popularity. The contraceptive that is pushed by HCWs is the long-acting reversible contraceptive (LARC), which is a transdermal, arm implant and lasts three years. If all women (married or not) engaging in sexual activity are counted when considering contraceptive prevalence, then that number drops dramatically. First, as leader of the family, a woman's husband is usually responsible for contraceptive decision making, something Hayes (this volume) found in southern Malawi as well. Religious affiliation affects this decision too, although even in this case, the husband is the likely trusted decision maker in the family for "interpreting" the contraceptive allowance according to their faith; this calls into question surveys that ask women whether husbands or religion inhibit their use. Since husbands are in charge, when women seek contraception at the public health clinic, nurses ask if they have received permission from their husbands. This is not a requirement, but HCWs told me stories of angry husbands taking IUDs out of women themselves and becoming verbally aggressive and threatening physical violence on HCWs if they did not remove contraceptive devices inserted without their permission. Thus HCWs, by informally requiring a woman receive her husband's permission, are attempting to protect themselves and these women from a potentially angry husband's response. Men sometimes refuse to allow contraceptives for a variety of reasons, most often because they desire more children or they fear their wife will have an extramarital affair if she doesn't have to worry about pregnancy. Other men are completely supportive, and the couple decides together how many children that they want and when to space pregnancies. The cause for concern, however, is not the men who do or do not support contraception; the problem is that women are not in charge of their own bodies, as a result of pervasive gender inequality.

With the exception of the rare adolescent girl with a sexually proactive mother, unmarried women have no *real* access to contraceptives unless they get pregnant first. The family planning section of the public health clinic is too public for girls to enter without some relative or neighbour seeing them in this small island community. Even if girls did approach, they would need to get parental permission, an unofficial policy. However, the HCWs with whom I spoke considered my inquiry strange because they rarely see an adolescent girl or unmarried woman seeking contraceptives. They do not exist there because their fear of "getting caught" or "being seen" is scarier than getting pregnant. Unmarried women and girls who give birth are asked about contraceptives, having been "caught" already.

For those who want to prevent unintended pregnancy, STIs, and HIV, the only places to access condoms on a regular basis in Chuuk are public health facilities or organizations supported by public health; in all cases, people must ask for condoms which, again, would reveal their sexual lives to people whom they likely personally know in the small island community (Smith). Counsellors explained that some boys and men will ask, but women rarely do. There are some youth and general outreach programs that pass out condoms but, in general, these events are sparse and inconsistent, as is the availability of condoms at the other access points. Thus, without true access to hormonal or barrier contraceptive methods, most girls become pregnant shortly after initiating sexual activity. Generally, these pregnancies are simply hidden until they cannot be hidden anymore. The girls, then, shame their family with the news of pregnancy and hope to be forgiven when the baby is born (Smith).

These barriers are all in addition to the logistical barriers of getting to Wééné. Some islands where nurses live have begun to bring contraceptive implant devices home with them to improve the access issue, but it is by no means solved in a systematic or universal way. This context is far from true "access" in my perspective, even if there are technically free contraceptives available, which connotes "access" for development targets such as MDG 5b. Thus, Chuuk is a perfect example of the ways in which quantitative counts and yes-no questions about "availability" and "access" represent very little, if anything, of the actual situation.

HOSPITAL CARE

Once a woman needs a sexual or reproductive health-related surgery or is in labour, she must find a way to get to the hospital or give birth on her home island or in her home on Wééné. If she does make it to the hospital, wait times for the few reproductive health doctors are long, the physical conditions of the hospital are terrible, and the outcomes in the hospital, unfortunately, reflect the lack of supplies, staff, and cleanliness in this deteriorating environment. In the hospital, many women have gestational diabetes and/or high blood pressure and need extra care from the relatively non-existent providers during childbirth. Horror stories of dead mothers and babies are known throughout the islands, prompting all those who can afford it to leave to seek surgeries and childbirth elsewhere. Although the HCWs are often doing the best that they can with the difficult conditions, these conditions do not allow their best to be good enough. Women who have experienced at least one birth are more likely to birth in the comfort and cleanliness of their own land and home (even on Wééné), but in cases of obstetric emergencies, they are often not close enough to the hospital to have a chance of survival.

So women leave. Sometimes they simply fly up to Guam to give birth and then return home as soon as they can travel with the newborn. Others decide to stay after the birth, recognizing the vastly different and improved opportunities in Guam, a U.S. unincorporated territory. Women cannot wait for international development agencies to implement policies when considering their health, the safety of their pregnancies, or even the quality of their children's education. They have to take it upon themselves to seek out a world outside the MDG framework, such as a U.S. territory, while the poorest are left behind to wait for improved quality and access.

DISCUSSION

Understanding the socio-cultural dynamics of reproduction and sexuality helps to explain poor health outcomes to some degree, such as not seeking health care when it is "available" because of social stigma surrounding sex. Chuukese women and men should not be considered any more static holders of a bounded culture than any group, however, and "culture" alone cannot be blamed for poor sexual and reproductive health outcomes. Colonizers brought with them STIs, a health care infrastructure not sustainable to treat those STIs and other SRHR needs, and a patriarchal ideology that reinforces and strengthens already-established male dominance, removing power from women.

Furthermore, the socio-economic system resulting from four centuries of colonization has created a need among Chuukese women to move to Guam, a place often hostile toward migrants, in order to feed their families and fulfill their health care needs. Hostile environments contribute to stress that, in turn, can contribute to poor birth outcomes in pregnant women and poor health outcomes for the general population. Furthermore, stress and discrimination contribute to Chuukese women's discomfort in accessing sexual health services in such a hostile environment (Smith). Chuukese women's reproduction is thus stratified not only in Chuuk but also in Guam and other U.S. jurisdictions (Smith). The Chuukese experience this social stratification in an entire region that has experienced colonial domination and second-class status from the U.S. and previous colonizers. Chuukese women carry the burden of a neocolonial, transnational, and unequal experience in their bodies, and their sexual and reproductive health outcomes reflect this burden.

This interconnected and multilayered analysis examines the complexity of social life integral to anthropological studies of reproduction. Do the current MDG goals reflect these same complexities? This is a scenario in which not only individual "cultures" perpetuating male dominance and sexual shame contribute to gender (in)equality and SRHR, but also contributing is social stratification, postcolonial and neocolonial poverty, and continuous transnational migration. I turn my attention to how these are reflected in MDGs 3 and 5.

MDG 3: GENDER EQUALITY AND THE "EMPOWERMENT" OF WOMEN

The MDG 3 focus on gender equality was an important stride yet as McPherson (this volume) argues, the way in which this particular goal was defined and perceived lacks depth of a true understanding of what gender inequality is and does. With an outdated perspective that simply educating girls will improve everything, measurements ensuring equal access to girls' and boys' education took centre stage. In Chuuk, girls do get educated, perhaps a bit less so than boys, but not by much. The issue in Chuuk is that the whole school system is deteriorating, so it is more an issue of the elite getting educated (in private schools) versus the rest, not girls versus boys. The secondary objectives for MDG 3, including women's participation in the labour market and political sphere, were developed in the same mindset—addressing three aspects of a woman's life that are most likely to explicitly contribute to economic growth—but not really addressing the inequalities that led to unequal participation in the first place. Ilcan and Phillips discuss the entire development framework as a rationality of powerful neoliberal governments with powerful governments imposing values of self-discipline, self-management, measurement, and tracking, as what is necessary for the goal of social transformation. The kind of transformation to be made, however, is one that makes developing countries *look like* those in power and standardizes the way in which all nations should *behave* (Ilcan and Phillips). Basically, it is the new colonialism to save the "savages" through institutionalization of neoliberal economic government processes, perpetuating a system of capitalism that does not stop, but rather generates social inequality. Specifically regarding gender, Mukhopadhyay explains that "as gender was institutionalized, the gap between intention and action grew," and the newly institutionalized concepts worked to produce "gendered citizens best suited to fulfill" neoliberal economic governments (357). Women's empowerment thus became "saving the colonized other" women, not to help increase the value of their established roles but to transform their labour to "serve the economic engine" (360). Thus, development agencies fund programs to teach individual women sewing, weaving, and other skills (in Chuuk) to contribute to their "culturally appropriate" microeconomic development, with minimal efforts to integrate them into the male-dominated government leadership or to dismantle the current systems—created by the also patriarchal U.S.—that continuously leave women out. Furthermore, the same capitalist governments guiding these goals often pull Chuukese women out of Chuuk because if they want to work, they often have to migrate to do so.

Another major concern regarding MDG 3 (and other goals) is that the entire structure of the MDGs places each goal in a "development silo" (Berer 10). If gender equality is one goal among many to end poverty, it makes the women of the developing world an "interest group" (Mukhopadhyay 363; Davids, Driel, and Parren). As an "interest group," gender is not "mainstreamed" as something that should be infused and examined for every MDG but is its own category to be discretely worked on, measured, and considered (Mukhopadhyay 363). Moreover, this discrete goal was too simple and left too many topics unaddressed, including marital relationships and dynamics, violence against women, women's place within families, and every other aspect of social and cultural life. Additionally, these targets focus on individual behavioural change, which continues to ignore the social structures and processes of power in which gender inequality is embedded (Davids, Driel, and Parren; Mukhopadhyay). An understanding of the complexities with which gender and culture interact differently across the world is non-existent in this goal; this, however, is a critique that could be leveraged against the entire MDG framework. Finally, the major goal of ending poverty, although important, completely leaves patriarchy unchallenged (Mukhopadhyay). As these goals are manifested in Chuuk, the patriarchal structure that sustains men's place is strengthened by any MDG-related work. Violence against women is not addressed; thus, the social sanctioning of such violence continues. The churches support men as leaders, which further contributes to this gender unequal environment. Yet "traditional culture" continues to be blamed for the entire scenario, with little attention to the colonial history, missionization, and the current neocolonial infrastructure in this struggling community.

MDG 5: IMPROVING MATERNAL HEALTH

The meaning of gender was also completely changed from the International Conference on Population and Development to the MDGs; its original intentions and transformative power were removed, and in many cases, the goals now actually perpetuate the gender stereotypes it was meant to dismantle (Mukhopadhyay). MDG 5, to reduce maternal mortality, is a perfect example of this perpetuation of stereotypes. Mukhopadhyay argues that the same simplification and de-politicization that occurred with MDG 3 happened to MDG 5. It was a grave disappointment to feminists and SRHR specialists for people's SRHR to transform into the simple goal "improve maternal health," with the only measurement being the maternal mortality rate (MMR). Although maternal mortality is an important indicator of SRHR, solely concentrating on it ignores other SRHR needs. It also removes and de-politicizes the perspective of maternal mortality as a symptom or manifestation of the greater issue of gender inequality (Mukhopadhyay). Finally, this simple goal removes the role of a woman as a social citizen, placing her only in her maternal role (Yamin and Boulanger). In Chuuk, a focus on a maternal role may be appropriate, given the value of motherhood in "empowering" women, yet it also perpetuates the inequality that stems from that gendered role for all women. Thus, the MDG 5 direction—as implemented in Chuuk—perpetuates the stereotype of women as mere reproducers and nothing else, *contributing* to gender *in*equality.

After much lobbying from UNFPA, a more comprehensive version of this goal was adopted in 2007: specifically Target 5b (Haslegrave; Yamin and Boulanger). Yet even this addition to ensure reproductive health access was a watered down version of the SRHR framework from the ICPD (Haslegrave; Yamin and Boulanger). This version was meant to appease those governments hostile to sexual rights or health including issues such as abortion access (Haslegrave). Because of this, what resulted were new health coverage indicators (contraceptive prevalence rate, adolescent birth rate, antenatal coverage, and unmet need for family planning) that continued to focus on biological reproduction. This focus on MCH-related programs leaves out all childless married women, unmarried women, teenage women and, all men (Sadik); it also creates yet another interest group—married, heterosexual women. Furthermore, even when "services" needs are met in this realm, MDG 5 continues to ignore how a woman's social standing (such as a woman's place in her household) is often the biggest contributor or deterrent to her *actual* reproductive and sexual health care access. As I have portrayed in Chuuk, gender roles shape women's sexual lives in profound ways, and women (and men) who do not fit the "hetero-married childbearing" category are completely left out of any attempt to meet this supposedly SRHR-focused MDG. This also contradicts other aspects of the same MDG, such as lowering the adolescent childbearing rate. As long as the health system in place caters to married women, adolescents will continue to get unintentionally pregnant in Chuuk.

A major critique of the MDGs is that they were simplified too much, often blamed on the attempt to standardize development for the entire world. Standardization—whether or not it is a function of the larger development engine to create "look alike" societies or not—oversimplifies goals to the point of changing their intentions (see Wentworth, this volume). As with most of the MDGs, gender and SRHR are complex and do not translate well to "goals," "targets" or "activities" (Davids, Driel, and Parren). Goals, targets, and indicators drive the agenda for MDGs and the complexities of the situation—globally and locally—are thus lost (Yamin and Boulanger). In this context, "activities" turn into workshops and trainings, cutting gender or SRHR into piecemeal presentations that teach a fraction of the original intent and leave participants "parroting slogans" that are "disembodied from the lived experience" (Mukhopadhyay 362). These buzz words are adopted, and gender and sexual inequality remain the same. I witnessed the overuse and misuse of such buzz words on a daily basis in Chuuk, when working with grassroots activists frequently "trained" by development and U.S. federal agency consultants. "Human trafficking" became a word for all violence against women and children; "challenges and lessons learned" was code word for any mistakes or poorly performing employees in these organizations, and "empowerment" meant making women feel good about themselves so that they might individually start to take responsibility for something (despite social pressures opposing such initiatives). Moreover, contraceptive access meant the contraceptives exist but only women who fit the "socially acceptable" stereotype or women who don't but are completely willing to shame their families (which may result in abuse) can get them. Finally, "stigma" was the catchall term for all negative energy surrounding HIV and AIDS, used to such a degree that the *word* stigma, I believe, actually generated *stigma* around STIs, HIV and AIDS.

In addition, the MDGs were never meant for national planning but the poorer, aid-dependent countries often adopted them outright because of their lack of negotiating power with the aid organizations working with the MDGs (Yamin and Boulanger). Yet, these same countries—such as the FSM—have the weakest data collection systems, making the data needed to measure the targets essentially impossible to collect (Yamin and Boulanger). In Chuuk, for example, twenty-two of the twenty-three inhabited islands have no electric power, computers, or internet, thus data collection is reliant on the paper-form reporting of inconsistently available health aides who may or may not understand the often internationally created English forms. The other data collected at the central public health office and the hospital are similarly subject to the HCWs who represent the only bodies available to work in Chuuk; they, thus, have complete freedom to do—or not do—their jobs and remain employed, and have many other duties included that can overwhelm even the most dedicated employees. This frustration often, unfortunately, takes the form of poor and sometimes hostile treatment of the patients, which gives them even less incentive to utilize the services. This scenario was strikingly common across the selections of the volume, from Wentworth in Vanuatu and Barlow in Papua New Guinea to Wogaing in Cameroon and Yakong in Ghana. More research with the specific goal of understanding these worker dynamics is needed, as all improvements are undermined when the staff are absent, not helpful, or, in the worst cases, verbally and physically abusive.

Furthermore, the same countries trying with great anxiety to meet the goals often work to meet them in the most efficient ways by focusing on urban or peri-urban communities (Yamin and Boulanger). The majority of women, mostly poor and rural women thus continue to have the least access to contraceptives (Sadik). This is like Chuuk, where "rural" means living outside of Wééné or living in the villages on the island of Wééné but far from Wééné health clinics. Access to the health centres, the hospital, or to health outreach programs is easier to accomplish for Wééné residents, which leaves the rest of the state at a great disadvantage. Outreach events *do* occur in other islands but with the cost and logistics involved in getting the few, overworked employees to these other islands, they are not frequent. In terms of hospital care and maternal mortality, MMRs continue to be a problem because of the delay in getting help for obstetric emergencies (individual decision delays); the delay in reaching the hospital because of distance and cost; and the delay in receiving adequate health care services because of a shortage (or absence) of skilled staff, which are all issues in Pacific Island states more broadly (Zaman 10).

Finally, the MDGs do not address migration or social stratification in terms of gender or SRHR. In Chuuk, particular clans have great power and status in the community and with that status, they disproportionately gain government jobs, control of the small private economy, and thus, money. These families have the resources to send their children off to better schools outside of Chuuk (or the best private schools within) and have the resources to support college education and U.S. medical care. Thus, women from these clans—even when living in Chuuk—have easy access to Guam through the collection of funds from their more affluent family members. Migration is bigger than just a product of the affluent, however, and families often muster up enough funds for one family member to get to Guam, only to have that family member find work and send money for the rest of the family. Many women then live in Guam, Hawai'i, or the mainland U.S. as adolescents or shortly after marriage and experience their first SRHR needs in these host contexts. Migration is increasingly a global phenomenon and is particularly relevant to the case of Micronesia. It is a topic that completely alters all discussions of "development" in the perceptibly "bounded communities" that the MDGs reflect. The MDGs do not and cannot reflect actual MMR if all women who can find the funds leave Chuuk to give birth; these women are not included in reports for Chuuk's birth outcomes despite often experiencing almost their entire pregnancy in Chuuk.

In short, the MDGs simply do not in any way reflect the reality of gender equality or the dynamics of SRHR at any level for Chuuk. As an anthropologist, I am interested in how and why the MDGs are so simplified as to not reflect the reality of the diversity of "developing countries," and I find it important to critique. As an applied anthropologist, I also find it important to consider solutions and alternatives to the current structure of MDG goals.

RECOMMENDATIONS AND CONCLUSIONS

Accountability rather than systemic change was the focus for MDGs (Yamin and Boulanger), and now it is time for systemic change. More anthropologists and other ethnographers should be consulted for revamping the framework, so attention to the social complexities can shine through future goals. In particular, I imagine this new framework could leave significant room for differences in various communities, both in needs and in approaches. Thus, the Sustainable Development Goals (SDG) framework of 2015 and beyond could focus instead on individual assessments of countries, with on-the-ground research and significant consulting with the actual community of interest, including not just government leaders but also grassroots organizations. In-depth research could highlight particular needs of that community, particular concerns, and strategies birthed out of participatory research and planning, then moving forward with setting goals.

Finally, gender is embedded in all social life and cannot be separated from it, making women an interest group. Feminism focuses on working from the ground up and dismantling power structures, so the original efforts were too global and top down to truly reflect a vision of creating gender equality. Future attempts to fight global patriarchy must do so with consideration for the structure and goals of feminism and the importance of considering its embeddedness in social life. Thus, *all* future goals must address gender. Additionally, future efforts to work toward a gender equal world must be participatory, incorporating multiple voices and encouraging grassroots involvement in the development *and* implementation of goals (Moser and Moser).

Many other recommendations are possible to draw from the Chuuk scenario described in this chapter and from the other chapters of this volume. The important message to draw, however, is more global: in-depth ethnographic research and local participation are vital to creating goals that "fit" the unique historical, socio-economic, political, and cultural elements of each "developing" country.

ENDNOTE

[1] Parallel cousins are children whose parents are the same sex; thus, their parents are brothers or their parents are sisters. The kinship system categorizes parallel cousins themselves as siblings, hence

subject to an incest taboo.

WORKS CITED

Alur, Pradeep, et al. "Epidemiology of Infants of Diabetic Mothers in Indigent Micronesian Population-Guam Experience." *Pacific Health Dialog* 9.2 (2002): 219-221. Print.

Baer, Hans A., Merrill Singer, and Ida Susser. *Medical Anthropology and the World System*. 2nd ed. Westport, CT: Praeger Publishers, 2003. Print.

Bautista, Lola Quan. *Steadfast Movement around Micronesia: Satowan Enlargements Beyond Migration*. Lanham, MD: Lexington Books, 2010. Print.

Benjamin, Jefferson B. *Community Perceptions of the Quality of Health Care Services in the Federated States of Micronesia*. Dissertation. University of Hawaii, 2000. Print.

Berer, Marge. "Key Messages in This Journal Issue." *Reproductive Health Matters* 21.42 (2013): 10-12. Print.

Browner, Carole H. "Situating Women's Reproductive Activities." *American Anthropologist* 102.4 (2001): 773-788. Print.

Caughey, John L. *Fa'a'nakkar: Cultural Values in a Micronesian Society*. Philadelphia, PA: University of Pennsylvania Publications in Anthropology, 1977. Print.

Colen, Shellee. "'Like a Mother to Them': Stratified Reproduction and West Indian Childcare Workers and Employers in New York." *Conceiving the New World Order: The Global Politics of Reproduction*. Eds. Faye Ginsburg and Rayna Rapp. Berkeley, CA: University of California Press, 1995. 78-102. Print.

Davids, Tine, Francien Driel, and Franny Parren. "Feminist Change Revisited: Gender Mainstreaming as Slow Revolution." *Journal of International Development* 26.3 (2014): 396-408. Print.

Dernbach, Katherine Boris. *Enacting Motherhood: Strategies of Grass-Roots Community-Building by Catholic Women in Chuuk, Micronesia*. Thesis. University of Iowa, 1998. Print.

Dernbach, Katherine Boris. *Popular Religion: A Cultural and Historical Study of Catholicism and Spirit Possession in Chuuk, Micronesia*. Diss. University of Iowa, 2005. Print.

Diaz, Angela. "The Health Crisis in the U.S. Associated Pacific

Islands: Moving Forward." *Pacific Health Dialog* 4.1 (1997): 116-29. Print.

Feasley, Jill C., and Robert S. Lawrence. *Pacific Partnerships for Health: Charting a Course for the 21st Century.* Washington, D.C.: National Academy Press, 1998. Print.

Fischer, Ann. "Reproduction in Truk." *Ethnology* 2.4 (1963): 526-540. Print.

Flinn, Juliana. *Mary, the Devil, and Taro: Catholicism and Women's Work in a Micronesian Society.* Honolulu, HA: University of Hawai'i Press, 2010. Print.

Federated States of Micronesia (FSM). "FSM Health Progress Report: 2008-2011." Ed. FSM Department of Health and Social Affairs. Palikir, Pohnpei: Government of the Federated States of Micronesia, 2012. Print.

Ginsburg, Faye, and Rayna Rapp. "The Politics of Reproduction." *Annual Review of Anthropology* 20 (1991): 311-43. Print.

Goodenough, Ward H. "Premarital Freedom on Truk: Theory and Practice." *American Anthropologist* 51.4 (1949): 615-620. Print.

Goodenough, Ward H. *Property, Kin and Community on Truk.* 1951. Second ed. Hamden, CT: Archon Book, 1978. Print.

Gorenflo, L. J., and Michael J. Levin. "Changing Migration Patterns in the Federated States of Micronesia." *ISLA: A Journal of Micronesian Studies* 3.1 (1995): 29-71. Print.

Government of Guam (GovGuam). "2011 Guam Statistical Yearbook." Ed. Bureau of Statistics and Plans. Guam: Office of the Governor, 2012. Print.

Haddock, Robert L., et al. "Lack of Prenatal Care—a Re-Emerging Health Problem on Guam." *Hawai'i Journal of Public Health* 1.1 (2008): 40-44. Print.

Hammar, Lawrence James. *Sin, Sex and Stigma: A Pacific Response to HIV and AIDS.* Anthropology Matters: Scholarship on Demand. Ed. Daniel Miller. Vol. 4.. Wantage, UK: Sean Kingston Publishing, 2010. Print. 6 vols.

Hanlon, David. "The 'Sea of Little Lands': Examining Micronesia's Place in 'Our Sea of Islands.'" *The Contemporary Pacific* 21.1 (2009): 91-110. Print.

Haslegrave, Marianne. "Ensuring the Inclusion of Sexual and Reproductive Health and Rights under a Sustainable Development

Goal on Health in the Post-2015 Human Rights Framework for Development." *Reproductive Health Matters* 21.42 (2013): 61-73. Print.

Hezel, Francis X. *Strangers in Their Own Land: A Century of Colonial Rule in the Caroline and Marshall Islands.* Pacific Islands Monograph Series 13. Honolulu: University of Hawai'i Press, 1995. Print.

Hezel, Francis X., and Michael J. Levin. *Survey of Federated States of Micronesia Migrants in the United States Including Guam and the Commonwealth of the Northern Mariana Islands (CNMI).* Palikir, Pohnpei: FSM Office of Statistics, Budget & Economic Management, Overseas Development Assistance and Compact Management, 2012. Print.

Hirsch, Jennifer S., Holly Wardlow, Daniel J. Smith, Harriet M. Phinney, Shanti Parikh, and Constance A. Nathanson. *The Secret: Love, Marriage, and HIV.* Nashville, Tennessee: Vanderbilt University Press, 2009. Print.

Ilcan, Suzan, and Lynne Phillips. "Developmentalities and Calculative Practices: The Millennium Development Goals." *Antipode* 42.4 (2010): 844-874. Print.

Jordan, Brigitte. *Birth in Four Cultures: A Crosscultural Investigation of Childbirth in Yucatan, Holland, Sweden, and the United States.* 4th ed. Long Grove, IL: Waveland Press, 1993. Print.

Kawamoto, Crissy T. "Chuukese Women Provide Insights into Cultural Barriers to Cervical Care." *Pacific Region Cancer Connection* (2009): 8. Print.

Kiste, Robert C. "United States." *Tides of Hisotry: The Pacific Islands in the Twentieth Century.* Eds. K. R. Howe, Robert C. Kiste, and Brij V. Lal. Honolulu, HI: University of Hawai'i Press, 1994. 226-257. Print.

Levin, Michael J. *The Status of Micronesian Migrants in the Early 21st Century.* Cambridge, Massachusetts: Population and Development Studies Center, Department of Public Health, Harvard University, 2010. Print.

Marshall, Mac. *Namoluk Beyond the Reef.* Westview Case Studies in Anthropology. Ed. Edward R. Fischer, Boulder, CO: Westview Press, 2004. Print.

Marshall, Mac, and Leslie B. Marshall. *Silent Voices Speak: Women and Prohibition in Truk*. Belmont, CA: Wadsworth Publishing Company, 1990. Print.

Moral, Beatriz Ledesma. *Conceptualization of Women, the Body and Sexuality in Chuuk (Micronesia)*. Diss. University of Basque Country, 1996. Print.

Moser, Caroline, and Annalise Moser. "Gender Mainstreaming since Beijing: A Review of Success and Limitations in International Institutions." *Gender & Development* 13.2 (2005): 11-22. Print.

Mukhopadhyay, Maitrayee. "Mainstreaming Gender or Reconstituting the Mainstream? Gender Knowledge in Development." *Journal of International Development* 26.3 (2014): 356-367. Print.

Pobutsky, Ann M., et al. "Micronesian Migrants in Hawaii: Health Issues and Culturally Appropriate, Community-Based Solutions." *California Journal of Health Promotion* 3.4 (2005): 59-72. Print.

Rogers, Robert F. *Destiny's Landfall: A History of Guam*. Honolulu: University of Hawai'i Press, 1995. Print.

Sadik, Nafis. "Sexual and Reproductive Health and Rights: The Next 20 Years. Keynote Address, ICPD Beyond 2014. International Conference on Human Rights 7–10 July 2013, Netherlands." *Reproductive Health Matters* 21.42 (2013): 13-17. Print.

Scheper-Hughes, Nancy and Margaret M. Lock. "The Mindful Body: A Prolegomenon to Future Work in Medical Anthropology." *Medical Anthropology Quarterly* 1.1 (1987): 6-41. Print.

Smith, Sarah A. "The Reproductive Lives of Chuukese Women: Transnationalism in Guam and Chuuk." Dissertation. University of South Florida, 2014. Print.

Wong, Vanessa S., and Crissy T. Kawamoto. "Understanding Cervical Cancer Prevention and Screening in Chuukese Women in Hawai'i." *Hawai'i Medical Journal* 69.6 Supplement 3 (2010): 13-16. Print.

Yamada, Seiji, and Ann Pobutsky. "Micronesian Migrant Health Issues in Hawai'i: Part 1: Background, Home Island Data, and Clinical Evidence." *California Journal of Health Promotion* 7.2 (2009): 16-31. Print.

Yamin, Alicia Ely, and Vanessa M. Boulanger. "Embedding Sexual and Reproductive Health and Rights in a Transformational Development Framework: Lessons Learned from the Mdg Targets and Indicators." *Reproductive Health Matters* 21.42 (2013): 74-85. Print.

Zaman, Wasim, ed. *ICPD and the Millenium Development Goals*. University of the South Pacific, Suva, Fiji: UNFPA Office for the Pacific and University of the South Pacific, 2009. Print.

Contributor Notes

Kathleen Barlow is professor of anthropology and museum studies at Central Washington University, Ellensburg, Washington. Prof. Barlow is a psychological anthropologist with particular interests in learning and culture, childhood, gender, and parenting. She has conducted local village-based and comparative regional research in the Lower Sepik region of Papua New Guinea, specifically the Murik Lakes, since the 1980s.

Philip Gibbs, a Divine Word missionary priest, has a doctorate in theology from Gregorian University, Rome, and a postgraduate diploma in anthropology from Sydney University, Australia. He has worked in Papua New Guinea since 1973 and his recent work includes promoting men advocates against gender-based violence. Currently, he is head of Governance and Leadership Department, Divine Word University, Madang, Papua New Guinea.

Nicole Hayes, Ph.D., is cultural anthropologist with a specialization in culture change. Currently, an adjunct lecturer at the University of Waterloo, Nicole's research explores how colonialism and globalization have placed the intimate relationships of poor Malawians on an increasingly transactional footing, creating a sexual economy based on competitive multiple concurrent partner sex.

Stephanie Hobbis is a co-supervised Ph.D. candidate in social anthropology and ethnology at École des Hautes Études en Sciences Sociales, Paris, and in social and cultural analysis at Concordia

University, Montréal. A Vanier Canada graduate scholar, her doctoral research explores state- and nation-building in rural and urban Solomon Islands (Lau Lagoon, Malaita; Honiara).

Naomi McPherson, Ph.D., is associate professor emerita, UBC Kelowna. She has conducted research in Bariai, West New Britain, Papua New Guinea since 1981, publishing on Bariai cosmology, ethno-obstetrics, traditional and cosmopolitan systems of maternal health, and birthing, and gender relations. With Michelle Walks, she co-edited *An Anthropology of Mothering* (Demeter 2011).

Nancy Pollock, Ph.D., teaches anthropology and conducts research on gender and health issues in Pacific communities and New Zealand. Her research on food security embraces the notion of good food as integral to women's household decision making and explores the health outcomes of ingested foods contaminated by radioactive fallout from U.S. nuclear testing in the northern Pacific.

Sarah A. Smith, Ph.D., is a feminist medical anthropologist and assistant professor in the Department of Public Health at the State University of New York at Old Westbury. Her dissertation research focused on the intersection of gender inequality, migration, and sexual and reproductive health, in particular examining Chuukese migrant women's lives in Guam, U.S.

Shauna LaTosky, studied cultural anthropology at the University of Victoria and received her Ph.D. in social anthropology from Johannes Gutenberg University in 2010. Since 2012, she has been a postdoctoral researcher at the Max Planck Institute for Social Anthropology in Germany. Her current research interests include pastoralism and the environment, local knowledge, comparative customary law, bridewealth, and marriage practices in southern Ethiopia.

Chelsea Wentworth, Ph.D. anthropology, master of public health, is assistant professor of anthropology at High Point University. Her research topics are critical medical anthropology, gender studies, maternal and child health, and Pacific Island studies. Since

2010, she has conducted research in Vanuatu with public health practitioners and families concerning infant feeding and childhood malnutrition.

Winnie William is from Nipa in the Southern Highlands Province, Papua New Guinea. She graduated as a registered nurse in Rabaul, PNG, in 1998 and has a Master's degree in nursing from Monash University, Melbourne (2008). Ms. William, a wife and mother of three, has been honoured as the Papua New Guinea Nominee for the 2015 U.S. Secretary of State International Women of Courage Award in recognition of her courage, dedication, and sacrifice to save the lives of women, often at great personal risk. At present, Ms. William is health secretary for the Catholic Diocese of Mendi, Papua New Guinea.

Jeannette Wogaing, Ph.D., is a lecturer in the Department of Anthropology at the University of Douala, Cameroon. A cultural and medical anthropologist, her research interests include traditional and contemporary patterns of motherhood and fatherhood in Cameroon, parenthood in the context of HIV, and women in prison.

Vida Nyagre Yakong, MSN, Ph.D. in Interdisciplinary Studies (anthropology and gender studies) from UBC Kelowna, is a lecturer and head of the Department of Midwifery, University for Development Studies, Tamale, Ghana. A cultural and medical anthropologist, her research focuses on the anthropology of reproduction, critical medical anthropology, rural women's and girls' empowerment, non-profits, and healthcare policy.